on what data will I gather + how
produce what materials/instrument
to assist IMG in accult

ABOUT THE AUTHORS

Ulla M. Connor, Ph.D., is the Barbara E. and Karl R. Zimmer Chair in intercultural communication, professor of English, and director of the Indiana Center for Intercultural Communication. Dr. Connor received B.A. and M.A. (*magna cum laude*) degrees in English philology from the University of Helsinki, an M.A. in English literature from the University of Florida, and an M.A. in comparative literature and a Ph.D. in English linguistics from the University of Wisconsin. Dr. Connor has held academic positions at a number of universities in the United States, and guest and visiting professor positions at Temple University (Japan), Lund University (Sweden), and Åbo Akademi University (Finland). She is also an elected member of the Finnish Society of Sciences and Letters. Dr. Connor has authored and coauthored 10 books and over 100 articles and book chapters, including *Contrastive rhetoric* (Cambridge University Press, 1996), and *Intercultural rhetoric* (University of Michigan Press, forthcoming). Results of her intercultural rhetoric research have been applied in the teaching of ESL and EFL students, intercultural business communication, and, most recently, the language of health care among U.S. immigrant populations.

Marisa Cordella, Ph.D., is senior lecturer in Spanish linguistics and convenor of the Spanish and Latin American Studies Program in the School of Languages, Cultures and Linguistics at Monash University, Australia. Born in Santiago, Chile, she obtained a diploma in translation studies in her home country, an M.A. in TESOL from the University of Canberra, and a Ph.D. in linguistics from Monash University. She has published and conducted research in the areas of intercultural communication, medical communication, interactional sociolinguistics, critical discourse analysis, pragmatics, teaching methodologies, and translation studies. Her joint research projects involve collaboration with colleagues from Australia and Chile. Her teaching commitments include units in the areas of pragmatics, discourse analysis, translation studies, and Spanish language for advanced learners. She is the author of *The dynamic consultation: A discourse analytical study of doctor–patient communication* (John Benjamins, 2004a).

Cheryl Hanau, M.D., is professor, Residency Program director, and chair in the Department of Pathology and Laboratory Medicine at Drexel University College of Medicine in Philadelphia. She received her M.D. from Jefferson Medical College, finished residency training in anatomic and clinical pathology, and completed a fellowship in cytopathology. Hanau has been a faculty member at Drexel College of Medicine since 1995. Along with her work as a pathologist, she has devoted much of her time to teaching medical students and residents, which has resulted in her receiving many teaching awards. Hanau's interaction with the ESL community began when she needed to find a way to improve English language pronunciation for several of her residents who were international medical graduates. She has presented at the international TESOL convention on the need for English for specific purposes programs for international medical graduates.

Barbara J. Hoekje, Ph.D., is associate professor of communication in the Department of Culture and Communication at Drexel University, where she directs the English Language Center. She received her Ph.D. in linguistics from the University of Pennsylvania and was a Fulbright Senior TEFL Lecturer in Mexico in 1994–1995. Her interests are in sociolinguistic approaches to language teaching, learning, and use, and she has published on international teaching assistants, testing, English language program administration, and English for medical purposes in *TESOL Quarterly*, *ESP Journal*, and the *RELC Journal*. Recent publications include (with M. C. Pennington) *Language program leadership in a changing world: An ecological model* (Emerald, 2010). She has developed orientation and education programs for international medical graduates in psychiatry, internal medicine, and pathology, and has consulted with the Educational Commission on Foreign Medical Graduates on issues of acculturation.

Joanna Labov, Ph.D., is clinical assistant professor of TESOL in the Department of Teaching and Learning at New York University, where she prepares student teachers to teach ESL and teaches graduate-level applied linguistics courses. Labov is a long-term TESOL professional with more than 20 years of experience in teaching English as a second language. She holds an M.A. in TESOL and a Ph.D. in educational linguistics from the University of Pennsylvania. Labov has traveled extensively internationally and in 2010 taught English at Wuhan University in China. Since 2001, she has worked with international medical graduates to improve their English pronunciation and communications skills. Labov has presented at the international TESOL conventions on topics related to international medical

ENGLISH LANGUAGE AND THE MEDICAL PROFESSION: INSTRUCTING AND ASSESSING THE COMMUNICATION SKILLS OF INTERNATIONAL PHYSICIANS

INNOVATION AND LEADERSHIP IN ENGLISH LANGUAGE
TEACHING   VOLUME 5

ENGLISH LANGUAGE AND THE MEDICAL PROFESSION: INSTRUCTING AND ASSESSING THE COMMUNICATION SKILLS OF INTERNATIONAL PHYSICIANS

Edited by

BARBARA J. HOEKJE
Drexel University

SARA M. TIPTON
Wayne State University

United Kingdom – North America – Japan
India – Malaysia – China

Emerald Group Publishing Limited
Howard House, Wagon Lane, Bingley BD16 1WA, UK

First edition 2011

British Library Cataloguing in Publication Data
A catalogue record for this book is available from the British Library

ISBN: 978-1-78052-384-2
ISSN: 2041-272X (Series)

Emerald Group Publishing
Limited, Howard House,
Environmental Management
System has been certified by
ISOQAR to ISO 14001:2004
standards

Awarded in recognition of
Emerald's production
department's adherence to
quality systems and processes
when preparing scholarly
journals for print

INVESTOR IN PEOPLE

area. Her chapter describes the development process of enhancing the skills of ESL faculty to better handle the specific needs of the ESP setting and to develop curricula and materials for workshops and courses. The section concludes with a chapter ("Pronunciation as life and death: Improving the communication skills of nonnative English-speaking pathologists") by Joanna Labov, an applied linguist, and Cheryl Hanau, M.D., a pathologist, who describe the development of a pronunciation course for nonnative English-speaking pathology residents. An innovative component of the course was the use of the real-world assessment task of autopsy dictations to measure the pathologists' improvement in intelligibility.

In assembling and editing this book, we have tried to keep in mind our various audiences. One key audience is our ESP colleagues, who we hope will gain ideas about different contexts, future trends, and resource development for medical communication. Another audience is medical educators in hospitals and other clinical settings, who could use the assessment tools as well as online resources, ongoing orientation, workshops, courses, and Webinars described and referenced in this collection to lend greater support to communication training in their medical education curriculum. Yet another audience is administrators of intensive English programs (IEPs), who can draw on the information provided in this volume to develop courses and the skills of faculty to meet the needs of the IMG population working in university or community hospitals in their geographical area. We also hope that this collection will be useful for IMGs who are preparing for their residencies and beyond, from studying for licensing exams to finding useful resources for when they begin and progress through their residencies. While there is no IMG author in our collection, their voices are expressed and their needs are discussed throughout, providing the thread that unifies the 12 chapters.

Overall, we hope that this collection will encourage further collaboration between ESP and medical professionals to work together to support the needs of international medical graduates. In addition, we hope program directors and medical educators will design more orientation programs and support tailored to the needs of new international doctors who enter their residencies. The forms of communication in their hospitals and clinics are not universal but rather culturally-bound and context-specific. Medical administrators and educators can consult with ESP and IEP specialists to design assessment, orientation, and educational components to proactively support the IMG experience.

ESP professionals should be prepared to meet global trends in English for medical purposes by contributing to cross-cultural perspectives on the language and practice of medicine and by taking the necessary steps to develop their own expertise with the required specialized content. As has been proven by those who assess and educate international graduate teaching assistants, ESP professionals are a valuable resource for knowledge, research, pedagogical applications, and advocacy for international students and workers. It is our hope that this collection allows the field of English for medical purposes to continue to grow—both expanding and maturing—to meet the needs of international medical graduates in the many contexts in which they study and work.

Barbara J. Hoekje
Sara M. Tipton

CONTENTS

PART III: COURSES AND CURRICULA

I dedicate this book to my colleagues in the ITA interest section, who created conditions in which our knowledge and practice could thrive, and to Greg Barnes and Yoko Koike, who have kept me in the Light.

Barbara J. Hoekje, Editor

I dedicate this book to Susan Eggly and Khaled Bachour, who introduced me to the world and experience of IMGs; to Rick Loftus, who provided vital feedback and constant support during the drafting process; to my parents, Thomas and Janice Tipton; and to the IMGs who continue to inspire me.

Sara M. Tipton, Editor

ACKNOWLEDGMENTS

We wish to thank Martha Pennington for her continued guidance and support. She values both education and innovation, and her vision for the series made this book possible.

We are grateful to our authors, who responded with enthusiasm and commitment from the beginning. We appreciate their generosity of spirit during the many cycles of editing that the manuscript has undergone.

Special thanks go to Katie Henninger, who managed the collection through the first round, and Reese Heitner, who saw the project through submission. We believe in the process approach to writing, but without their editorial support, we would have lost track of the process.

As coeditors, we share an understanding of the work we do with ITAs, IMGs, and intensive English programs. When we started the project, we hoped, but didn't know as we do now, that we would work so smoothly together, kind through the end, with each providing the necessary inspiration in turn as needed. We are deeply grateful for this.

Barbara J. Hoekje
Sara M. Tipton

graduates and ESL. In 2010, Labov published her dissertation, *The acquisition of English Short A and E by second language learners: The roles of vowel height, duration and task for German learners of the English Short A and E contrast* (Lambert Academic Publishing, 2010).

Lia Logio, M.D., is professor of medicine at Weill Cornell Medical College, where she serves as vice chair for education in the Department of Medicine. She is a practicing general internist, having obtained both her bachelor's and medical degree from Johns Hopkins University. She has worked collaboratively with linguists on helping international medical graduates acculturate to the U.S. health-care system, including participating in the development and pilot testing of the Interpersonal Communication Assessment tool. Her main focus is in graduate medical education with recent work on patient safety education, inter-professional collaboration, and communication standards in health care.

Marie McCullagh, M.A., is senior lecturer at the University of Portsmouth in the United Kingdom, where she teaches on a range of ESP and EAP courses. Since 2005, she has provided training on doctor–patient communication skills to international medical graduates and native English-speaking doctors within the National Health Service, and is also an ESOL examiner for Trinity College London. She holds a master's degree in language teaching and materials development from Leeds Metropolitan University. She is author (with Ros Wright) of *Good practice: Communication skills in English for the medical practitioner* (Cambridge University Press, 2008).

Catherine O'Grady, Ph.D., is an ESP teacher and researcher. Following her career with the New South Wales (Australia) Adult Migrant English Service (AMES), where she specialized in the development of intercultural communication programs in medical contexts, she has taught clinical communication for organizations, including the Royal Australian College of General Practitioners. She has recently completed her doctoral studies in applied linguistics at Macquarie University. She holds a master's in applied linguistics from the University of Sydney and a TESOL diploma from Macquarie University. Her publications include *Finding common ground: Cross cultural communication strategies for job seekers* (National Centre for English Language Teaching and Research, 1994) and *Diversity: An educational resource for junior doctors and other health professionals* (published jointly by the Postgraduate Medical Council of New South

Wales and AMES, 2000). Working closely with medical educators, she has developed and taught clinical communication courses for international medical graduates seeking local registration, for recent graduates about to enter the medical workforce and for international medical graduate psychiatrists working in remote locations.

Susan Olmstead-Wang, Ph.D., is assistant professor at the University of Alabama, Birmingham, where she teaches dissertation strategies and writing for the graduate school and linguistics courses for the M.A. in English as an international language in the School of Education. She received her Ph.D. in English and applied linguistics at the University of Alabama, Tuscaloosa. As coordinator of the English Language Program at Johns Hopkins University-School of Advanced International Studies, she developed language policy and taught advanced second language writing. She is author of the article "Medical doctors using authentic Web cast lectures to learn lexical phrases" published in *Authenticity in the language classroom and beyond: Adult learners* (TESOL Publications, 2009) and international coordinator for the Kaohsiung Medical University English Language Project.

Carol Piñeiro, Ed.D., is senior lecturer in the Center for English Language and Orientation Programs at Boston University, where she designed and taught summer courses in English for health and medical professionals. During the academic year, she teaches English for international business and seminars for international teaching fellows. She holds a master's degree in TESOL and a doctorate in educational media and technology from Boston University and was director of the English Program in Madrid at the Instituto Internacional en España in 2006–2008. She is a writing consultant for students in the MIT/Universidad de Zaragoza master's in logistics program and a language coach at the Sloan School of Management at MIT. She received a Fulbright Scholar Award for 2012 for teaching and research in Santiago, Chile. Her interests include incorporating technology into language teaching, and she has written several articles on the topic for TESOL publications.

Laurie Lipsig Pylitt, M.H.P.E. is associate professor in the College of Pharmacy and Health Sciences at Butler University in Indianapolis, Indiana, currently serving as the Director of Assessment for the College. She is a certified physician assistant, who has a master's of health professions education degree from the University of Illinois Health Science Center in Chicago. In her former position as the education coordinator of the Indiana University Family Medicine Residency, she worked extensively with resident physician trainees, representing five continents, the majority of whom trained outside of the United States. She identified unique cultural and interpersonal communication challenges faced by these foreign-trained physicians and then spearheaded a partnership between the Indiana University Family Medicine Residency and the Indiana Center for Intercultural Communication aimed at facilitating the successful assimilation of these internationally trained physicians into the norms of U.S. society and its health-care system.

William Rozycki, Ph.D., is professor and director of the Center for Language Research, University of Aizu, Japan. He earned his Ph.D. from Indiana University and has taught ESL and technical communication at the university level in the United States, as well as EFL in industry and academia in Korea and Japan. He is a coeditor (with Ulla Connor and Ed Nagelhout) of *Contrastive rhetoric: Reaching to intercultural rhetoric* (John Benjamins, 2008) and has also copublished in *Communication and Medicine* and the *Asian Journal of English Teaching*. From 2003 to 2008, Rozycki served as director of the Indiana Center for Intercultural Communication training program for international medical residents at Indiana University Health.

Sara M. Tipton, M.A., is lecturer in the English Language Institute at Wayne State University, where she coordinates the testing and training of international teaching assistants and teaches intensive English classes as well as graduate-level writing. She holds a master's degree in linguistics and a TEFL-TESL certificate from Ohio University, and was a Fulbright Senior TEFL Lecturer in the Slovak Republic in 1999–2000. In her goal to support international medical graduates in improving their oral and written communication skills, she has tutored prospective and practicing international interns and residents in metropolitan Detroit since 1996. She has also taught scholarly writing skills to graduate students at the Wayne State University School of Medicine since 2000. She has presented at TESOL on international teaching assistant and international medical graduate topics and published in the *Journal of Applied Linguistics*.

Marta van Zanten, M.Ed., Ph.D. candidate, is research associate at the Foundation for Advancement of International Medical Education and Research, the foundation of the Educational Commission for Foreign Medical Graduates® (ECFMG®). She holds a B.A. from the University of

Waterloo, Canada, and an M.Ed. from Temple University in Philadelphia, and is currently a Ph.D. candidate in health studies at Temple University. She has published on international medical graduate issues, including accreditation processes of international medical schools, the impact of accreditation on student outcomes, doctor–patient relationships, spoken English proficiency, and cross-cultural communication skills, and she has twice received the Research in Medical Education (RIME) Outstanding Paper Award. She was involved in the development and implementation of the spoken English proficiency and communication and interpersonal skills evaluation components of the ECFMG Clinical Skills Assessment® (CSA®) and the ® (USMLE®) Step 2 Clinical Skills.

Gerald P. Whelan, M.D., FACEP, is director of the Acculturation Program at the Educational Commission for Foreign Medical Graduates® (ECFMG®). As faculty in emergency medicine at the University of Southern California Medical Center, he became involved in assessment with the American Board of Emergency Medicine, serving as president in 1996–1997. That same year, he came to ECFMG to lead a team in developing the first high-stakes medical performance assessment to be implemented in the United States, the Clinical Skills Assessment® (CSA®). He subsequently moved on to begin developing resources to assist international medical graduates in their acculturation to U.S. medicine and culture. He is coauthor of *The international medical graduate's guide to U.S. medicine and residency training* (ACP Press, 2008) and has published in *Medical Teacher*, *Medical Education*, and *Academic Medicine* as well as developing extensive Web-based resources for international medical graduates and graduate medical education faculty and staff.

MaryGrace Zetkulic, M.D., is a board-certified physician in internal medicine. She is chief of General Internal Medicine and associate program director for the Internal Medicine Residency Program at St. Peter's Hospital in New Brunswick, New Jersey. She is assistant professor of medicine at Drexel College of Medicine. She received her medical education at the University of Medicine and Dentistry of New Jersey. She previously was the third- and fourth-year medicine clerkship director at the University of Medicine & Dentistry of New Jersey-Robert Wood Johnson Medical School and served to develop the ECFMG® development acculturation website.

INTRODUCTION

We began our professional careers in ESL and applied linguistics in the 1980s with the testing and education of international graduate teaching assistants (ITAs), nonnative speakers of English who teach undergraduate students while pursuing graduate degrees at U.S. universities. During the following two decades, that subfield of applied linguistics/ESL and English for specific purposes (ESP) matured and developed its own research base, disciplinary content, and pedagogy, as well as its own interest section within the TESOL organization, creating a framework for investigating the interaction of culture, language, and pedagogy among international graduate students and teachers in U.S. higher education. At the same time, both of us began to receive inquiries from medical educators and administrators about "communication issues" related to international medical graduates within U.S. hospitals and residencies. International medical graduates—or IMGs—had some similarities in their educational profiles to ITAs, in that they were admitted into U.S. graduate medical education to complete their medical residencies but had received their undergraduate and medical education in other countries. The inquiries were reminiscent of the early conversations about international teaching assistants and their communication difficulties, with requests to "fix this problem" being a recurrent theme.

In our initial sessions with IMGs, we applied the frameworks and expertise we had developed through ITA work to the medical setting. In particular, as we had used a cross-cultural framework to analyze the language and pedagogy of U.S. higher education, so we also approached the language and practice of medicine in U.S. medical education as a culturally organized activity. In some cases, we found that "fix this problem" referred to a mismatch of "ways of speaking," to go back to Dell Hymes' (1974) fundamental concept, that is, the ways of using language in specific contexts rather than issues of pronunciation or grammar per se. The seriousness of the language issue facing international doctors could not be overstated. The competency of doctors was questioned on the one hand; on the other, clear communication about patients' healthcare was at risk. At the same time that IMG communication was becoming more visible to us in the United States, another trend was taking place—the spread of English for medical purposes

(EMP) worldwide. This included both the flow of international doctors into English-speaking countries such as the United Kingdom, Australia, Canada, and the United States, as well as the shift to English as a medium of instruction in medical education and professional settings worldwide.

Despite the magnitude of these trends, we were aware of few resources for those in the ESP community working with IMGs to assist in their communication. We sought ways to collaborate with those sectors of the medical community who were addressing communication issues from their own frameworks of practice. At the 2008 TESOL Convention in New York City, we organized a panel, "Assessing and instructing communication skills for international physicians," moderated by Barbara Hoekje, with presenters Sara Tipton, Mara Blake-Ward, Martha van Zanten, and MaryGrace Zetkulic, M.D. Our audience that day included ESP professionals also working with international doctors and English for medical purposes in the United States and elsewhere. We then began the journey of assembling this book from many of the presenters in that panel and other authors responding to a call for papers in the ITA and ESP interest section listserves of the TESOL organization and related international professional organizations. The volume, *Discourse and Performance of International Teaching Assistants*, edited by Carolyn Madden and Cynthia Myers (TESOL, 1994), was a model for the present volume. We were fortunate to find in Martha Pennington's series on Innovation and Leadership in English Language Teaching a suitable place to publish our book and an editor who saw the potential of our collection.

Our volume, *English Language and the Medical Profession: Instructing and Assessing the Communication Skills of International Physicians*, consists of 12 chapters organized in three main sections. Taken as a whole, the book covers settings within the United States, the United Kingdom, Australia, and Taiwan and includes the perspectives of physicians and medical educators, testing specialists, ESP specialists, and applied linguists. It is both a practical and a theoretical collection, providing resources to support IMGs on several levels and in a range of pedagogical and real-world contexts, from individual consultations to workshops and courses, and from initial preparation for licensing examinations to on-the-job settings. The book offers an extensive bibliography, including Web links to all aspects of supporting and educating the IMG, as well as reproducible feedback sheets and resources for lesson design and workshop planning.

We begin in *Part I: Perspectives on Communication and Acculturation* by providing three different lenses through which to examine issues of communication for international doctors. In the first chapter ("International medical graduates in U.S. higher education: An overview of issues for ESP and applied linguistics"), Barbara J. Hoekje uses a sociolinguistic framework to examine issues related to IMGs in U.S. graduate medical education and practice. Following approaches developed for international teaching assistants in U.S. universities, she proposes an English for specific purposes and applied linguistics research agenda in order to situate IMG issues within a cross-cultural perspective on medical discourse, education, and communication. In the following chapter ("Steps along the way: A personal retrospective on the development of the U.S. ECFMG acculturation program"), Gerald (Gerry) P. Whelan, M.D., who developed the IMG acculturation program for the Educational Commission on Foreign Medical Graduates® (ECFMG®) in the United States, describes the development of this key resource for the preparation and orientation of international doctors during their initial stages of entry into U.S. graduate medical education. In the third chapter ("Teaching the communication of empathy in patient-centered medicine"), Catherine O'Grady examines empathy in doctor-patient communication in clinical settings in Australia. She under-scores the communication of empathy as an interactional achievement and shows how the use of transcripts of authentic discourse of doctor-patient communication can be used in educating international medical graduates and novice clinicians in how to use empathy as a key resource in patient-centered medicine.

Part II: Qualifications and Competencies introduces the significant topic of the necessary competencies for medical practice and the various methods used to assess them both before and after the start of residency. First, Marta van Zanten ("Evaluating the spoken English proficiency of international medical graduates for certification and licensure in the United States") describes the historical background and development of the Clinical Skills (CS) examination. While Van Zanten discusses issues of CS test reliability and performance from an institutional perspective, the following chapter ("The Clinical Skills (CS) test: IMG preparation and perception") by Sara M. Tipton presents a perspective on the CS test from the point of view of a consultant assisting IMGs who are preparing for the test. Tipton represents the concerns not only of the consultant but also of the IMGs preparing for the test.

As an initial licensing test for medical practice in the United States, the United States Medical Licensing Examination® (USMLE®) provides an initial measure of language competency in a clinical context. In the next chapter ("Assessing cultural knowledge among international medical graduates in the United States"), authors William Rozycki, Ulla M. Connor, Laurie Lipsig Pylitt, and Lia Logio, M.D., a team of collaborating ESP and medical professionals, describe the development of an instrument to proactively assess cultural knowledge of clinical norms in family medicine among first-year residents. The second section concludes with a chapter ("By the bedside: Lessons about communication from an internal medicine program director") by MaryGrace Zetkulic, M.D., a program director in internal medicine at a small urban hospital in the northeastern United States. In response to her need for a comprehensive but logistically manageable diagnostic tool for both clinical and communication skills for USMG and IMG residents, she developed a one-station Objective Structured Clinical Examination (OSCE) test to be implemented on an ongoing basis as part of the training of residents in the hospital setting.

Part III: Courses and Curricula reports on curriculum and course development initiatives around the world to address the needs of IMGs. Susan Olmstead-Wang ("Developing curriculum and strategies for a Chinese-language medical university in Taiwan adopting English as a medium of instruction") begins with the description of the processes of faculty development in one department of a medical university in Taiwan as it began to institute English as a medium of instruction together with a greater problem-based learning pedagogy. Within the collection, Olmstead-Wang's chapter is unique in describing an EFL context in which English has become a medium of instruction in medical education. In the following chapter ("Overcoming language and cultural differences in medical encounters: The use of a language and culture training course (LACT) in educating IMGs in Australia"), Marisa Cordella discusses the development of a language and culture course for IMGs in Australia. She begins with the intercultural communication issues of the medical encounter, describing the various roles that a physician plays and the concomitant "voices" of these roles as doctor, educator, and fellow human being. Her curriculum builds upon these voices through reflective exercises that help speakers develop awareness of their own and others' communication. The following chapter ("Addressing the language and communication needs of IMGs in a U.K. context: Materials development for the doctor-patient interview") by Marie McCullagh focuses on IMG education in the United Kingdom. McCullagh describes the research that led to the development of the text, *Good Practice* (McCullagh & Wright, 2008), reflecting upon the materials and the transferability of information about the doctor-patient interview to communication in other settings.

The final two chapters return to U.S. contexts. Carol Piñeiro ("Courses for health and medical professionals") describes the broadening mission of a U.S. university-based intensive English program (IEP) to include English for medical purposes for international medical professionals in the Boston

PART I
PERSPECTIVES ON COMMUNICATION AND ACCULTURATION

CHAPTER ONE

INTERNATIONAL MEDICAL GRADUATES IN U.S. HIGHER EDUCATION: AN OVERVIEW OF ISSUES FOR ESP AND APPLIED LINGUISTICS

Barbara J. Hoekje

ABSTRACT

This chapter reviews the literature on language, culture, and communication issues in IMG education and practice. An English for specific purposes (ESP)/applied linguistics research agenda on these topics is proposed in order to situate IMG issues within a cross-cultural perspective on medical discourse, education, and communication. It is proposed that the flow of international medical graduates (IMGs) into U.S. graduate medical education has characteristics similar to that of international graduate teaching assistants (ITAs) coming into U.S. universities from the 1970s, and that much can be learned from the perspectives and frameworks developed by ESP and applied linguistics in that case.

English Language and the Medical Profession: Instructing and Assessing the Communication Skills of International Physicians
Innovation and Leadership in English Language Teaching, Volume 5, 3–19
ISSN: 2041-272X/doi:10.1108/S2041-272X(2011)0000005007

INTRODUCTION

The second half of the twentieth century ushered in unprecedented growth and widespread availability of higher education in the United States on a scale unknown in its own history and in the world generally (Lemann, 1999). Not only did returning GIs take advantage of postwar scholarship opportunities, but international students and scholars sought the expanding access to higher education offered by both private and public universities in the United States (Bevis & Lucas, 2007). Many international students entered graduate programs in the fields of engineering, mathematics, computer science, and business, with funding from the U.S. universities in the form of teaching assistantships and, increasingly, postdoctoral fellowships (National Academy of Sciences, 2000). Graduate medical education (GME) in the United States also attracted increasing numbers of students from around the world both as doctors and as researchers (Astor, Akhtar, & Matallana, 2005; Hallock, Stephen, & Norcini, 2003; Mullan, 2005). This trend has continued virtually unabated. By 2006, international medical graduates comprised 25.7% of the physician workforce in the United States, up from 17.1% in 1970 (American Medical Association, 2008, p. 394).

The response of U.S. higher education to the influx of international graduate students initially showed little planning or policy (Goodwin & Nacht, 1983). Rather, the entering international students created pressure within the existing system of U.S. higher education in the areas of their needs. Particularly visible in the university were the pressures caused by the graduate students' role as teaching assistants. As graduate teaching assistants (GTAs), they were expected to instruct undergraduate students in lectures, labs, recitations, and office hours. The courses they taught were often introductory science courses required for distribution credits of nonmajors throughout the university. As was the usual practice in the academy in the early 1980s, little preparation was given to GTAs—international or American—beginning their teaching responsibilities despite the demands of their role (Nyquist, Abbott, Wulff, & Sprague, 1991).

Thus, the international GTAs, who had excelled in other educational systems relying on large lectures, professorial authority, deep but specialized subject matter mastery, and knowledge of written English, were severely underprepared for teaching American undergraduates who came to class with vastly different backgrounds (Smith, Byrd, Nelson, Barrett, & Constantinides, 1992). The undergraduates expected personalized, interactive forms of teaching, sympathy for their unspecialized but broad subject mastery, a friendly "captain of the team" type of authority, and unaccented North American English.

When problems of communication arose between the international GTAs and the undergraduates, language was most often blamed although cultural differences also received attention. As the "foreign TA problem" escalated in public awareness, lawsuits were filed against universities on behalf of undergraduate students (Brown, Fishman, & Jones, 1990) and states developed legislation mandating language fluency (see, inter alia, Pennsylvania State Senate Bill No. 539, 1989, amended 1990).

In response to this fray of mismatched cultural expectations and legal battles, higher education administrators turned to English language specialists to establish programs in language, culture, and pedagogy addressed to the international GTAs' perceived needs (Bailey, 1983; Bailey, Pialorsi, & Zukowski/Faust, 1984; Young, 1989). Within the field of applied linguistics, the dominant model of language use—"communicative competence" (Canale & Swain, 1980)—was applied to the specific context of ITA education (Hoekje & Williams, 1992). Curriculum was developed around spoken language discourse (Pickering, 2001; Wennerstrom, 1989), cultural issues such as student/teacher roles and the expectations of the classroom (Pettigrew, 1998; Pialorsi, 1984), and the forms and functions of academic discourse (Madden & Myers, 1994; Rounds, 1987; Shaw, 1994; Tanner, 1991; Tyler, 1992; Williams, 1992).

The case of the international GTA within U.S. higher education provides a useful introduction to the situation of international medical graduates within U.S. graduate medical education. Many of the historical conditions that attracted international students to the United States for graduate study in departments of science and engineering and other fields also drew international doctors into advanced medical study. For historical reasons and those related to the institutions of medical education and practice, however, the profile of the international medical graduate has only recently become more prominent within U.S. graduate education.

The practice of medicine is now increasingly subject to patient advocacy and legislative scrutiny. New accreditation standards for both graduate medical education and hospitals increasingly emphasize communication and cultural competency. In this context, the necessary preparation for IMGs for the practice of medicine in U.S. hospitals must become more comprehensive in scope. Yet, like universities whose model of graduate teaching assistantships was based on assumptions about a domestic population, the institutions of medicine have generally not adjusted their educational design for an international population.

This chapter will argue that IMG training and orientation has much to learn from ESP and sociolinguistic approaches developed in response to issues raised by international teaching assistants within U.S. higher education. Language use seen within a communicative competence framework allows consideration of formal, discourse, sociolinguistic, and strategic competencies. The influence of culture, broadly speaking, is key to understanding expectations about doctor and patient roles, the nature of the medical encounter, and the legal context of hospital practice (e.g., patient privacy). The medical encounter can be understood as fundamentally cultural in nature.

This chapter reviews the literature on IMGs in U.S. graduate medical education and provides an overview of language, culture, and communication issues related to their practice of medicine. The chapter proposes an ESP/applied linguistics research agenda on medical discourse, culture, and language to be used for orienting IMGs to U.S. graduate education and practice.

THE ENTRY OF INTERNATIONAL MEDICAL GRADUATES INTO U.S. HIGHER EDUCATION

International medical graduates began to enter the United States in significant numbers following World War II. The Exchange Visitor Program established by the United States Information and Educational Exchange Act of 1948 (the Smith–Mundt Act) allowed international doctors from a wider range of countries to enter graduate medical programs (American Medical Association, 2007, p. 3). According to popular sources, the post-World War II United States had become a "medical mecca" drawing foreign doctors to the United States to train (Plight of foreign doctors, 1960). The Fulbright–Hays Act of 1961 established the exchange visitor visa (the J-1 visa), which allowed doctors to engage in educational and cultural exchanges (American Medical Association, 2007, p. 4). Because of high failure rates on examinations within the United States, international applicants were required to pass tests before receiving exchange visitor (J-1) visas (Plight of foreign doctors, 1960). The precursor to the Educational Commission for Foreign Medical Graduates®️ (ECFMG®️) was established in 1956 to oversee standards and testing for doctors educated outside the United States. This organization merged with a visa oversight organization to become the current organization in 1974 (American Medical Association, 2007, p. 4). By the academic year 1959–1960, 9,457 foreign physicians from 92 countries were training in U.S. hospitals (Institute for International Education, 1960, p. 13).

Today, licensure for all physicians regardless of site of training requires passage of the United States Medical Licensing Examination® (USMLE®) Steps 1, 2, and 3 (USMLE, 2009). Steps 1 and 2: Clinical Knowledge (CK) are administered via computer in testing centers around the world. Step 2: Clinical Skills (CS) is an in-person performance examination, administered in five test centers in the United States, which examines language proficiency, interpersonal skills, and clinical knowledge using standardized patients as raters (Boulet, McKinley, Whelan, van Zanten, & Hambleton, 2002; van Zanten, 2008; van Zanten, Boulet, McKinley, & Whelan, 2003). Step 3 is the final licensing test for independent practice within the United States and is administered at computer test centers in the United States and its territories.

The growth in IMGs corresponded to the rapid growth and demand for qualified physicians in the United States. In 1983, the number of places allotted for residency training exceeded the annual graduation rate of USMGs by 40% (American Medical Association, 2007, p. 5). In 2006–2007, 26% of the 104,879 residents in the Accreditation Council for Graduate Medical Education (ACGME)-accredited training programs were IMGs (American Medical Association, 2007, p. 5).

The flow of students into U.S. higher education in the sciences and medicine has become a feature of the modern quality of globalization: "the flow of technology, economy, knowledge, people, values, and ideas … across borders" (Knight, 2003). Other major recipient countries of international physicians include Canada, the United Kingdom, and Australia (Astor et al., 2005; Mullan, 2005; Rao et al., 2007).

RESEARCH ON FOREIGN NATIONAL PHYSICIANS

Reports about foreign-born physicians started to appear in medical professional journals in the early 1970s, especially in key specialties. A special issue of the journal *Psychiatry* (1971) was devoted to foreign medical graduates (e.g., Char, 1971). Studies on foreign-born psychiatrists continued for the next two decades, identifying concerns, including the influence of culture on learning psychiatry, issues of performance, integration of international doctors into the training program, and issues related to the psychiatrists' own identity and adjustment. An annotated bibliography in these areas is provided by Rao et al. (2007).

From a workforce perspective, Salsber and Forte (2002) examined physician trends from 1980 to 2000, focusing on the role of IMGs in filling workforce shortages in the United States. An extensive literature exists on workforce issues, flow, and migration patterns for IMGs in the United States. Their role has been seen ambivalently: both as a "safety net" for physician shortages in rural and other underserved areas but also as downward pressure on opportunities for U.S.-born applicants to medical schools, for example, the articles in Rao et al. (2007).

By the 1990s, there were larger changes in medical education and the practice of medicine in the United States, and a new focus on the importance of communication skills for doctors emerged (e.g., Fisher & Groce, 1990; Hydén & Mishler, 1999; Maynard, 1991; Mishler, 1997; Ong, de Haes, Hoos, & Lammes, 1995). Good communication skills were shown to increase patient satisfaction, compliance, and better health outcomes (Silverman, Kurtz, & Draper, 2005, p. 8).

In 1999, the ACGME established new standards for graduate medical education programs which required residency programs to train their residents for competencies in six skill areas: (1) Patient Care, (2) Medical Knowledge, (3) *Interpersonal and Communication Skills* [emphasis added], (4) Professionalism, (5) Practice-Based Learning and Improvement, and (6) System-Based Practice (see ACGME General Competencies). The standard in (3) Interpersonal and Communication Skills was for skills "that result in effective information exchange and teaming with patients, their families, and other health professionals" (Accreditation Council for Graduate Medical Education, 2009). The significant inclusion of interpersonal and communication skills as one of the core competencies required in graduate medical education resulted from an increasing awareness of the contribution of communication to patient diagnosis, compliance, and satisfaction.

Hospitals concerned about safety standards also needed to adhere to hospital accreditation standards. The Joint Commission on the Accreditation of Healthcare Organizations ("JCAHO" or simply "The Joint Commission," see www.jointcommission.org) publishes standards for accreditation for a variety of institutions, including hospitals. The 2009 National Patient Safety Goals (NPSG) for hospitals include communication-based goals such as improving the (1) accuracy of patient identification, (2) effectiveness of communication among caregivers, and (3) safety of using medications with attention to labeling medicines (The Joint Commission on Accreditation of Healthcare Organizations, 2008a).

Within a hospital setting, intimidating and disruptive communication behaviors by physicians or other staff have also been implicated in compromising the "culture of safety" in a hospital (The Joint Commission on Accreditation of Healthcare Organizations, 2008b). The seriousness with which communication is viewed as a safety issue by The Joint Commission cannot be overstated. In fact, in its annual report on U.S. hospital safety (2007), communication was seen as the most important root cause of serious "sentinel events" such as medication errors and wrong site surgery: "Inadequate communication between care providers or between care providers and patients/families is consistently the main root cause of sentinel events. Other leading root causes include incorrect assessment of a patient's physical or behavioral condition and inadequate leadership, orientation or training" (The Joint Commission on Accreditation of Healthcare Organizations, 2007, p. 47).

The Joint Commission has strongly stated communication standards for providing access to culturally and linguistically diverse patients as well. In short, there has been an increasing emphasis on the role of effective communication in health-care education and hospitals, explicitly linked to accreditation standards both in graduate medical education and in hospital and other health-care organizations.

OVERVIEW OF IMG ISSUES AND THEIR IMPLICATION FOR ESP/APPLIED LINGUISTICS RESEARCH

Introduction

The issues faced by IMGs with regard to their practice as doctors in health-care settings (Kramer, 2005; McMahon, 2004; Schuster, 2000), their studies as graduate students within U.S. graduate education, and their experiences as immigrants transitioning into U.S. life (Schuster, 2000) have been increasingly well-documented. In these various arenas, language, communication, and culture play a significant role. The first step in examining the issues and dynamics of language and culture in IMG communication is to identify the various subgroups of the IMG population and the terms of reference used to describe them.

Terms of Reference for IMGs

Throughout the research literature, the term *international medical graduate* or *IMG* is used to refer to different populations. Technically, the term refers to all doctors who graduated from a medical school located outside the United States or Canada; this category includes both U.S. citizens and citizens of other countries. In many venues, however, the term *IMG* is used to refer only to international doctors, that is, doctors who are citizens of other countries, sometimes referred to as "foreign nationals," or "foreign-born physicians." Medical institutions such as the American Medical Association and the National Board of Medical Examiners®, which oversees the U.S. medical licensing exams, tend to use the technically correct term, that is, it is the medical school which is international; for these agencies, the jurisdiction of the U.S. accrediting bodies is the significant issue.

The term *international medical graduate* replaced the earlier term *foreign medical graduate* (FMG) in a general renaming trend throughout the 1990s (the preferred term for international teaching assistant shifted from *foreign teaching assistant (FTA)* to *ITA* in the same time period). It is likely that the intent of the renaming was generally to de-emphasize the term *foreign*, which includes the meaning of "strange," and "other" in English.

Within U.S. graduate medical education, various populations can be distinguished: (1) doctors from other countries who went to medical school outside the United States, (2) U.S. citizens who went to medical school outside the United States, and (3) U.S. citizens who went to medical school in the United States. There are also students from other countries who went to medical school in the United States, but this population is currently small (Bishop, 2008).

It is difficult in the literature at times to know which population is being referred to. For example, the American Medical Association (AMA) has an IMG section in which all IMG members of the association (both U.S. and foreign national citizens) are automatically enrolled (American Medical Association, 2009). Yet at times, the AMA IMG section literature itself distinguishes between these two subsets of graduates of foreign medical schools, as in the following statement: "*IMGs* are more willing than *U.S. IMGs* or *U.S. medical school graduates* to practice in remote, rural areas through J-1 visa waiver requirement" (American Medical Association, 2007, p. 5). There are references elsewhere in the same document to a subset of IMGs "*born outside the United States*" (American Medical Association, 2007, p. 9, emphasis added). For the purposes of this chapter, these different populations will be differentiated, with the term, *international medical graduate (IMG)*, used more restrictively, that is, to designate only doctors from other countries who attended medical school outside the United States or Canada. Even with this more restrictive reference, however, the diversity in background and experience among doctors of other nationalities practicing medicine inside the United States is extensive and resists "simple categorization" (Rao et al., 2007, p. 70).

More accurate and specific identification of the relevant subsets of IMGs is key to identifying core issues relevant to their preparation and training. Both U.S. and international medical graduates experience differences in medical school education that may influence their ability to perform successfully in U.S. residencies (McMahon, 2004). In addition, international physicians face visa requirements and immigration decisions that U.S. citizens do not face in choosing to practice in the United States. In both groups, there are wide ranges in individual experience: IMGs may have many years of experience in the United States or have special language and cultural ties with local U.S. patient populations, while U.S. nationals may have had very little exposure to the local cultures where they do their residencies.

Language

Language impacts the practice of medicine in specific ways. With the ITAs, seeing language as an interrelated set of competencies allowed issues of register, sociolinguistic appropriateness, discourse, and strategic competence to be addressed as well as pronunciation and grammar (Hoekje & Williams, 1992). In the case of medical communication, such larger frameworks of analysis will be useful as well. To begin with, the terms *native* and *nonnative* speaker of English do not begin to describe the varieties of English used by doctors. U.S. national doctors may be first generation immigrants who moved to the United States as older children and whose English remains imprinted with the sounds and grammar of a first language. Those from other countries where English is a national language may have extensive control of a world variety of English with very few differences from the U.S. variety—or a world variety of English with substantial differences in phonology, grammar, and lexicon from U.S. English. For most doctors raised outside the United States, colloquial forms of U.S. spoken English are unfamiliar; they must learn the conversational register and local references to talk informally with patients. Monolingual English speakers from one geographic area of the United States also may not understand the local expressions and pronunciation of the patient population where they do their residencies. Hoekje (2007) describes the language usage covered in an acculturation course for first-year residents in psychiatry whose first experience of U.S. patient care was with an urban population in the northeast United States:

> [C]ourse goals include familiarizing doctors with the language of the patient community. Over time, we have compiled a set of terms, many of which were first suggested by IMGs, including slang terms for body parts, illnesses and symptoms ("throw up"), drugs ("wet") and drug use, sexual activity and orientation ("come out," "rubber") (this has a different meaning in the United Kingdom), as well as behaviors ("roughhouse") and attitudes ("diss" (disrespect)). They also include euphemisms ("I have a problem with my thingy") and child language ("pee pee"). (p. 337)

Eggly, Musial, and Smulowitz (1999) found that doctors' English language skills can affect patients' perceptions of their competency. In this study of patient satisfaction of a largely female, elderly African-American population, judgments in a number of areas varied significantly based on IMGs' English language proficiency as measured by the Test of English for International Communication (TOEIC) and the SPEAK test. Doctors' first languages included Arabic, Farsi, Mandarin, Spanish, Tagalog, Hindi, and Marathi. Key areas such as the doctor's perceived friendliness, care in examination, and competency were shown to correlate significantly with spoken English (Eggly et al., 1999, p. 204).

Some negative bias toward accent may be mitigated due to the high status of doctors. Using a matched guise test design in which undergraduate students listened to doctors' statements, Rubin, Healy, Zath, Gardiner, and Moore (1997) investigated the effect of a doctor's ethnolinguistic accent upon students' judgments of the doctor, comprehension of the doctor's speech, and intention to comply with the doctor's instructions. In that study, the results showed a limited effect of ethnolinguistic status upon undergraduates' judgments of the doctor's personality but not upon comprehension or outcomes of intention to comply. The researchers proposed that the high status of physicians might mitigate the effect of ethnolinguistic markers in doctors' speech.

The interaction of international medical graduates with the diverse patient populations of the major urban areas where they initially practice and the largely rural areas where they participate in visa waiver programs after licensure has not received much attention. The complexity of minority or immigrant, limited-English proficient patients in communication with nurses and other health-care workers of different immigrant or foreign national backgrounds has been described in several health-care contexts in the United States and Canada (Bosher & Smalkoski, 2002; Cameron, 1998; Duff, Wong, & Early, 2002). Further research in this area for international medical graduates working with such patient communities would be valuable as it could help portray the reality in which many IMGs work.

In addition to patients, residents interact with medical students, staff, and attending doctors, and may face preconceptions or bias in these cases (Schuster, 2000). How do IMGs' interactional skills support or interrupt others' preconceived notions? What are the dynamics of the conversations of shared culture versus nonshared culture doctors and other speakers? For these questions, identifying the subgroups of the IMG population and their interaction with various patient and staff groups is a necessary first step.

Forms and Functions of Medical Discourse

An inventory of the forms and functions of language use in health-care contexts is needed similar to the research on forms and functions of academic discourse. Health-care communication in the United States takes place within a medical discourse that encodes specific ways of knowing, ways of seeing, and ways of talking (Ainsworth-Vaughn, 2001; Atkinson, 1995; Engeström, 2005; Good, 1994; Good & Good, 2000; Hoekje, 2007; Kleinman, 1995; Konner, 1987; Scollon & Scollon, 2001). Students in U.S. medical schools are acculturated into this system from the first year as they listen to lectures and discuss the evidence for disease at the cellular level. In the last two years of medical school, they participate in clinical practice in the hospital and begin to learn the specific genres of clinical practice such as morning rounds and case presentations. Through all these processes, U.S. medical students begin to internalize or acquire the particular language usage of their role as doctor. Gee (1990) refers to this as the acquisition of the secondary "Discourse" (capital D) of their role. For Gee (1990), this secondary Discourse entails both verbal (language) and nonverbal (body language, manner, dress) ways of enacting a role; speakers are legitimized as doctors because they can appropriately enact through both verbal and nonverbal means the Discourse of doctors.

The entering IMG has not had these years of acculturation in this Discourse but instead will have had other educational and occupational acculturation experiences, including different cultural expectations about the roles of doctor, nurse, and patient (Whelan, 2006). The new IMG will also have expectations of the forms of language to use in his or her work as a doctor. Specific discourse forms such as the case presentation may be unfamiliar and require coaching (Tipton, 2005, 2008). Ways of talking with patients may require a new communicative competency in the sense of

Hymes (1974)—new discourse forms that encode different underlying norms of interaction and interpretation.

Communication Tasks

While many studies of communication between doctors and patients exist (e.g., Fisher & Groce, 1990; Hydén & Mishler, 1999; Maynard, 1991; Mishler, 1997; Ong et al., 1995), the specific dynamics of the interactions between international doctors and their patients rarely emerge; the study by Erickson and Rittenberg (1987) is an exception as they focus on issues related to hierarchy and control in conversation. Compared to the language needs of ITAs managing classrooms with multiple speakers, the task of doctors talking to patients is principally dyadic (Ong et al., 1995). The medical interview itself is premised upon the need to ask open-ended questions as well as having the listening competency to understand the language of patients from a much wider range of socioeconomic backgrounds than is typically found among university undergraduates. Comprehension tasks of doctors include being able to understand patients who are in pain or who are using medication.

Tipton (2005) classifies IMGs' communication tasks into two broad areas following Lingard, Schryer, Garwood, and Spafford (2003): talking with patients and talking about patients. She describes the resident's communication tasks in a typical day:

> Examining and interviewing patients, discussing patients with colleagues, giving instructions to patients and other healthcare professionals, leading discussions with patients and their families, telephoning social services and other physicians, consulting with physicians in other specialties, teaching medical students, writing patient care notes, dictating discharge summaries, delivering formal morning report and research presentations, and presenting cases to their supervising or faculty physician, the attending physician. (Tipton, 2005, p. 396)

In their analysis of the dynamics of professional communication, Sarangi and Roberts (1999) discuss medical practice using Goffman's (1959) concept of "frontstage" and "backstage" settings. In her work as a consultant with IMGs, Tipton (2005) reports that some IMGs find tasks which might be considered "frontstage," such as talking to patients, easier than "backstage" tasks, such as case presentations and other communication activities that take place outside the presence of the patient but in the presence of supervising faculty.

For both frontstage and backstage settings, more basic research is needed on the organization of key tasks and the communicative competency required to perform medical communication tasks in terms of their linguistic, sociolinguistic, discourse, and strategic components. Pronunciation instruction will need to target the most critical words and phrases in high-stakes communication tasks (Labov & Hanau, 2005; this volume). Research on medical discourse must highlight the nature of dyadic interpersonal communication in clinical settings and the role of listening, in particular. Key genres such as the case presentation (Tipton, 2005) will be necessary for international doctors to master as they begin to practice in a U.S. context. The team approach to health care may require more communication skills on the part of the doctor in negotiating meetings between the patient, family members, social workers, and others. Information about medical forms and functions can provide the basis for IMG preparation programs just as knowledge about the forms and functions of academic discourse laid the groundwork for instructing ITAs in appropriate pedagogy for lectures, recitations, and other instructional contexts.

Spoken Language Assessment

Assessing the comprehensibility of medical communication raises important issues in the area of language evaluation. What forms of prior assessment are sufficient to predict adequate communication in on-the-job settings? The relationship of entry-level language skills to the specific workplace-based talk of the clinic or hospital has yet to be completely understood. Those who have passed the test may have reached a threshold level but still be referred for later communication support work (Blake-Ward, 2008). In research by Eggly et al. (1999), even those IMGs with very high level English skills had reduced levels of patient satisfaction and a continuing identification of language skills as a primary weakness by faculty and colleagues. In another study, Boulet et al. (2002) found that program directors reported deficiencies in diagnosis and management, history taking, and physical examination, even among those residents having passed the Clinical Skills Assessment CSA (CSA®), a prior form of the Step 2 (CS) exam administered by the ECFMG. While one-half to two-thirds of these residents improve within four months of training (Boulet et al., 2002, p. S34), this still leaves a substantial population with identified skills deficiencies well into the residency period. At the same time, an entry test that sets the bar too high will screen out too many applicants. As it is, some test-takers believe that the CS test is harder than on-the-job communication (Tipton, 2008; this volume).

The unified approach taken by the USMLE in screening medical applicants can be distinguished from the language screening approach taken until now with ITAs. The USMLE Step 2 (CS) Clinical Skills exam is required for all applicants regardless of national origin or language status, thus avoiding the necessity of defining who must be screened for language in terms of "native" versus "nonnative" English speakers, a distinction increasingly challenged by applied linguists (e.g., Pennycook, 1998). In the Step 2 CS exam, both medical knowledge and language are evaluated in a performance test format.

Workplace assessments such as those conducted by Zetkulic (2008; this volume) are designed for all first-year residents without differentiating background and provide ample opportunity for all to hear supervisory feedback and internalize appropriate communication. One outcome of an inventory of health-care communication needs may be the development of new rubrics for assessing and instructing interpersonal communication skills in the course of dyadic clinical encounters.

Culture

Culture remains an important component in any assessment or instructional setting for international doctors. As established in ITA education, *culture* was defined widely to include such aspects as the values of U.S. education, the forms and functions of academic discourse, roles of faculty and students, and attitudes and expectations of American students (Smith et al., 1992, pp. 40–41). In medicine, culture broadly defined can include underlying values about the nature of illness and health, expectations about doctor and patient roles, the forms and functions of medical communication, and institutional and professional values.

Focusing on the experience of IMGs transitioning to practice in the United States, Whelan (2006) describes the following cultural issues in the U.S. practice of medicine:

> The structure and hierarchy of American medicine, the role of nurses and other healthcare colleagues, the concepts of informed consent and shared decision making, issues of confidentiality and documentation—these are but a few of the broader topics that need to be clearly explained in a context where IMGs not only receive information but also have the opportunity and time to ask questions and to discuss their understanding of these issues. (p. 177)

The work of Whelan and others at the Educational Commission for Foreign Medical Graduates (ECFMG) has led to important resources for

IMG acculturation based upon extensive interviews with IMGs about their experience and needs in entering U.S. residencies: Focus areas include the doctor–patient relationship, the coordinated services provided by the health-care team, the nature and importance of documentation, and confidentiality and informed consent (Educational Commission for Foreign Medical Graduates, 2009a). The structural organization of hospital rooms shapes the nature of doctor–patient interaction, and the naming practices of medicines are different (McMahon, 2004).

The medical encounter itself admits culture in multiple ways—from the expectations and experiences of patients from various backgrounds; to the approach of the doctor in the diagnostic interview based on his or her professional training and experiences with patients; to the organization of the space, time, and resources allotted to the medical encounter within the institution; and finally, to the language and culture of the country (and region of the country) in which the institution is located. All these different levels of context bring further cultural elements into doctor–patient interactions.

Culture informs both the register of technical medical communication as well as the larger cultural patterns underlying communication generally throughout the United States. The use of common names of medicines derives largely from their widespread use in popular culture, for example, Tylenol rather than acetaminophen (Hoekje, 2007). "Professionalism" as an ethic is highly reinforced (Alguire, Whelan, & Rajput, 2009). For example, doctors are advised to respond to patients' expressions of anger in nondefensive ways (Educational Commission for Foreign Medical Graduates, 2009b).

The effect of culture in medicine has also been seen in physicians' diagnostic and treatment decision-making processes. Gumperz (1982a) raised classic issues about the role of culture in doctors' expectations and treatment in the case of a Filipino doctor charged with perjury in relation to a child's death. In this case, the doctor's culture-bound conceptualization of child abuse was seen as a possible factor in the treatment decisions pursued. As another example, Kales et al.(2006) report that, even after years of practice in the United States, internationally trained doctors show differences compared to U.S.-trained doctors in rates of diagnosing depression among the elderly. Many other examples can be given of differing cultural frames of reference applied by international doctors practicing in unfamiliar U.S. contexts, including areas relating to occupational hazards, sexual practices, and dietary traditions. It is worth emphasizing that American doctors without prior experience with a particular patient population or geographic area may also be unaware of key issues in some specific contexts.

Curricular Support for IMGs

Elsewhere (Hoekje, 2007), I have proposed that support for IMGs is especially important at three points in their U.S. graduate medical education: (1) upon arrival when immediate needs are pressing; (2) early in the first year when residents begin to meet patients and prepare academic work in a new educational system; and (3) the final years of residency as doctors prepare for licensing and independent practice. Short-term orientation programs specifically designed to address immediate needs and prepare the ground for later coursework are extremely valuable for new IMGs. Mentoring programs such as the international advisors network of the ECFMG can provide important professional and logistical preparation even before the doctor relocates (Educational Commission for Foreign Medical Graduates, 2009c; Whelan, this volume).

In addition to short-term orientation programs, longer-term educational programs allow IMGs time to interact, view, and begin to internalize discourse forms such as case presentations through the scaffolded interaction needed to learn the "Discourse" of physicians (Gee, 1990). The opportunity to provide information that will address the negative perceptions of attending faculty and supervisors who have little experience with IMGs is also important as such perceptions may be widespread (Schuster, 2000). Programs that provide opportunities for IMGs to gain clinical experience such as the eight-week surgical residency training program described by Horvath, Coluccio, Foy, and Pellegrini (2004) may be useful in providing opportunities for IMGs to learn both clinical knowledge and cultural information. Information about other curricular approaches that have been found useful in providing acculturation support is now appearing, such as a film-based approach to teaching American culture (Sierles, 2005).

CONCLUSION

The entrance of large numbers of international graduate students as teaching assistants into North American universities created the need for a comprehensive, pedagogically based research agenda in ESP and applied linguistics. As it was carried out, this agenda enlarged our view of what was initially framed as an issue of language and cultural deficit (the "foreign TA problem") to our current understanding of the U.S. classroom as a place of specific discourse forms and culturally based (not universal) academic practices.

A research agenda for ESP/applied linguistics can inform orientation and education programs for international medical graduates as well. Medical encounters are fundamentally cross-cultural by virtue of the experiences and expectations of the patients and the doctors and the structures of the institutions in which medical practice takes place. Language use is not a simple matter of pronunciation and grammar but a contextualized set of practices within these settings. As hospitals move to address standards in communication, culture, and patient-centered care, ESP and applied linguistics research can provide insight about the ways these dimensions interact.

ESP specialists and applied linguists can highlight the discourse forms and cultural assumptions of U.S. medicine and advocate for increased cross-cultural expertise in medical education generally. Case studies are needed to differentiate the IMG experience so that the term "IMG" is more than an umbrella category used to refer monolithically to the experience of all members of the category. Studies are needed on the socialization process of U.S. doctors such as that of Konner (1987); such studies illustrate the profoundly cultural basis of the value system into which the U.S. doctor is acculturated. Other studies such as that of Fadiman (1997) are also needed to illuminate the cultural meaning of illness within diverse communities in the United States. Studies of medical practice in countries outside the United States such as the research of Ibrahim (2001) on the practice of medicine in Egypt will also inform our understanding of the cultural nature of medical practice.

To conclude, U.S. graduate education has enrolled international students in substantial numbers for more than half a century, yet it is only recently that globalized perspectives and frameworks of analysis for this context of cross-cultural exchange have emerged. ESP and applied linguistics established important research that contributed to the current understanding of the cultural context of U.S. undergraduate classrooms and the forms and functions of classroom academic discourse. This wider cross-cultural framework is one that ESP and applied linguistics can contribute to U.S. medicine as well.

CHAPTER TWO

STEPS ALONG THE WAY: A PERSONAL RETROSPECTIVE ON THE DEVELOPMENT OF THE U.S. ECFMG ACCULTURATION PROGRAM

Gerald P. Whelan

ABSTRACT

*The Educational Commission for Foreign Medical Graduates®
(ECFMG®) Acculturation Program arose out of a recognition that
doctors arriving from other countries to train in the United States wanted
and needed assistance in many areas both professional and personal.
Direct contact with examinees in a pilot project followed by focus groups
with IMGs and training program staff guided the evolution of a now
comprehensive array of resources and services.*

INTRODUCTION

It was the spring of 1996. I was well into my third decade in emergency
medicine (EM), the still very new medical specialty that I had been drawn to

English Language and the Medical Profession: Instructing and Assessing
the Communication Skills of International Physicians
Innovation and Leadership in English Language Teaching, Volume 5, 21–42
ISSN: 2041-272X/doi:10.1108/S2041-272X(2011)0000005008

years before it was recognized. Probably because I got in on the ground
floor (I finished my residency in 1975, but it would be 1979 before EM
would be formally added to the roles of the American Board of Medical
Specialties), I had gone farther and faster than perhaps I would have
otherwise. I had been a residency director and associate director of one of
the largest emergency departments in the country. I was also just about to
begin my term as President of the American Board of Emergency Medicine
(ABEM). I was very well versed in all aspects of EM and most of Graduate
Medical Education (GME) in general. Yet throughout my career to that
point, I had had only minimal contact with international medical graduates
(IMGs), in those times known as FMGs (foreign medical graduates). EM
was a very popular specialty for U.S. medical students, and IMGs were
rarely encountered in EM programs. Therefore, it was somewhat ironic that
I would see an ad for a position with the Educational Commission for
Foreign Medical Graduates® (ECFMG®), an organization of which I had
previously been only vaguely aware. More ironically perhaps, I responded
to it, and so began a journey that would take me to a whole new world of
medical education and a new and very different set of challenges. In this
chapter, I will recount both my personal journey and the development of the
ECFMG's Acculturation Program, a major new initiative to develop
resources and support for international medical graduates coming to the
United States.

IMGs AND THEIR JOURNEYS

International medical graduates (IMGs) are by definition graduates of
medical schools outside of the United States and Canada. Those who choose
to pursue U.S. Graduate Medical Education (GME) programs, particularly
those who are not U.S. citizens, must embark on a real, physical journey
from their homeland to the United States. Depending on where they are
coming from, it can be a long, arduous, and expensive journey. However, in
addition to this actual physical journey, there is another journey on which
they must embark, and it may in fact be more challenging than their
physical travels. This is a cultural journey, leaving the culture of their home
country and arriving in a new culture that may be very different and often
perplexing. It also involves a journey from the culture of medicine where
they have learned and practiced it, or where they first began their studies, to
a U.S. medical culture that can be quite challenging in its complexity and
high technology. For many, the journey forces them to leave positions of

professional esteem as practitioners of their art and begin again the first steps in the hierarchy of American medicine. They also often must journey from a privileged place in their society wherein their judgments would rarely, if ever, be questioned by a patient to a practice of medicine characterized by shared decision-making and even challenges to their authority. Moreover, for those who make these journeys with spouses, children, or families, there is a shared challenge of resettling those who have no role in medicine per se but who find themselves in a world where even the most common aspects of daily living may be unfamiliar and confusing. Challenging journeys, all!

As I made the quantum geographical and professional leap from emergency medicine in California to ECFMG in Philadelphia, I was oblivious to almost all of these issues. I had been recruited to lead the team that would develop and implement a new examination specifically for IMGs, the Clinical Skills Assessment® (CSA®). This was an entirely new direction for me. But first, some background on the Educational Commission for Foreign Medical Graduates or ECFMG.

THE EDUCATIONAL COMMISSION FOR FOREIGN MEDICAL GRADUATES

Medical schools outside the United States and Canada vary in educational standards, curriculum, and evaluation methods. Since its inception in 1956, ECFMG has been assessing the readiness of IMGs to enter supervised Graduate Medical Education (GME) programs, residencies, and fellowships, in the United States. It currently does so by a series of examinations and by primary source verification of medical education credentials and transcripts. It is the sole agency within the United States on which medical licensure and credentialing bodies rely for this certification. Certification by ECFMG does not ensure the IMG a position in a U.S. GME program but rather is one of the basic prerequisites for entry. It is the responsibility of the individual IMG to apply for and successfully obtain a position. This is a highly competitive process. There are a finite number of entry level GME positions offered each year, and the vast majority are filled by graduates of U.S. medical schools (USMGs). Some programs rarely accept or even interview IMGs, particularly the more competitive programs in the more competitive specialties. As a result, IMGs often must seek positions in specialties less popular with USMGs such as primary care and psychiatry and often in less prestigious programs in community rather than university settings. Just the application process itself can be daunting, especially for someone unfamiliar with U.S. GME, applying from abroad, possibly with a limited budget, and often still facing challenges with English as a second language.

Even when an IMG succeeds in obtaining a GME position, there are still many challenges. From the first day in the new program, the IMG is thrown into an environment of medical education and practice that may be very unfamiliar, with quite different procedures, priorities, and ways of relating to faculty, peers, other members of the medical team, and even patients and their families. The new arrival is inundated with policies, protocols, and pharmacopoeia which dictate highly complex rules, regulations, and requirements in areas that the IMG may never before have even considered a part of medical practice: confidentiality, Medicare regulations, and documentation—not to mention encountering complex electronic information systems. And when they leave the hospital after their first exhausting shifts, IMGs find no respite but, on the contrary, face a whole other set of challenges having to do with daily living in the United States— finding housing, getting finances established, getting drivers licenses, and learning where and how to shop for food and other necessities. If accompanied by a spouse and/or family, the IMG must face all the issues of getting them settled as well—schools, day care, employment for a spouse, and many other details of establishing a home in a new and different country. It is a tribute to the resilience and commitment of IMGs that with few exceptions, they come through these challenges successfully and find their places in American medicine and American society where they become a major resource in providing care, often for the neediest.

THE CLINICAL SKILLS ASSESSMENT (CSA)

For most of its history, ECFMG functioned primarily as an administrative agency. It administered (but did not design or score) examinations; tracked individual applicants' progress; collected and verified medical educational credentials; and, when all requirements were met, issued a Standard ECFMG Certificate. The National Board of Medical Examiners® (NBME®) had primary responsibility for examination development. That changed in 1996 when I was recruited to lead a small team already in place to develop and implement a new examination just for IMGs. This examination was created to address concerns regarding basic clinical skills such as taking a medical history, performing a physical examination, and communicating with patients. While it was required that these areas be addressed in U.S. medical schools, there was no way of assuring that IMGs had received instruction or training in these critical areas. Therefore, the logical solution was to assess them using a valid and reliable performance examination. The Clinical Skills Assessment (CSA) used Standardized Patients (SPs), laypersons trained to portray an assortment of patients with different medical problems. As the IMG examinee moved through a series of simulated encounters and medical examinations, the SPs were trained to assess not only their medical knowledge and skills but also their communication skills and spoken English proficiency. For the first time, ECFMG staff had direct responsibility for development of its own examination materials as well as administering and scoring the CSA.

Like all the examinations, CSA needed to go through a series of pilot studies. As part of that process, my colleagues and I had the opportunity to interview scores of IMGs individually and in focus groups immediately following their participation in pilot examinations. Although we initially focused primarily on what we considered to be the obvious issues surrounding the examination (timing, level of difficulty, clinical relevance, fidelity of the SPs, etc.), it soon became apparent that these encounters between IMGs and simulated American patients presented even more subtle challenges, including nuances of vernacular language, customs of meeting and greeting, nonverbal culturally based behaviors, gender roles, and other aspects of a physician–patient interaction in a new and often very different cultural context. In addition, we could not help but develop an increasing awareness that there were many other issues with which IMGs had to struggle to get into and succeed in U.S. GME programs.

When live testing began, the CSA was administered at a single test center in Philadelphia, and IMG applicants had to come to the center and spend approximately eight hours taking the exam and interacting with ECFMG staff and SPs. There were then as many as 36 IMGs coming to the test center at the ECFMG facilities every day and although we were unable to interview them in the context of such a high-stakes examination, their very presence added to the personal dimension that had begun to show itself during the pilot studies. Despite a number of outreach initiatives earlier on, in prior years communication with IMGs had been primarily limited to letters, e-mails, or phone conversations. There was now a steady stream of very real people, spending considerable time on site. The CSA staff, myself included, began to gain a heightened appreciation of the human and personal dimensions of these physicians struggling to achieve their goals of coming to America and entering U.S. GME programs. It started to become more obvious that they had needs beyond simply being directed through the certification process.

The next chapter in the story was somewhat but not completely serendipitous. The National Board of Medical Examiners (NBME), and the Federation of State Medical Boards (FSMB), the organizations responsible for development of the United States Medical Licensing Examination® (USMLE®) had been exploring the development of a clinical skills examination for U.S. medical students (USMGs) for some time. Noting the success of the CSA for IMGs, collaboration with ECFMG was proposed to develop a single clinical skills examination that would be required of both IMGs and USMGs and that would become part of the USMLE series. The collaboration moved ahead and in the process it became clear that a new entity would have to be created to continue the development and implement of the examination that would come to be known as the USMLE Step 2 Clinical Skills (CS) examination. And, just as importantly, it would require a new Executive Director coming from outside of both ECFMG and NBME. A highly qualified physician was recruited and has ably taken and held the reins of the newly formed Clinical Skills Evaluation Collaboration (CSEC) since 2006. As a result, having effectively put myself out of a job, I could now turn my full attention to an idea that had been germinating since my first serious contact with the IMG community—the idea that we could do much more to ease the journey and transition of IMGs, that we could develop resources and services and make them freely available, that we could create ... an acculturation program!

THE ECFMG ACCULTURATION PROGRAM

Needs Assessment

The logical place to begin such an initiative was with a needs assessment. The first step was to invite several residency program directors (PDs) from the greater Philadelphia area who had significant numbers of IMGs in their programs to get their input into what resources might be most useful for IMGs. A group of about a half dozen local PDs gathered at ECFMG Headquarters and with no preset agenda, they were asked what problems they typically encountered in dealing with their IMGs and what resources or services might help the individual IMG and the program to deal with those issues. Expressed priorities seemed to be for materials that would help the

IMG better understand the workings of the culture of American medicine, particularly as it might differ from their home countries. An essential piece of that would need to include issues of communication. But perhaps the most prescient recommendation coming from the group was that IMGs would need to have access to useful resources well before arriving in the United States and perhaps even before initiating the ECFMG certification process. It was not immediately clear how that might be accomplished, but it was certain that the Internet would play a role in evolving this accessibility.

Since I had no formal staff, I was fortunate to recruit some assistance from other ECFMG staff as well as a local university-based sociolinguist experienced in working with IMGs (Barbara Hoekje at Drexel University), and I formed an informal "A Team," which then met with focus groups of IMGs in GME programs. Our limited resources restricted us to the local greater Philadelphia area and to a limited number of specialties. We recognized that this carried some risk of skewing results but that we would have to defer more in-depth exploration of unique regional or specialty issues. Thus, recognizing that the perfect is the enemy of the good, we began where we could. In the first year of these outreach efforts we visited four area hospitals and met with a convenience sample of 5 to 15 IMG residents and program staff in departments of medicine, pediatrics, and psychiatry. In some of the sessions, we requested to meet with the IMGs without staff present to minimize inhibitions, but in retrospect we did not hear substantially different things with or without staff present.

Primary Areas of Concern for IMGs

What we heard emerging from all those conversations was that there were at least two broad areas that were of concern to newly arriving IMGs. The first related to all the issues of learning the U.S. health-care system and U.S. graduate medical education, and the other regarded settling in to living and working in American culture and dealing with what came to be known as "survival issues"—the details of accommodations, finances, driving, and a host of other daily activities. For those who were accompanied by spouses or family, there were additional issues, including schools for children, employment for spouses, and integration into American social life.

The highest and most immediate priority for most IMGs was to learn how to function in their new roles as resident physicians or fellows. They had to learn to integrate the two concurrent aspects of being a physician in training in the U.S. health-care system, namely, being simultaneously students and health-care providers. These are highly interwoven activities in U.S. GME, and for many this was a significant change from the way medical schools and health-care facilities operated in their home countries. They had to learn the discourse of interacting with not only physician faculty, but also peers and a wide range of other health-care professionals. Although American GME obviously has some degree of hierarchy, to many IMGs the relatively relaxed and informal way that attending physicians and residents interact in the United States seemed far removed from the way professors or supervising doctors were approached (or not) in their prior education and training. Many of the categories of other health-care professionals they encountered were previously unknown to them or had significantly different roles and stature than those they had dealt with in their home countries, the most notable being nurses, who in their home cultures were subordinate to physicians but in the United States routinely questioned or challenged physicians' (especially junior residents') assessments, judgments, and orders.

Physician–patient interactions and patient expectations were also often quite different from what the IMGs had been used to. The typically unquestioning and totally compliant patients they had encountered in their homeland were rarely seen; instead, patients often questioned physicians and wanted to participate in decisions regarding their management and care. The role of families, particularly with respect to elder patients, was again often very different than in their home cultures and frequently left some IMGs confused and uncertain how to proceed. Similar confusion all too often occurred regarding how to reference religion in dealing with illness and bad news, and issues surrounding domestic violence, substance abuse, and sexual health.

Many other complexities of the U.S. health-care system were also initially quite baffling: health insurance provisions and requirements, documentation and access to electronic medical records and radiology files, and rigid restrictions and requirements regarding confidentiality and patient information, to cite just a few.

These were all issues that needed to be addressed in program orientations for new residents, but to do so would take days of indoctrination and that time simply was not available for most. Hospital administration mandated that certain topics, usually those relating to hospital finances and liabilities, would take precedence for the sparse time available for orientation before IMGs began their first clinical rotations, with the result that some of the most fundamental issues noted above got short shrift (or no shrift). The result was that for most IMGs, learning in these areas took place on the fly and the source of learning was most often the residents one or two years ahead of them. Another very practical resource, but only for those wise enough to realize it, were those same nurses who questioned and challenged them; if approached appropriately and collegially, they could be an excellent source of learning the day-to-day issues and practices of the wards, units, or clinics where many of them had been working for years.

In a similar vein, formal orientation and assistance in addressing the "survival issues" previously identified was also inconsistent and much had to be garnered from peers who had recently gone through the process themselves.

Program Directors and Staff Concerns

Although there was less direct exchange with PDs and staff than IMGs themselves in these meetings, a parallel set of concerns emerged from the PDs and other staff who supervise, train, and work with IMGs. Communication issues were high on their lists, in some cases due to accent, rate of speech, or unfamiliarity with U.S. medical terminology or jargon, but in others due to unfamiliarity with the discourse models of doing patient rounds ("rounding"), case presentations, or presentations at conferences. Conflicts with nursing and other medical support staff sometimes arose out of misunderstanding or ignorance of the roles and capabilities of the various members of the interdisciplinary health-care team, the concepts and the models of which were often very new to many IMGs. Authority and gender issues also sometimes muddied these relationships and, when they occurred, needed to be sensitively yet effectively addressed. In addition, IMGs coming from cultures where there was great deference to elders or authority needed to be actively encouraged to be more outspoken and responsive in exchanges on rounds and in conferences, lest their silence be mistaken for ignorance or disinterest.

The need for meticulous, timely, and accurate documentation in medical records and charts was also an area that may not have been prominent in many IMGs' previous experience and training. An understanding and respect for not only the obvious but the more nuanced elements of patient confidentiality and informed consent was also often challenging for those coming from health-care systems that may not have recognized or encouraged these values.

Drafting a Plan: Goals and Objectives

With this initial input as to the range of information, resources, and services that were wanted and needed by IMGs and the staffs of the GME programs

Table 2.1.   ECFMG Acculturation Program Goals and Objectives.

Goal

To assist newly arriving international medical graduates (IMGs) in adjusting
more quickly and easily to learning and practice within the U.S. medical
education system, and working and living in the United States.

Objectives

To identify the core issues relating to acculturation for IMGs and monitor
issues as they evolve

To develop resources, including model syllabi for IMG orientation
programs that can be used by IMGs, Program Directors, and others

To make these resources widely and freely available via the ECFMG
Web site and other means to any and all interested users

To provide appropriate services to facilitate communication between IMGs
and those who can best advise and assist them

To develop and disseminate faculty development materials and other
educational resources for those who supervise, teach, and work with
IMGs to enhance understanding of the challenges, backgrounds, and
issues relating to IMGs

To collaborate with individuals, institutions, and organizations that are
developing resources in acculturation and related areas

To serve as a clearinghouse for a range of materials, programs, and
resources that may be useful to IMGs and those with whom they work and
interact

they would be entering, a set of goals and objectives for the overall
Acculturation Program was drafted, presented to ECFMG leadership, and
accepted as the direction the program would take. These are shown in Table 2.1
and are published on the Web site www.ecfmg.org/acculturation/goal.html.

Development of the IMG Advisors Network (IAN)

Although developing specific resources for IMGs would be an ongoing
priority, it was clear from all our focus groups that there was a wide range of
issues, particularly with respect to coming to the United States and getting
settled, that would be difficult to exhaustively address by resource

development alone. Questions in these areas are best answered individually. Since it was not feasible to have them all answered by Acculturation staff (me), the first step in the Acculturation Program was the implementation of an IMG Advisors Network (IAN). Focus group participants indicated that often the best sources of practical advice and guidance for them on arrival were the IMG residents a year or more ahead of them in the GME process. They had just or at least recently come through the same process and challenges facing the new IMGs, so the experience and what they had learned by way of solutions was still fresh in their memory. However, in this informal arrangement newly arriving IMGs had no access to these "advisors" until they had actually arrived in the United States and in their programs. Many of the issues needed to be addressed before then and a lead time of even a few months could make a big difference in making the transition smoother and less harried. What we envisioned was a one-on-one advisor relationship that could begin as soon as IMGs gained acceptance into a GME program, in many cases well before they even left their home countries. Therefore, we set about identifying a cadre of IMGs who would be willing to serve as such advisors to newly arriving IMGs. The main criterion was a willingness to contribute in this way; beyond that we merely required that the advisor be in or had completed a U.S. GME program and had a medical license (training license acceptable) in at least one U.S. jurisdiction. Invitations were sent out through ECFMG publications, notably *The ECFMG Reporter*, an electronic newsletter that reaches tens of thousands of IMGs and international students. We also solicited support to get the call for volunteer advisers out from several other medical organizations, notably the American Medical Association as well as from several specific medical societies, including among others, the American Association of Physicians of Indian Origin and the Association of Pakistani Physicians of North America.

Advisees were initially limited to IMGs who were being sponsored by ECFMG for their initial J-1 Exchange Visitor Visa. This limited the potential pool of advisees to approximately 1,500, a manageable number for a pilot program. Furthermore, since applicants for J-1 sponsorship must have achieved ECFMG certification and received a formal offer for a GME position, the issues for which they would likely be seeking advice would be limited to those having to do with traveling to the United States, getting settled into suitable accommodations, getting started with the actual training program and a myriad of the aforementioned survival issues—drivers licenses, credit cards, schools for children, and similar issues. It was felt that these were the areas where advisors would be most comfortable and where there was the least potential for misinformation having serious consequences, as might be the case regarding certification or immigration status issues.

IMGs who became eligible for participation as advisees in IAN by virtue of their applying for initial J-1 sponsorship by ECFMG received one or more e-mail invitations with instructions on how to enroll in the program. They were directed to the Acculturation pages of the ECFMG Web site, where they found an in-depth description of the program. Those who were interested could then proceed through a registration process after which they could search the roster of advisors based on medical specialty, country of medical school, gender, family status, year of graduation, and location of practice or program in order to find the best possible match. They could select up to three advisors and could compose brief introductory remarks to each. The advisors were then notified by the IAN program that they had been requested to serve as an advisor for a particular advisee and could see the potential advisee's profile and personal statement. They were provided an e-mail address for the advisee, and it was their responsibility to establish contact. Communications between advisors and advisees were not monitored by ECFMG although there were options to copy the IAN program if they so chose.

The program was launched in December of 2006. From that time until March of 2007, over 100 advisors were recruited. That March date is significant because it is when the National Resident Matching Program (NRMP) annually announces the matching of applicants with GME programs, and it is after that time that the vast majority of J-1 visa sponsorship applications are submitted to ECFMG, triggering the invitation to eligible IMG advisees. The program appeared to run smoothly in support of the class of IMGs beginning training in June 2007, but since we had no ability to monitor communications between advisors and advisees, we administered a survey of advisors, advisees, and nonparticipants who had been invited but did not opt to participate.

The numbers after that first "season" of IAN were relatively modest, with 87 advisees and 130 advisors registered. At that point, we did not have the technical capabilities to track the actual numbers of matches. Of the 43% of advisees who responded, 60% thought the program functioned very well or adequately while 67% felt the information they had gotten was very or somewhat useful. As expected, the issues most addressed were the "survival issues" but approximately half also had questions about "down the road" issues like applying for fellowships, obtaining waivers, and other visa issues.

The biggest areas of dissatisfaction were in not finding a suitably matched advisor or not getting any response from the advisors, unfortunately 20% of respondents.

Of the 60% of advisors responding, 87% felt the program worked well while 97% felt very comfortable in answering questions and giving advice; 95% said they would continue as advisors. The biggest complaint from the volunteer advisors, approximately half of respondents, was that they had never been requested to serve as an advisor.

The survey also included those who had been invited to participate as advisees in IAN but did not choose to do so. Interestingly, there were 389 such respondents to the survey. About one-third did not recall being invited, and another third already had good sources of advice and information. However, 90% of respondents said that in retrospect they might have benefitted from having an advisor.

Based on this initial positive response to the pilots, the IAN program was adopted as an ongoing service of the ECFMG Acculturation Program. However, continuing dialogue with IMGs made it clear that although they were appreciative of assistance in getting settled into GME programs and living and working in the United States, there was also perhaps an even more urgent desire to get information and advice relative to the process of applying to GME programs and trying to find a position. Restricting IAN participation to physicians who had already received a program affiliation and offer of J-1 sponsorship not only limited the number of IMGs who could participate but precluded initial advisee–advisor contacts prior to the IMGs actually obtaining a U.S. GME position. As a result, in late 2009 a significant change was made in eligibility for advisees. The program was opened to IMGs who had registered in the Electronic Residency Application Service (ERAS®) and the National Resident Matching Program (NRMP). This significantly broadened the potential pool of IMGs advisees although it was still limited to those seriously engaged in the application process for any given year. In addition to increasing the number of potential advisees, this change introduced a significant qualitative difference in the program. Now in addition to seeking information about coming to the United States and getting settled in their programs and personal lives, significant numbers of advisees still in the process of applying for GME positions could pose very different questions for advisors—selection of medical specialty, selection of programs to apply to, preparation of application materials, including personal statements, interview strategies, and many more. In addition, there were a number of advisees who had been unsuccessful in obtaining GME positions and were seeking advice on remediating their application profile.

Since this may have represented a significant change from the role for which advisors had initially volunteered, they were given an option to restrict their advice to only acculturation issues or to only application issues. The overwhelming majority of advisors who responded indicated a willingness to provide advice and information in both areas.

The IAN program continues to expand and is now a permanent part of the ECFMG Acculturation Program. As of the closing months of 2010, there were over 600 advisors and almost 1,800 advisees; of those advisees, over 600 are actively engaged in communicating with one or more advisors. As the program becomes better known and established, it is anticipated that it will continue to grow. IAN not only provides a real and practical (and free) service to IMGs, but is also creating a virtual IMG community where ECFMG has an increasingly positive presence in enabling IMGs to actively talk to and help each other. And although it has not yet been studied, it is hoped that some of these advisor–advisee matches will lead to lasting mentorships and even friendships. (Current information on the IAN program can be found online at www.ecfmg.org/acculturation/ian.html.)

Resource Development

Meanwhile, back at ECFMG, with the IAN program up and running, it was time to begin developing other resources. Remembering that program directors had urged that resources be available to IMGs early on, even before leaving their home countries, it was obvious that a Web site, or more specifically, a set of Web pages on the ECFMG Web site needed to be developed and dedicated to acculturation resources.

The first resource to be developed was focused on the culture of U.S. medical practice and was entitled "The One Dozen Most Important Things You May Not Have Known, Understood, or Realized about American Medicine." This was a series of video vignettes with supporting text material providing overview, analysis of the videos, and discussion questions regarding the focus of the video on topics, including the physician–patient relationship, the role of family, confidentiality, gender issues, informed consent, professionalism, and others. I was the primary author of these scripts based on my years as faculty in GME, and they were also reviewed by several physician colleagues at ECFMG. Conveniently, ECFMG had the in-house resources to produce these videos, including a very able audiovisual team, staff with experience in theatrical production and a whole cohort of actors, that is, our extensive cadre of SPs, many of whom had significant acting experience. We also had the resources for postproduction editing allowing us to create a final product that was professionally finished and served our purposes very well. The goal of producing these videos and supporting documentation was to provide a resource that could be used either by individual IMGs for self-study or by programs as part of IMG orientations. (These materials can be accessed and downloaded at www.ecfmg.org/acculturation/dozen.html.)

A second resource simultaneously developed was specifically oriented toward the jargon of medical practice, "Medicalese." This is a glossary of American medical jargon and slang as commonly used in U.S. hospitals and medical facilities, including approximately 60 terms that even fluent English speakers from other countries might not recognize. The material also includes caveats about the propriety of using these terms cavalierly or in front of patients and strongly discourages the use of any terms that would ever be perceived as disrespectful or belittling of patients. (Access Medicalese at www.ecfmg.org/acculturation/glossary.html.)

Launching the Web Site

We now had the Acculturation Program Goals and Objectives developed in support of the initiation of the program, as well as the "One Dozen Things" and "Medicalese." But how would we make them available to IMGs and programs? The obvious answer would be the Internet. They needed to be posted on our Web site where they could be freely accessed by any and all interested parties whether IMGs, PDs, or anyone else. This also fulfilled the request that our original focus group of PDs had made to make materials available to IMGs even before they left their home countries.

With the help of a very able and meticulous Communications staff at ECFMG, all of these materials were edited and proofed, and on February 11, 2008, they were posted on a new section of the ECFMG Web site, www.ecfmg.org/acculturation, accessible either directly through that URL or linked through the ECFMG homepage. It was also established as policy from the outset that all of these materials were to be offered to the public free of charge. These materials can also be modified to suit the users' specific needs, as long as an attribution to ECFMG as the original developers is given.

Launching our Web pages would obviously be of no use unless they were publicized. ECFMG has an electronic newsletter, *The ECFMG Reporter*, that is distributed periodically to tens of thousands of IMGs at all phases of the application and GME process. We used this vehicle for our initial announcements but also enlisted the cooperation of several medical education organizations, the American Medical Association, and a number of specialty and ethnic medical societies to broadcast the news as widely as possible.

At the time the Web pages were launched, we had no convenient way of tracking use, but anecdotally the "One Dozen Things" was receiving a very positive reception, and I personally participated in a number of workshops for IMGs offered by specialty societies where the materials were very successfully used for spirited group discussions. Although not initially an option, after a few months the materials were made available not only for viewing on the Web site but for downloading as well. (Downloads are available at www.ecfmg.org/acculturation/downloads.html.)

The Interdisciplinary Health-care Team

Among the issues that continue to surface in focus group discussions with IMGs and program staff was the confusion that often arose regarding the capabilities and roles of the myriad of health-care professionals that were encountered in U.S. health-care facilities, many of which were completely unfamiliar or did not even exist in the IMGs' home countries. Hence, the Acculturation Program began development of another Web-based resource having to do with the Interdisciplinary Health Care Team (IHCT). Profiles were developed for 10 categories of people who made up this comprehensive team, and included not only doctors but nurses, other direct care providers, therapists, and several other categories, including patients and families.

Within each category there were several different kinds of team members. Each one was described through answers provided to a standard set of questions which included (using Registered Nurses as an example) who a registered nurse is, what a registered nurse does, and several other questions providing information on education and training, supervision, day-to-day activities, licensure or certification, types of patients typically served by this type of provider, and how they may get involved with the management of the patient. In all, some 35 different profiles were compiled for people as diverse as respiratory therapists, chaplains, and ward clerks.

The information for each of these roles was compiled from direct consultation with the national professional organizations (where such existed) who responded to the template questions and provided contact links for further information which are also appended to the profiles. Where such organizations did not exist, I developed profiles which were locally reviewed. Overarching the directory of health-care providers included in this resource is an essential element to provide context for the IMG reader, namely, an overview of the fundamental concept of the interdisciplinary health-care team and the teamwork that it involves. It pointedly addresses the role of the physician, especially the junior physician just beginning training, in interacting respectfully and effectively with the many classes of colleagues that might be encountered in a typical U.S. hospital clinic. (This material is available at www.ecfmg.org/acculturation/ihct/index.html.)

In addition, the IHCT section contains a description and discussion of the role of consultants, especially physician consultants, vis-à-vis the role and continuing responsibility of the physician providing primary care to the patient. IMGs new to the U.S. medical system might be intimidated by consultants or might mistakenly feel that they can abrogate responsibility for the patient to the consultant. This section of the IHCT tries to clarify and explain that often delicate balance (see www.ecfmg.org/acculturation/ihct/consultants.htm).

What's In a Name?

Another area where some IMGs have difficulty is in the vernacular language used in meeting, greeting, and addressing people encountered in the medical setting and beyond. Actually, IMGs themselves rarely recognize this as a problem, but it is noted by colleagues, nurses, and other staff and patients. These verbal foibles and misusages generally do not compromise significant communication and are often accepted by native speakers of English as a somewhat humorous wrinkle in dealing with people from another country, language, or culture. Nevertheless, albeit unconsciously or even subliminally, these minor errors tend to undermine the IMG's credibility and make him or her appear less competent. Therefore, to attempt to address this particular challenge, we developed a simple interactive program, "What's in a Name?" Users are presented a mix of simple scenarios—greeting a new patient or a child, addressing colleagues and nurses, taking telephone calls— and are presented options as to what words or phrases would be most appropriate. Erroneous choices provide explanations as to why they might not be the best choice and redirect the user to try again. Correct answers provide the option of directly moving on to the next item but exploration of other choices is encouraged simply to enhance learning. The program is primarily designed for self-assessment; there is no sign-in required, and no score is generated. This was a simple program to design and create, and it might serve as a prototype for other self-assessments in other areas relevant to acculturation (see www.ecfmg.org/acculturation/whatsinaname.html).

The IMG Survival Guide Template

The idea for this recently developed resource came from participants in a series of Webinars more fully described below. There was wide recognition that compendia of useful local information, often called "Survival Guides," can be very helpful to newly arriving IMGs in navigating not only the policies and procedures of their new institution but also the locale in which they, and often their families, are living and working. These concerns encompass all of those issues identified early on as survival issues. However, the actual creation and production of a guide to reflect and contain the mass of local information needed to be of practical use could be a daunting task. Following a Webinar with GME staff, one of the programs that had participated submitted a copy of the local survival guide which they had developed for their institution and locale. It was quite extensive and comprehensive. Using that document somewhat as a model but more as an inspiration, work began on developing a survival guide template. The final product was a freely editable document covering a broad range of issues related to getting settled in a local community as well as some basic policies and procedures of the individual program. Each section contains generic information on the topic, some suggestions for customization, and suggestions for specific contact information such as local addresses, telephone numbers, and Web sites. A hospital policies and procedures section includes lists of equipment, guidelines for writing orders and prescriptions, suggestions for dealing with difficult situations, including whom to contact, and several other topics. There are also two appendices, one a list of Web sites of "U.S. English Idioms, Slang and Expressions" and the other "An Annotated Suggested Reading List for IMGs, IMG Applicants, and Spouses."

On May 12, 2010, the "IMG Survival Guide Template" was posted on the Acculturation Web pages of the ECFMG Web site with a brief description and rationale for use. The document can be freely downloaded as can instructions for customizing the template to produce either a hard copy or electronic survival guide. A copy of the survival guide that served as the model is also available. Users are encouraged to edit and modify the document as they wish and to generate their own cover materials in order to present their survival guide as a publication of their own institution. In the first five months of its posting, approximately 100 copies of the documents were downloaded. Unfortunately, no tracking mechanism was in place to allow follow-up to see if and how successfully programs had used the template. At this writing, that functionality is being added to ECFMG's Web site, and follow-up of users' experience will surely lead to improvements and refinements of this resource. Again, this model, that is, an editable template, may well have application in other areas of the growing acculturation agenda. (Learn more about and download the template and supporting documents at www.ecfmg.org/acculturation/survivalguide.html.)

Real-Time Communication

In addition to providing freely accessible resources on its Web site, and actively managing the IAN program, direct contact with all stakeholders is essential to keeping the program vibrant and in touch with the IMG and GME communities. At the outset of the program, ECFMG did in fact offer a one-day orientation program to local IMGs, at least in part to explore firsthand some of the issues and challenges in conducting such programs. One of the biggest obstacles to doing so is finding a workable date for residents from the various programs since they have variable starting dates and extensive commitments for orientation at their institutions. The same factors appear to be obstacles to IMG orientation throughout the GME landscape and, based on polls conducted during a recent Webinar, only a small percentage of programs actually conduct IMG-specific orientation.

Reference has been made to Webinars, real-time online meetings where participants from far and wide can listen, speak, and simultaneously view materials. This is a very practical and user friendly way of assembling various groups of stakeholders to exchange ideas and share problems and solutions. A nationwide group of GME program directors and staff has been evolving and is becoming an invaluable resource not only for consultation but hopefully for increasingly collaborative work. There are now regularly scheduled Webinars on a variety of topics of interest to this group and attempts are continually being made to widen participation.

The IAN Advisory Council

While the group referenced in the previous paragraph helps us keep in touch with program directors and staff, we have also established a group more representative of IMGs themselves. Drawing on volunteers from the advisor ranks of IAN, 20 individuals representing a spectrum of specialties, countries of origin, and locations in the United States as well as a mix of gender and family status was formed into an IAN Advisory Council which now serves regularly, again primarily by Webinars, as a consultative and work group reflecting the IMG perspective.

Getting Out in the IMG and GME Communities

It is the intent of the program also to periodically participate in various focus groups to try to continuously monitor the IMG community and stay abreast of any changing concerns, issues, or priorities. As alluded to earlier, I have also participated in a number of orientation programs offered by specialty societies (Psychiatry and Family Medicine to date) and presented various components of the program at national and international medical education meetings.

Collaboration

It has always been the intent of the Acculturation Program to collaborate with other organizations, groups, and individuals who share our goals of assisting IMGs in accessing, entering, and transitioning to GME programs and life and work in the United States. Although there was some limited collaboration in the aforementioned IMG orientation programs offered by specialty societies, to date the most significant collaboration has been with the American College of Physicians (ACP) in authoring *The international medical graduate's guide to U.S. medicine and residency training* (Alguire et al., 2009). This is a quite comprehensive 228-page reference to all aspects of the process of pursuing and entering GME training in the United States, and learning to function in the U.S. health-care system and live and work in the United States. Published by ACP in hard copy and electronically, there is a link to more information on this resource on the Acculturation Web pages.

Going Forward

The ECFMG Acculturation Program would not have been possible without the generous support of many people at ECFMG and without access to its extensive resources. We intend to continue to develop new programs, develop and collect new materials useful for both IMGs and program staff, and pursue active collaboration with a range of organizations and individuals with interest and stakes in the process of IMG acculturation.

More importantly, our hope is that we are at least beginning to highlight the importance of active—even better, *pro*active—efforts to identify and respond to the needs of all involved in the IMG experience. Our work has not been based on extensive research or massive databases. Our mode has been to ask and listen, and then seek creative and accessible resources and services to address the needs and desires identified. Especially important is the recognition of how necessary and feasible are orientation and training resources targeted to individual programs and individual IMGs. Time and resources are scarce in every GME program, but a personalized orientation and welcome for each IMG is a worthwhile investment with very rewarding returns.

Our work has been more than anything else intuitive. The committed men and women who comprise the GME program staffs that teach and train IMGs clearly have the best perspective on what is wanted and needed in their own backyards. We will continue to make resources available, but they can only be improved by use and modification at the local level. We invite, we challenge, we cajole—whatever it takes! Meaningful efforts at acculturation and the genuine welcoming that those efforts bespeak are the least we can offer the IMGs who have worked so hard to gain a place in this health-care system in which we all take such pride.

IN CLOSING

My personal journey to the world of the IMG journey has taken me from a time in my medical education career when the entire universe of IMGs was barely on my radar to a profound understanding of the myriad challenges and opportunities in the world of IMGs. In the process, I have gained a profound respect and admiration for these men and women, who often must struggle to overcome seemingly insurmountable obstacles to find their places in U.S. GME and U.S. medicine. I have come to experience firsthand that they are bright, dedicated, and committed to the highest standards of medical practice. And I have also come to admire and respect the program directors and staffs that work so hard and tirelessly to make them a part of their programs and institutions. I consider it a privilege to have had the opportunity to work with and meet so many dedicated people and can only hope that the work that ECFMG has allowed me to do through the Acculturation Program will have some lasting and meaningful impact on the IMG journey.

The overarching mission of ECFMG is to protect the American public by ensuring the qualifications of the IMGs it certifies as eligible for entry into U.S. GME and ultimately into the larger U.S. health-care system. At one level, the efforts of the Acculturation Program to assist IMGs and ease the hardships of their journeys may be seen inherently as simply doing the right thing. More directly consistent with ECFMG's mission, and particularly with respect to the IAN program, the efforts to provide IMGs with advice, guidance, and information concerning the GME application process (not unlike that available to USMGs from their medical schools) may direct them to programs and specialties to which they are most appropriately suited—and arguably may lead to selection of better qualified and motivated applicants, who logically would then make better residents and physicians. And I would submit as not at all arguable that IMGs who begin training with a better understanding of the complex health-care system they are entering and who are more comfortable with their new roles and lives in and out of the hospital can better and sooner concentrate on learning medicine and providing caring, effective, and safe care to the patients they tend. So after my very long journey, which is far from over, and a rather long chapter, which mercifully is over, hopefully we are all on the same page!

CHAPTER THREE

TEACHING THE COMMUNICATION OF EMPATHY IN PATIENT-CENTERED MEDICINE

Catherine O'Grady

ABSTRACT

Empathy is a recurring theme in teaching clinical communication within the profession of general practice. Drawing upon analysis of the discourse of a challenging primary care consultation, this chapter describes how clinically effective empathy is interactionally accomplished. In light of this analysis, particular challenges facing some IMGs in communicating empathy are discussed. A pedagogical approach is suggested that makes use of authentic discourse data as a means to enhance the ability of doctors to communicate empathy in their interactions with patients.

INTRODUCTION

Empathy, described as the capacity to place oneself in another's shoes and to sense the patient's private world as if it were one's own (Bellet & Maloney, 1991; Rogers, 1961), is a salient theme that animates discussions about clinical communication within the medical profession of general practice.

English Language and the Medical Profession: Instructing and Assessing the Communication Skills of International Physicians
Innovation and Leadership in English Language Teaching, Volume 5, 43–72
Copyright © 2011 by Emerald Group Publishing Limited
All rights of reproduction in any form reserved
ISSN: 2041-272X/doi:10.1108/S2041-272X(2011)0000005009

The communication of empathy is considered by practitioners to be an overarching skill that is at the heart of caring and central to achieving patient-centered care (Frankel, 2009). Empirical studies tie the doctor's display of empathy to desirable clinical outcomes, including better quality of clinical data emerging in the consultation (Beckman & Frankel, 1984), increased patient satisfaction, enhanced patient–doctor trust, adherence to treatment decisions, and improved health status (Stewart, 1995; Stewart et al., 2000). Accordingly, empathy is a recurring theme in teaching and assessing clinical communication. This chapter is informed by data from a study that includes ethnographic observations of clinical training and assessment in the Australian general practice context (O'Grady, 2011). In that context, general practice registrars,[1] who are qualified doctors working toward a career in general practice, undergo an extended educational program that combines on-the-job training with classroom-based learning. The program culminates with an examination that assesses their readiness for unsupervised practice. Both medical educators who implement the training program and medical examiners who assess a registrar's capacity for unsupervised practice frequently invoke the concept of empathy in their feedback to registrars on their communicative performance, with comments such as "make more empathic statements," "excellent communication skills, empathy and concern," "very good empathy with patient." In the world of general practice, empathy is a key construct through which practitioners perceive and evaluate communicative expertise.

But what is empathy? How is it conceptualized by clinicians? How is it actually accomplished in interaction? Might the communication of empathy present particular challenges for some international medical graduates? When conceptualized as a disposition or capacity that doctors bring to their encounters with patients, empathy pertains to individual doctors to varying degrees, regardless of their language and cultural background. Irrespective of background, some doctors may be intrinsically more empathic than others. But when empathy is conceptualized as an activity that doctor and patient jointly accomplish through interaction, the effective communication of empathy may present special challenges for doctors functioning in a new language and in an unfamiliar social and clinical culture.

With reference to ethnographic interviews with medical educators and examiners, as well as to the professional literature, this chapter begins by considering how empathy is understood within the medical profession. Drawing upon close analysis of the discourse of a challenging primary care consultation, the chapter then illustrates how empathy is actually achieved in situated interaction. In light of this analysis, communicative challenges are identified that may arise for some international medical graduates as they strive to perceive and to respond to patients' cues for emotional support in clinically effective ways. The chapter concludes by describing how empathy is currently taught and offers for consideration a pedagogical approach that makes use of authentic discourse data as a means to assist doctors to improve their ability to communicate empathy in their interactions with patients.

The interview extracts, training observations, and clinical case study that illustrate this chapter are drawn from a broader study conducted by the author to meet Ph.D. requirements (O'Grady, 2011). Empathy and its accomplishment was a central focus for that study.

EMPATHY AS DISPOSITION

Within the profession of general practice, empathy is sometimes perceived as a disposition that pertains to the doctor rather than as action that is taken by the doctor. Consider the following extract from an interview with a medical examiner at the Royal Australian College of General Practitioners (RACGP)[2] that formed part of my Ph.D. research:

> I really think it's [empathy] something you may well be born with. It's like any facility. You can improve on your natural ability but if you haven't got that natural ability, you're really up against it. You can learn and you can become better at doing it but like if you're a good sprinter that's great and you can improve on that but if you're a lousy sprinter ... (O'Grady, 2011, p. 82)

The implicit assumption that underlies this examiner's view is that some individuals are by nature more empathic than others. Empathy is conceptualized as an intrinsic capacity that one has naturally and can improve upon. It is a disposition or personality trait that the doctor brings to a consultation, rather than an aspect of mutual understanding that is achieved jointly by doctor and patient through their interactions with each other.

A more active, coconstructed conceptualization of empathy emerges in the following extract from an interview with a senior medical educator responsible for preparing general practice registrars, both locally and internationally trained, for unsupervised medical practice:

> I think one of the things I found interesting was one of the registrars who'd just started working. [Quoting registrar] "It's funny but most of my patients sit down and start to cry." So what is it in the consultation that allows the patient to feel so comfortable that they would unload such an emotionally disturbing element to a perfect stranger? And yet to other doctors that would never have happened. Some people might say "I don't ever have depressed patients in my surgery." But is it because they don't pick up on the cues or is it

because those patients choose to go elsewhere because of some personality trait that they have or [is it because] linguistically that environment has been set up and that problem is never even presented because there has been a barrier set up? (O'Grady, 2011, p. 83)

As this medical educator ponders the reasons why emotions might rise to the surface in one consultation rather than another, she appears to suggest that empathy may be situated and coconstructed and not simply a matter of a doctor's pre-existing disposition. She alludes to a particular and locally produced interactional context that might be conducive to a patient's offering some perceptible cue to an emotionally disturbing situation, and to the doctor's contribution to the achievement of empathy through the action of picking up on and responding to such a cue. Thus, while she conjectures that an empathic personality is a contributing factor to accomplishing empathy, she also seems to suggest that empathy is an activity that patient and doctor jointly achieve, or fail to achieve, through interaction.

This perception resonates with a model of empathic communication from within the medical world that has been influential in teaching clinical communication (Suchman, Markakis, Beckman, & Frankel, 1997). In this model, derived empirically from observation and analysis of recorded and transcribed general practice consultations, empathy is framed, not as an intrinsic capacity or disposition, but as an interactional process.

EMPATHY AS INTERACTION

In developing their empathic communication model, Suchman and his colleagues (1997, p. 680) drew upon observations of a large number of clinical interactions. Focusing on interactional sequences initiated by a patient's cue for emotional support, they found that patients rarely talk about their emotions directly and without prompting. Instead, they provide clues to their underlying feelings, thus presenting the doctor with a potential opportunity for empathic communication.

Through the doctor's attentive listening that includes use of acknowledgment tokens that encourage the patient to continue, a context is created wherein patients can more readily express and elaborate upon their emotions and concerns, to which doctors, in turn, can respond with empathic understanding. The model also incorporates the finding that empathic opportunities can be missed or not taken up by the doctor through responses that terminate any further elucidation of the patient's emotional concerns. While these theorists acknowledge that a doctor's intrinsic capacity and motivation to attend to the emotional experiences of others are essential preconditions for the achievement of empathy, their study and the model that it generates focus on empathic communication as an interactional accomplishment.

But models are necessarily reductionist. It is in their nature to abstract from and leave behind the complex interactional reality that they purport to represent. In generating their model, Suchman and his colleagues were focused on drawing general conclusions from a large collection of interactional sequences extracted from context. Their interest did not lie in the broader interactional context that gives rise to a patient's cue for emotional support or in the consequences of empathy in the ensuing interaction. Their focus was on the doctor's moves in an empathic sequence rather than on the fine-grained detail of how empathy is collaboratively constructed by both patient and doctor together.

Questions remain as to how such a model might play out in practice, and these questions are particularly pertinent for educators working with internationally trained medical graduates. What is the nature of those subtle, indirect clues that patients tend to offer to their underlying emotional and life-world concerns? What are the actions of doctors that encourage patients to elaborate on their feelings and concerns? What characterizes an effective empathic response that resonates accurately with the patient's emotions at a particular moment, and, as a consequence, functions to open up communication about delicate matters of possible clinical significance? The answers to these questions are relevant for all doctors but may be of particular value for nonnative English-speaking doctors who are less familiar with the nuances of language and other ways of meaning through which effective clinical empathy is achieved in English-speaking contexts.

In order to describe how empathy is actually accomplished *in situ*, I will now turn to analysis of the discourse of three extracts from a transcribed videorecorded consultation that was submitted for examination by an experienced medical practitioner seeking membership of the RACGP.[3] The consultation represents a case type considered by practitioners to be among the most communicatively challenging and, as a consequence, among the most revealing of communicative expertise, that is, a case where underlying psychological and emotional issues are not immediately evident in the patient's stated reason for visiting the doctor. A particular challenge in such a clinical situation is to accomplish empathy at critical moments so as to create an interactional climate wherein deeper issues can emerge to be addressed. RACGP examiners rated the candidate doctor in this encounter as an "excellent" communicator, referring specifically to her empathy with the patient.

In presenting the results of this analysis, I would like to suggest that discourse analysis, by making visible and available for discussion the actions that doctors and patients actually perform to accomplish empathy in specific situations, offers a resource for discussion and reflection that is of value for educators and their students. Further, as will later be discussed, pedagogical approaches that make use of transcriptions of authentic interaction might usefully augment current practices for teaching the communication of empathy.

EMPATHY IN ACTION: A CASE STUDY

The patient in this consultation is a 58-year-old woman who initiates the interaction with a request for advice about ovarian cancer screening. She has had a single panic attack in the past and the doctor is aware of this. As the consultation unfolds, the likelihood of more pervasive anxiety and serious depression begins to emerge.

Across the opening turns of the consultation, doctor and patient have discussed the symptoms that have led to the patient's request for cancer screening. The doctor has displayed nonjudgmental sensitivity to the patient's voiced concerns and has gone on to share the biomedical reasoning that would lead her to attribute the patient's symptoms to a pre-existing and benign condition. By turn 104, where the following extract begins, concern about ovarian cancer has been put to rest and the doctor moves to open up discussion about other issues.

Extract 1[4]

104	D:	All right ((redirects gaze from computer screen to patient, reorients upper torso toward patient)) so how are you apart from that (.) that's one worry
105	P:	Um pretty good but : ((fall rise tone)) you know when I came last time I told you I had (.) you said I had you thought I had a panic attack :
106	D:	Yeah ((fall rise tone)) ((sits back from the desk, takes hands off paper records and places them on lap, focuses gaze on the patient))
107	P:	And I still sort of get that feeling (.)# inside : h ((shrugs shoulders))
108	D:	((leans forward elbows on desk and hands cupping her face))

109	P:	[((shrugs shoulders again))
110	D:	[It's a rotten thing °rotten°
111	P:	.hh
112	D:	Tell me about the feeling
113	P:	(..) ((indicates chest)) Um # seem ok during the ## day
114	D:	Yeah
115	P:	But when I get into bed at night not relaxed # # it ° sort of goes chooooo ((gestures to indicate fluttering feeling over chest and abdomen)) ((slight shrug))
116	D:	What's your head doing in that time
117	P:	(.) That seems to be ok just sort of ((pats stomach and chest)) in here sort of thing ((shifts posture quickly in seat))
118	D:	So is your heart beating strangely ((enacts beating gesture across own heart))
119	P:	A little bit yeah
120	D:	mm

This sequence constitutes "a critical moment" (Candlin, 1987) in the consultation, a moment when emotionally sensitive and clinically significant information is being gingerly broached by the patient and when an insensitive response on the doctor's part could lead to her retreat. At turn 105, the patient raises the topic of panic attack obliquely as a reported concern that she attributes to the doctor rather than as her own assessment of her symptoms: "you said I had you thought I had a panic attack: ." In this way she works to distance herself from ownership of the condition.

From the perspective of medical educators who were invited to comment on this transcribed interaction, this is a moment where the direction of the consultation could turn, leaving the true nature and extent of the patient's symptoms unexplored.[5]

> The risk here for the doctor I think is going down the diagnosis pathway and saying "yes I think you had a panic attack, this is a panic attack," but, this doctor doesn't do anything other than leave an opening to go on, concentrates on the feelings and this allows progression. (O'Grady, 2011, p. 178)

As this educator notes, the doctor's attentive silence and bodily actions (106) encourage the patient to continue. At turn 107, the patient offers her symptoms vaguely, tentatively hedging their certainty with the particle *sort of*. Apologetic shrugs, pauses, voice quavers, and intake of breath are visual and vocal perturbations that appear to underline her conversational discomfort with the topic. These subtle vocal and nonvocal signs suggest feelings of disquiet. In the terms of the model of empathic communication (Suchman et al., 1997), they constitute an *empathic opportunity*.

In response, the doctor acts empathically to acknowledge the patient's discomfort by heightening her engagement, reorienting her body toward the patient, and intensifying her gaze (106, 108). Then, as the patient shrugs apologetically once more (109), the doctor transforms the patient's down-graded assessment of her experience with an utterance that seems to resonate with its true intensity: "It's a rotten thing, rotten" (110). With a small intake of breath (111) the patient receives and acknowledges this assessment. This accurate, empathic formulation by the doctor, resonant with feelings that the patient was unable or unwilling to voice, displays both cognitive understanding of the quality of the patient's experience and emotional engagement. It is an expert empathic response that achieves "emotional resonance" (Halpern, 1993) because it accurately reflects the intensity of the patient's feelings. In so doing, it functions to diffuse the patient's embarrassment and discomfort. The patient's experience of panic attack is now out in the open as a matter that can be interpersonally but professionally discussed.

From turn 112, there is a consequent shift in frame to franker discussion. The doctor deploys a command-like utterance, "Tell me about the feeling," that is hearable as a personal request and displays a personal as well as professional interest in the patient's symptoms. This occasions a response in which the patient provides a more detailed clinically useful description of her symptoms. It ushers in a series of more focused diagnostic questions and responses through which the character and intensity of her experience of panic attack begin to emerge.

From this extract, it can be seen that achieving clinically effective empathy is not simply about perceiving, appreciating, and expressing understanding of a patient's feelings. Effective empathy is consequential, and particularly in cases such as this, empathy has clinical work to do. Empathic formulations that articulate feelings which the patient has been unable to explicitly voice, together with the interactional consequences of such formulations, are one set of resources that doctor and patient deploy to put the interaction onto a new footing so as to accomplish a gradual transition to increasingly delicate topics, such as debilitating panic attacks and, as emerges later in this consultation, significant depression.

EMPATHY AS MULTIMODAL ACTION

Extract 1 also illustrates that empathy is accomplished by the simultaneous deployment of a range of semiotic resources. As Kendon (1986) points out, "in interaction we do more than form strings of words. We also employ our bodies in visible actions that have an indissoluble connection with what is said" (p. 4). In this interaction, gaze, body orientation, posture, and gesture function in concert with wording to intensify engagement with the patient at critical moments.

Gaze and body orientation are interrelated, and the body can be seen as an organization of segments, each of which can be oriented in different directions. It is the lower parts of the body, that is to say, the legs and torso, that are relatively more stable and so more strongly communicate participants' frames of dominant orientation with the action going on and with each other (Kendon, 1990; Mehrabian, 1967). In this consultation, as in most general practice encounters, the doctor is engaged with both the patient in person and "the patient inscribed" (Robinson, 1998) in computer records and files. Often, the doctor's engagement with records is accompanied by dominant body orientation toward the computer. Doctors may turn their gaze toward the patient periodically, but keep their legs and torso squarely toward the desk. This communicates the doctor's dominant engagement in the impersonal, noncollaborative action of dealing with records.

However, this doctor, considered by her examiners to be particularly empathic, frequently enters records with her right hand while legs and torso continue to align with those of the patient. Often, this body orientation is maintained as she reads records as well. Her body alignment consistently communicates that she is in interpersonal contact with the patient and poised for mutual talk.

Then, at critical moments, she moves strategically to intensify her engagement with the patient. For example, at turn 106 through a series of interrelated actions she signals readiness for full collaboration with the patient, repositioning her body away from the desk, realigning head and torso, and focusing her gaze on the patient's face. This engagement is intensified further from turn 108 as she leans forward, cupped hands framing her gaze. It is these semiotic actions that herald and accompany her crucial empathic reformulation of the patient's experience, intensifying its impact and enabling the patient to present relevant but emotionally sensitive information for the purpose of diagnosis.

As this extract suggests, and as noted by the medical educator quoted below, effective empathy is likely to be a complex, multimodal accomplishment.

I was just thinking about your analysis of the elements that flesh out empathy. There's no one single point where the doctor has done the single empathic thing. There's a set of behaviors that involve language, posture, silence ... (O'Grady, 2011, p. 179)

In addition, as further analysis of this encounter will affirm, empathy is a cumulative activity. It does not consist in a single, empathic response on the doctor's part. Rather, it involves constant monitoring of the unfolding interaction and continuing responsive action.

EMPATHY AS A CUMULATIVE ACCOMPLISHMENT

At this point in the consultation, the full extent of the patient's emotional and psychological difficulties has not been made accessible to the doctor. Gradually, as the consultation continues to unfold, doctor and patient collaborate to produce delicate moments that reveal more about the patient's emotional experiences. Empathy is an ongoing accomplishment and these sequences cumulatively and progressively contribute to a more detailed picture of the patient's symptoms and thus to the achievement of a mutual understanding about the true nature of her condition.

Across a number of turns leading up to the sequence set out in Extract 2 below, the patient has struggled against loss of emotional composure. As illustrated in Extract 1, voice quaverings and dysfluencies, such as reduced grammatical forms involving the omission of subject pronouns (113, 115), have betrayed the patient's efforts to conceal her distress as she responds to the doctor's diagnostic questions.

113   P: (..) ((indicates chest)) Um # seem ok during the ## day
114   D: Yeah
115   P: But when I get into bed at night not relaxed # # it ° sort of goes
           chooooo ((gestures to indicate fluttering feeling over chest and
           abdomen)) ((slight shrug))

At turn 115, the patient substitutes words with gesture to visually display her symptoms in a "descriptive and verb like" way (Beach & LeBaron, 2002, p. 624), in what appears to be an attempt to avoid speech so as to maintain composure and emotional control.

From turn 124, there is a shift to more explicit emotional talk in which the patient at first describes and then displays tearfulness that is indicative of her level of sadness and is, as a consequence, of therapeutic and clinical significance. This shift in frame is occasioned by a collaboratively produced empathic sequence, initiated by a gesture from the patient that offers a clue to her bewilderment and concern.

Extract 2

124	D:	... just just tell me more [cause
125	P:	[((patient shrugs in bewilderment))
126	D:	((left hand stretches out toward the patient, palm open and fingers splayed)) You look worried like you're
127	P:	((left hand stretches out toward doctor palm open and fingers splayed)) Um (..) I try not to think about it and I try not the tears when I talk the tears come um I don't know ((shakes head)) ##I don't (.) I just sort of get all ((gestures over stomach)) and I thought when you get into bed you should be relaxed:
128	D:	° yeah°
129	P:	And um I just sort of hh (.) I don't know I sort of feel like everything's jumping around inside ¦ It's all (.) and ((shrugs))# I don't know (.) I suppose ##I don't know and #I don't know if it's nerves or what it is (.) ### I don't know
130	D:	What are your nerves like at the moment
131	P:	((shrugs)) um (.) ## I'm fine most of the time and I think it's just um >when I was here last time I told you about< the dog [it's sort of been since then
132	D:	[yeah
133	P:	And I don't know if that's what it is (.) I think that's what's brought it on:
134	D:	°Yeah°
135	P:	((crying)) # ## and I'm trying to get over [it but I'm not:
136	D:	[((doctor reaches for tissues, takes two and hands them to the patient))
137	P:	((takes tissues, sniffs)) I'm sorry ((dries eyes with tissue))

Note that at turn 124, the doctor again deploys a command-like question, mitigated by *just*, that serves both to encourage elaboration and to communicate personal interest in the patient's symptoms: "just just tell me more." While the doctor's invitation to talk obtains only a bewildered shrug in response, this action in turn evokes an empathic response on the doctor's part that is enhanced semiotically by the accompanying openhanded gesture with which she reaches out to the patient (126). At turn 127, the patient receives this response with a mirroring gesture that is a recognizable "re-performance" (Beach & LeBaron, 2002, p. 625) of the doctor's action and is thus expressive of strong affiliation. This coconstructed empathic sequence is effective and consequential, and it evokes the patient's disclosure of the delicate matter of the tearfulness that comes when she talks about her symptoms (127).

Note also the patient's self-repetition of the phrase "I don't know" (127, 129, 133), which constitutes a coherent theme across this sequence. Repetition is evaluative and expressive of attitude (Labov, 1972; Tannen, 1989), and the evaluative effect of this accumulation of repeated phrases, accompanied by voice quavering, shrugs, and head shakes that signify increasing distress, is to emphasize the intensity of the patient's bewilderment at her symptoms and their cause. Across this sequence, the doctor responds with softly voiced acknowledgment and agreement tokens (128, 132, 134) that display empathic attentiveness and so encourage the patient to continue.

At turn 131, in an elaboration of her response to the doctor's question about her nerves, the patient refers to the death of the family dog. She goes on to associate this event with the onset of her symptoms so as to offer an account for their cause (133). The emotive topic of the dog that the patient herself has introduced triggers a reaction that occasions her emotional release, and at turn 135 the patient begins to cry. In a consultation in which the patient has worked to at first conceal and then control her underlying emotional distress, this tearful release is a moment of clinical significance that makes available to the doctor signs that are indicative of the patient's level of sadness. It is also a moment of interpersonal significance occasioning the doctor's display of sensitivity to the patient's tearfulness as she extracts tissues from the box and offers them to her (136).

Yet still, the full extent of the patient's experience of anxiety and depression remains hidden. As the consultation proceeds, the patient continues to invoke matters from the "life-world" (Mishler, 1984), that is, from the social and emotional context of her illness, such as grief over the loss of the family dog, and biomedical factors, such as menopause, to account for her symptoms and to minimize psychological causes. Further, she continues to be evasive about the pervasiveness and frequency of the episodes of anxiety and tearfulness that she is experiencing. How is this elusive information that is crucial to an accurate diagnosis of the patient's condition to be brought into the discourse? What part might the communication of empathy play in this disclosure?

At turn 249, where the final extract in this consultation begins, the doctor has just attended to the medical and administrative tasks of taking the patient's pulse and updating the patient's records on the computer. This done, she moves to re-engage with the patient in person so as to seek out this diagnostic information.

Extract 3

249 D: ((removes hand from patient's wrist)) That's good ((types into computer)) how often do you feel ((turns away from computer whilst gesturing toward her own heart and touching her chest)) (0.3) ((directs full gaze on patient's face)) churned up
250 (0.5)
251 P: # It didn't sort of happen last night :
252 D: ((nods slowly and sustains gaze on patient's face over next turn))
253 P: And it sort of happened (..) it's (..) we've been home (.) a week and a bit (.) it's happened a few times since I've been home (.) because I made this appointment to see you before I went away because I knew it'd be a while before I could get in and I thought well (.) I'm going to speak to you about it
254 D: Yeah ((leans forward toward patient, leans on elbow supporting face in her hand))
255 P: Because I've been sort of upsetting me :
256 D: Yeah
257 P: What about in the daytime (.) how often do you feel a bit (..) teary or sad
258 D: (0.3) ((twisting tissue in hand)) # ° a couple of times °
259 D: A day :
260 P: ((nods)) .hhhh
261 D: (1.0) ((gazes at patient's face)) ... (.) why don't ((leans forehead into hand then raises face to gaze at patient's face)) uuhh :
262 P: .Hh hhh ((begins to cry, takes off glasses)) ## sometimes ## it [just comes out]
263 D: ((extracts two tissues from box and hands them to the patient))[It's rotten (.) it's absolutely rotten]
264 P: ##I don't know why I'm doing it =
265 D: = yeah

At turn 249, as the doctor shifts posture to disengage from the computer and to re-engage with the patient, she simultaneously gestures toward her own heart and touches her chest. Typically, it is patients who self-touch during medical interviews as an adjunct to or substitute for verbal description of their symptoms (Heath, 2002). But in this consultation (see also 118, Extract 1), self-touch on the doctor's part functions to display empathy as the doctor registers on her own body the symptoms that the patient had previously described.

Further, in referring verbally to these symptoms, the doctor chooses to use the metaphorical expression *churned up* over a less marked "core vocabulary" item (Carter, 2004) such as *anxious* or *upset*. As Carter points out, such expressive metaphors lend "an affective contour" (p. 117) to what is being said and are thus expressive of greater intimacy and intensity. Here, the doctor's empathic self-touch, gaze, and body orientation as well as her expressive lexical choice combine to accomplish increased interpersonal engagement between doctor and patient at this sensitive moment.

The impact of this contribution from the doctor is evident in the significant moment of silence that it evokes and that the doctor allows (250), and in the quavering, cracking voice quality that accompanies the patient's hedged, evasive response (251). At this critical moment, the doctor refrains from speech. Once again (see also Extract 1), she makes use of attentive silence to encourage further disclosure, a feature of effective empathic communication that educators commenting on this transcription consider to be a marker of experience and expertise:

She uses silence. I mean there's just a resounding silence. To me that just reeks of someone who's learned from experience that you don't rush in, you let it run for awhile. (O'Grady, 2011, p. 192)

Encouraged by the doctor's slow attentive nod and sustained gaze (252), the patient tentatively elaborates, at first hedging: "and it sort of happened," and then disclosing that she had experienced symptoms of anxiety "a few times" in a little over a week (253). Interestingly, the patient also discloses that this matter has been on her mind for some time. It is an issue that she had intended to discuss with the doctor. Yet, up until this point in this long consultation, the pervasiveness, intensity, and frequency of her symptoms have remained hidden.

At turn 257, the doctor continues to pursue her medical agenda with a diagnostic question about the frequency of the patient's daytime bouts of tearfulness and sadness. But in doing so, she simultaneously works to sustain a relationship of intimacy with the patient by foregrounding a personal rather than a professional identity. *Teary* and *sad* are words from the life-world that realize a personal voice. By choosing these familiar words over more technical and hence distancing terms such as *low in mood* or *depressed*, the doctor maintains her engagement with the patient at this crucial moment.

The patient's response (258) is delayed, an indication of her discomfort with this question; and by manipulating the tissue in her hand, she displays her efforts to maintain composure. Then, with quavering voice, she offers a barely perceptible and unfinished fragment that implies but fails to specify the frequency of her tearful episodes: "# ° a couple of times °." At turn 259, the doctor collaborates to assist the patient to complete this fragment. With an upwardly inflected utterance, she infers and seeks confirmation that these bouts are a daily occurrence. At turn 260, the patient completes this sequence to confirm with a nod and drawn out intake of breath that this inference is correct. The pervasiveness of her symptoms is now out in the open.

The doctor's bodily action (261) as she momentarily buries her face in her hand before appealing to the patient with an upwardly inflected "uuhh:" appears to express a mixture of frustration at the patient's reticence and empathic concern. This prompts a second emotional release from the patient and, at turn 262, following an intake of breath, she again begins to cry. In response to this tearful display, the doctor again acts empathically to offer tissues (263). Her move accompanies a verbal empathic response that is a reprise of her expert reformulation of the patient's earlier hedged and downgraded assessment of her experience (110). This time, however, the formulation is intensified by marked word stress and the addition of the "mood adjunct" (Halliday, 1985) *absolutely*: "It's rotten (.) it's absolutely rotten." Thus, the doctor's response can be seen to resonate with the patient's heightened emotional distress and to display understanding of the intensity of her disturbing symptoms at this moment of full disclosure.

ACCOMPLISHING EMPATHY: A COMMUNICATIVE CHALLENGE

Close analysis of the discourse of this consultation has demonstrated that the communication of clinically effective empathy is a complex, coconstructed, interpersonal, and interactional process that is likely to be challenging for all doctors, and particularly for nonnative English-speaking doctors functioning in an unfamiliar clinical culture.

The achievement of empathy involves constant monitoring of the interaction as it unfolds, and the ability to perceive and to respond to cues for an empathic response that are frequently implicit and indirect. As evident in the transcribed interactions presented in this chapter, such cues include subtle visual and vocal perturbations, such as an intake of breath, a barely perceptible shrug, or a quavering voice, that signify a patient's emotional disquiet. They might also include actions that downplay the significance of what the patient is saying, such as hedging or minimizing, or laughter tokens that take a light-hearted stance toward matters of concern. Under the dual burden of communicating in a second language and pursuing a clinical diagnosis, some IMGs are likely to focus on the explicit meaning of what a patient is saying and to overlook implicit clues to a patient's underlying feelings and concerns.

Prosodic cues, such as marked word stress or shifts in pitch direction, may be especially challenging for IMGs. As Gumperz (1982b) points out, in moment-to-moment interaction, we cannot express in words all that we mean and all that listeners need to attune their talk to in response. Rather, subtle "contextualization cues" (Gumperz, 1982b, 1999), which are often prosodic and often produced and interpreted without conscious thought, function to cue listeners to infer what is intended by speakers and to respond accordingly. But in cross-cultural encounters where participants may not have knowledge of the same prosodic conventions, these barely perceptible cues may pass unnoticed. As an illustration, consider the following extract from a roleplayed consultation that I observed at a clinical communication training workshop for IMGs.

The nonnative English-speaking doctor in this role-play was interviewing a patient believed to be experiencing postnatal depression. He was assessing the patient's mood and had arrived at a point where he wished to explore possible thoughts of suicide or self-harm.

Training Role-play Extract 1

D: ... please tell me Margaret have you ever thought of harming yourself
P: No doctor no (.) I've never thought about harming my<u>self</u> ((rise–fall tone))
D: Good good but you're feeling sad (.) for how long have you been feeling sad

The roleplaying patient's use of marked stress on *self*, together with a rise–fall tone, marked departure from a simple statement of fact. This prosodic contextualization cue, probably produced without reflection, was a signal to the doctor to explore the patient's intention and to infer her hidden concern that she might harm her child. It invited an empathic response that would display the doctor's perception and understanding of the patient's fear and thus encourage her to elaborate. But here, doctor and "patient" did not share communicative background and did not share the same inferential processes. The doctor did not recognize the prosodic convention and could not infer the patient's intention. This competent IMG went on to follow protocols for interviewing a patient exhibiting signs of postnatal depression. At a later stage in the role-play, he asked about the patient's feelings toward her child. However, at this particular moment in the interaction, he was unable to perceive and to respond to the subtle prosodic contextualization cue that carried a clue to her state of mind.

Formulating an empathic response that resonates accurately with a patient's emotions may also pose special difficulties for nonnative English-speaking doctors. IMGs practicing and studying in the Australian health system come from a wide range of places, including the Indian subcontinent, Malaysia, Singapore, other Asian countries, and the Middle East (Pilotto, Duncan, & Anderson-Wurf, 2007). Many have received their medical education, wholly or in part, through the medium of English. They are generally comfortable with the language of medicine and competent in deploying a professional voice, but less familiar with everyday English (McDonnell & Usherwood, 2008; Pilotto et al., 2007). Thus, they may not have ready access to a wide repertoire of lexical and discursive choices that can be drawn upon in order to construct a verbal empathic response that is appropriate, personalized, and effective in its local interactional context.

Furthermore, patient-centered clinical models that require a doctor to enter empathically into the world of the patient may be unfamiliar to many IMGs. As a teacher of internationally trained medical graduates, I am aware that many doctors come from medical cultures where time constraints, extremely limited resources, and a more doctor-centered approach to practice function to prioritize biomedical matters over a patient's emotional and life-world concerns. As these doctors acculturate to a new medical culture, they generally embrace principles and models of patient-centered care that consider psychological and social aspects of a patient's illness along with biological processes. Nevertheless, doctors trained in a strictly biomedical model are sometimes reticent to engage empathically with patients for fear of directing the interaction away from a more medical agenda, of bringing matters into the discourse of the consultation that they feel ill-equipped to handle, or of overstepping what they see as appropriate professional boundaries between the world of the doctor and the world of the patient.

Such reticence is not restricted to doctors trained overseas. Medical educators participating in the study that informs this chapter suggest that locally trained doctors making the transition from hospital-based medicine to primary care are also challenged by the communicative demands of patient-centered care. In hospital settings, a traditional doctor-centered diagnostic model prevails, involving doctor-directed question–answer sequences that tend to marginalize emotional and life-world concerns. Novice doctors, regardless of background, may require focused training in order to develop the capacity to engage in responsive, empathic interaction.

TEACHING THE COMMUNICATION OF EMPATHY: SOME OBSERVATIONS FROM CURRENT PRACTICE

Medical educators participating in the study that informs this chapter refer to "reflecting" as a key strategy for communicating empathy. Through accurately reflecting a patient's feelings, the doctor's understanding of the patient's emotion can be made explicit. In this way, it is argued that empathy can be achieved. In training, many educators provide registrars with a repertoire of exemplar phrases, drawn from practice and considered to carry empathic value, so as to assist their students in developing the ability to reflect a patient's emotions and situation:

> I actually give everybody it doesn't matter if they're from overseas or not I actually give them a list of empathetic sort of statements and um you know when you actually use certain things and so on, and nonverbals. I spend a whole tute [tutorial] a whole hour on empathy and then they've actually got some tools that they can use. (O'Grady, 2011, p. 86)

However, modeling and memorizing a repertoire of stock phrases that have been extracted from the particular interactional context wherein they have a specific meaning and effect, and using these phrases in a new situation, can prove to be problematic. While lists of phrases might appear to be a useful resource, particularly for doctors who are less familiar with English, such an approach can lead to a standardized response that is inappropriate in a specific interaction. As educators themselves acknowledge, recourse to preconceptualized phrases risks undermining the creativity and responsiveness that is a hallmark of effective empathic communication. The repetition of a learned and rehearsed response can in fact communicate the exact opposite of empathy, as this educator seems to suggest:

> But to give you an example of how it [use of standardized empathic statements] can backfire. One of the things I teach is *That must be hard for you*. [Referring to a registrar] "If you use the phrase 'That must be hard for you' just one more time I'm going to strangle you. You need to be more adaptable. It can't just be by numbers." (O'Grady, 2011, p. 87)

Use of standardized forms of language that do not accurately reflect the patient's emotion at the moment of interaction can be received by the patient as a sign of lack of engagement and attention, and as a failure by the doctor to fully grasp and to fully understand his or her true position or state of mind. Such routine phrases can suggest detachment, undermine the emotional resonance that arises out of accurately reflecting the patient's feelings, and run counter to the achievement of empathy. Clearly, the capacity to communicate empathy needs to be developed in context and by way of interaction.

Role-plays of clinical scenarios represent one highly valued and established method that educators use to contextualize the teaching of empathy. This method is illustrated below by way of ethnographic observations of a clinical communication workshop conducted for general practice registrars by a medical educator in Sydney. Yet, role-play cannot reproduce the challenges of authentic interaction. As Stokoe (2011) points out, interaction is not actually "simulateable." Within the role-play activity, doctor and "patient" orient to different interactional contingencies than they would in a "real" consultation in which the patient is truly sick and vulnerable. Role-plays are "essentially educational devices rather than exact representations of doctor–patient interactions" (De La Croix & Skelton, 2009, p. 695). It follows that role-play as a teaching method might be usefully complemented by providing novice doctors and IMGs with opportunities to engage closely with transcriptions of authentic clinical interactions wherein empathy is achieved.

Using Role-play to Teach Empathic Communication:
Observations from Registrar Training

The following vignette captures the use of role-play in a training workshop that was videorecorded and transcribed as part of my Ph.D. research. The session, which addresses clinical communication, including the communication of empathy, was facilitated by an experienced medical educator. Participants comprised both locally and internationally trained registrars who were on day release from their clinical attachments in general practice clinics. Observations of this session draw attention to both the value and the limitations of role-play as a teaching–learning mode in developing the capacity to communicate empathy.

Early in the session, by way of a PowerPoint presentation, registrars were presented with a model for implementing the patient-centered clinical method. Strategies for eliciting patient's ideas and concerns were discussed, empathy as the action of perceiving and communicating understanding of a patient's feelings was considered, and participants and educator generated a repertoire of empathic statements for responding to patient's cues for emotional support. Opportunities were then provided to apply these principles and strategies through participation in a series of clinical role-plays.

The following extracts are from a transcription of one such role-play designed with the theme of empathy in mind.[6] The "patient" had been briefed to begin the consultation with a display of anger at having been kept waiting for her appointment. It emerges that her anger masks fear that she may have diabetes, a fear that is compounded by a family history of amputation related to unmanaged diabetes, and the fact that the clinic had failed to get back to her following an earlier blood glucose test. By way of an apology, the registrar has succeeded in defusing the patient's anger. As we join the role-play, he has just consulted the computer records to locate the results of the patient's earlier glucose test.

Training Role-play Extract 2

97   R: I've checked your results what did the doctor say were you fasting at that time
98   P: Yes
99   R: Your blood sugar is a bit higher than normal
100   P: Oh no re:ally > does that mean I'm diabetic : will I have to take injections : will that impact on my work : <
101   R: I can't tell you (..) it won't impact on your work I can tell you that but if you've got diabetes yes or no I can't tell you now
102   P: Well would somebody get back to me this time :
103   R: Well what happens (.) you'll need to come back again I know it's very difficult for you you're a very busy person and time is very valuable for you

At turn 100, the "patient" responds to news of her test results with an utterance that suggests dismay. Successive questions, delivered with increased velocity, are indicative of her underlying anxiety and constitute a cue that is designed to elicit the registrar's empathic response. However, while the registrar attends to the propositional content of the patient's questions (101) and protects rapport by upholding her image as a busy person (103), he does not appear to have grasped the principles of empathic communication and fails to offer an empathic response that displays understanding of the patient's fears. This prompts the educator to intervene as follows:

Training Role-play Extract 3 (Educator Intervention)

104 Ed: Let's pause here a lot of material there so um the patient made a whole list of concerns and um ah worries there was about three or four just bang bang bang straight in a row and um I agree you dealt with that nicely

105 P: ((nods))

106 Ed: But if we're to practice what we were talking about this morning what's some sort of empathic statement you can make after being told a:ll my worries

107 R: ((2.0))

108 Ed: ((directs gaze to observing participants)) Do you remember that part of the consultation (.) something we could say just to sort of make a connection

109 R: Reassure her like

110 Ed: Can we reassure her :

111 R: Like she was worried about her job that it will affect her job

112 Ed: Yeah something more general than that can we sort of =

113 R: = We are not sure we are not sure that she has diabetes

114 Ed: Yeah but again we don't know we're right at the front end of this consultation there's a lot of information we need to bring together before we can actually work out what needs to happen in the future but she's presenting with an enormous amount of concern and um and apprehension so (.) you need to practice an empathic statement

115 R: I need to know about her personal life is she smoking and other =

116 Ed: = yep we need we're going to get to all that but I just want a statement that will just make her know that she's being listened to

117 Prt: I understand your concerns

118 Ed: I understand your concerns

119 Prt: Or you seem very concerned about these things I think maybe a statement to reflect back to her that you've heard what she's saying under all these questions

120 P: ((nods)) mm yeah

121	Ed:	So you've got many concerns (.) that's a lot of concerns yes you're very concerned (.) I can understand your concerns I mean you have to personalize it and make it work for you (.) empathic statements from a list don't work so well
122	Ed:	((directs gaze to observing participant)) What would you say Anne
123	Prt:	It depends on the patient but I'd probably say something like you've obviously got a lot of concerns we'll make sure we address all of these today
124	Ed:	Mm it's an empathic statement plus a sort of a way forward as well

Clearly, role-play is a useful teaching and learning device that provides educators and registrars with the opportunity to jointly construct empathic responses in context-sensitive ways. Empathy is perceived by this educator as an interactional accomplishment, and, across the sequence, he works with the registrars to construct an empathic statement that might display recognition of the patient's concerns at this particular moment. Further, he is wary of stock phrases that are inappropriate in a specific local interactional context and can run counter to the achievement of empathy. At turn 121, he enjoins the registrars to personalize their statements, "empathic statements from a list don't work so well." But despite this concern to contextualize empathic responses and to avoid simple replications of preconceived phrases, the teaching of empathy appears to be narrowly focused on the doctor's contribution to the interaction.

Yet, as discourse-analytical findings that have been set out in this chapter have shown, the achievement of empathy is a complex, coconstructed, multimodal, and cumulative process that goes beyond a single, verbal empathic statement on the doctor's part. Empathy in action involves ongoing monitoring of a patient's changing emotional state and the perception of clues to that state that are frequently indirect and implicit in nature. It involves empathic responses to these implicit cues that resonate accurately with the patient's feelings at a particular moment and the patient's receipt of these responses as acknowledgment that they feel understood. Further, clinical empathy is purposeful and consequential, engendering trust, opening the way to a more effective therapeutic relationship, and bringing matters of clinical significance into the discourse.

In light of this complexity, it would appear that training practices might be enhanced by providing opportunities for registrars to closely examine authentic patient–doctor interaction. How can transcriptions of interactions that display how empathy is actually achieved be usefully incorporated into communication training to complement role-play? As a response to this question, I will now propose a model for teaching the communication of empathy that makes use of discourse-analytical findings.

TEACHING THE COMMUNICATION OF EMPATHY: USING TRANSCRIPTIONS TO COMPLEMENT ROLE-PLAY

The sample training session for registrars and novice doctors that is set out below follows a procedure for working with transcriptions that was developed by Candlin, Maley, Crichton, and Koster (1994) for use in communication training in legal contexts, and has also been proposed by S. Candlin (1995) for use in the context of nurse education. The procedure is experiential and participatory and facilitates joint reflection on transcribed interactions with a view to behavioral change. It follows a pedagogically phased cycle of *awareness, knowledge, critique,* and *action* originally developed by Auerbach and Wallerstein (1984) for use in ESL contexts in the United States.

Phase 1: Awareness

This phase involves consciousness-raising about the nature of empathy and its clinical importance. Participants are encouraged to share what they know about empathy so as to enhance their understanding of the topic. They are invited to reflect briefly on their experiences of clinical situations, either authentic or simulated, where empathy was invoked, on how they responded, and on the impact of this response. Concerns they might have about engaging with patient's emotions and life-world issues are elicited and acknowledged. The discussion is consolidated with definitions of empathy that focus on empathy as an interactional accomplishment that has consequences for the clinical direction of a consultation. Synthesizing definitions of empathy drawn from the work of Frankel (2009), Mercer and Reynolds (2002), and Suchman et al. (1997), empathy is an activity that involves (1) the doctor's accurate perception of the patient's feelings, (2) the effective communication of that understanding back to the patient, and (3) the patient's receipt of that understanding as acknowledgment that their feelings and situation have been accurately understood. Clinical empathy is effective and consequential. It involves not only the ability to perceive and respond to the patient's feelings, but the ability to act on that understanding in a helpful and therapeutic way.

Transcriptions of empathy in action, such as Extracts 1, 2, and 3 from the consultation presented in this chapter, are then provided to participants. Registrars examine these transcripts, first individually and then collectively in small groups in order to consider what is going on.

As registrars examine the transcribed interactions and discuss them with their peers, they are likely to notice that the doctor's empathic responses go beyond the stocks of preconceptualized phrases that circulate in discussions and appear in training texts. They might see and appreciate that these responses are carefully designed to display sensitivity to the quality and intensity of the patient's experiences. Their awareness of empathy as a multimodal accomplishment might also be enhanced as they appreciate the role of silence in encouraging the patient to elaborate, and of body orientation, gaze, and gesture that function in concert with wording to intensify engagement with the patient. Their attention might also be drawn to the nature of the patient's cues for emotional support that are seldom explicit, frequently nonverbal and include shrugs, voice quavers, and barely perceptible signs such as an intake of breath.

Phase 2: Knowledge

In this phase, new knowledge is brought to bear on the task of describing, interpreting, and explaining more precisely what it is that is going on in the transcribed interactions. As educators join with participants to discuss the transcripts, they introduce pertinent explanatory concepts to facilitate a more in-depth analysis of the interaction. In this way, they gradually build a shared analytical language that might later provide a resource for joint reflection on the registrars' own communicative performance in role-plays or real-world encounters.

For example, the concept of "emotional resonance" (Halpern, 1993) might be usefully introduced to capture the combination of cognitive understanding of the patient's experience of panic attack and emotional engagement that is displayed in the doctor's expert empathic responses (see 110, 263). By describing the doctor's expert empathic responses as "designed for the recipient" (Drew & Heritage, 1992), educators might focus the atten-tion of registrars on the context-sensitive nature of effective empathic com-munication that stands in contrast to the preconceptualized, rote-learned response. At such moments, educators might also encourage the participants to generate alternative responses to the patient's cues for emotional support. Such an activity would be of particular value to IMGs, expanding their repertoire of empathic responses as they develop the capacity to create empathic responses in context-sensitive ways.

During this phase educators could fruitfully broaden discussion beyond a focus on the doctor's empathic responses to consider empathy as a sequential, coconstructed and consequential accomplishment. With reference to Extract 2 for instance, they might direct attention to the empathic sequence that is instigated by the doctor's sensitively designed question (124) and culminates in the patient's disclosure of the delicate and clinically significant matter of her tearfulness (turn 127).

124   D: ... just just tell me more [cause
125   P: [((patient shrugs in bewilderment))
126   D: ((left hand stretches out toward the patient, palm open and
            fingers splayed)) You look worried like you're
127   P: ((left hand stretches out toward doctor palm open and fingers
            splayed)) Um (..) I try not to think about it and I try not the
            tears when I talk the tears come um I don't know ((shakes head))
            ##I don't (.) I just sort of get all ((gestures over stomach)) and I
            thought when you get into bed you should be relaxed:
128   D: ° yeah°

Here, close attention to the design of the doctor's question (124) would build and refine the registrars' knowledge of question design and its effects. Participants, both IMGs and locally trained, would come to appreciate that such a formulation is not simply an open question that functions to elicit information or to invite elaboration. Rather, such a question type also has interpersonal effects. In choosing this form, the doctor conveys a personal as well as a professional interest in the patient and her symptoms, thereby evoking the subtle bewildered shrug (125) that represents a clue to the patient's emotional state and a cue for emotional support.

As the registrars take note of the doctor's empathic response (126), appreciating how wording and gesture combine to intensify its effect, and, as they notice the affiliative mirroring gesture that it evokes in the patient, the registrars' perception of empathy as a mutual and responsive accomplishment will be heightened. Further, as they consider the consequences of empathy in encouraging the patient to disclose sensitive details of her symptoms, their appreciation of empathic communication as an effective clinical tool is likely to be sharpened.

Phase 3: Critique

In this phase, registrars are invited to examine the interactions more closely in order to critique the strategies that the doctor deploys. They are asked to consider why particular strategies were chosen, to evaluate their effectiveness in the context of the interaction, and to consider what alternative actions might have been taken and to what effect.

For example, with regard to Extract 1, they might be asked to consider the doctor's response to the patient's hedged, guarded allusion to her experience of panic attack (105). Educators participating in the study that informs this chapter have suggested that this doctor's action at this critical moment in the consultation contrasts with the likely response of a novice doctor, and is a marker of experience and expertise.

> I look at this and I see experience, 'cause we deal with registrars all the time. You said you thought I had a panic attack. A registrar would say "well yeah" or "we'll talk." This doctor doesn't do *any*thing other than leave an opening to go on, [she] concentrates on the feelings and this allows progression. "And I still get that sort of feeling" (107). Again an opportunity where an inexperienced person I guess in *my* experience would rush in and say something and again the doctor uses body language, doesn't fill the space, refuses to fill the space with noise, uses their body, does a number of things. (O'Grady, 2011, p. 312)

In order to bring the expert practice of their experienced colleague into sharper focus, registrars would be encouraged to critique the doctor's actions by considering such questions as:

• Why did this doctor choose to respond as she did?
• What was the effect of her attentive silence?
• What if she had responded by sharing the reasoning behind her diagnosis of likely panic attack?
• What impact might this choice have had on the interaction?
• How might this choice have altered the trajectory of the consultation?

By interrogating the practices of their more experienced colleagues in this way, in the company of mentors and peers, it is envisaged that novice doctors as well as doctors trained in a different medical culture would build knowledge about the mechanisms whereby effective empathy is accomplished, as well as confidence to try out new behaviors, including attentive silence, in their own practice.

Phase 4: Action

In this final phase, registrars consider what they have learned about the accomplishment of empathy through their analysis of transcribed interactions. They reflect on how this new knowledge will be brought to bear on their own practice as they try out new behaviors in both roleplayed and real-world consultations and as they evaluate their impact and effect. They are also encouraged, with the consent and permission of patients, to undertake the recording and transcribing of critical moments from their own interactions with patients in the future as a means to reflect on their developing practice.

A CLOSING COMMENT

Close analysis of the discourse of transcribed consultations makes visible the lived, *in situ* practices of experienced members of the professional community of general practice as they interact with patients in specific, communicatively challenging encounters. But transcriptions cannot provide novice doctors and IMGs with models to emulate or scripts to follow. Each clinical encounter is unique, and empathy is accomplished through responsive, coconstructed interaction. Action, both verbal and nonverbal, that is appropriate and effective at a particular moment in one consultation may not readily apply in another.

Nevertheless, transcribed interaction offers doctors of all backgrounds the opportunity to see, in fine-grained detail, what others do. As Schön (1983) suggests, professional expertise, including communicative expertise, develops gradually and cumulatively as practitioners build up a repertoire of experiences, images, actions, and examples that guide and inform reflection-in-action in subsequent situations. In this way, over time, practitioners develop a faculty of "professional judgment" that can be relied upon to inform their choices in unforeseen situations.

Through engaging with transcriptions that represent real-world practice and through learning to see, appreciate, and critique what others do to accomplish empathy, doctors of all backgrounds might augment the repertoire of communicative resources available to them as they make communicative choices in the complex and challenging situations that make up clinical practice.

NOTES

1. In the Australian medical environment, the term "registrar" refers to a qualified medical officer who is working under supervision in a particular medical context, such as a general practice clinic, while preparing for an examination for admission into a specialist medical college, such as the Royal Australian College of General Practitioners.

2. The Royal Australian College of General Practitioners is a professional organization representing members of the medical profession who are working in or toward a career in general practice. It is the body responsible for assessing doctors' skills and knowledge and for supporting ongoing professional development.

3. To attain membership of the RACGP, experienced practitioners have the option of submitting recordings from their practice to the College for assessment. The transcribed extracts analyzed for this chapter represent one such consultation.

4. The key to transcription conventions that are used throughout this chapter is set out in Appendix 3.1.

5. The research methodology for my Ph.D. research included a number of collaborative workshops in which participating medical educators and examiners engaged with my analysis so as to bring practitioners' perspectives to bear on findings and to consider the relevance of these findings to practice. This extract is from one such workshop.

6. In the training transcriptions R refers to the registrar taking the role of doctor, P to the actor playing the patient, Ed to the medical educator and Prt to other registrars participating in training.

ACKNOWLEDGMENTS

I wish to acknowledge the Royal Australian College of General Practitioners for their support and involvement in the research project that informs this chapter and for permission to make use of the data that appears (for details, see O'Grady, 2011). I also wish to acknowledge the medical educators, examiners, registrars, and patients who participated in the project, as well as my Ph.D. supervisor at Macquarie University, Professor Emeritus Christopher Candlin, for his valuable input and advice.

APPENDIX 3.1 TRANSCRIPTION SYMBOLS

[	A square bracket indicates the point at which a current speaker's utterance is overlapped by the talk of another.
(1.0)	Numbers in parentheses indicate silence between turns at talk. The number indicates the length of the silence, for example, (1.0) indicates a silence of a second.
=	Where the turns of two different speakers are connected by two equal signs, this indicates that the second followed the first with no discernable silence between them, or was "latched" to it.
(.)	A dot in parenthesis indicates a micropause that is hearable but not measurable.
(words)	Words within parenthesis indicate the transcriber's best guess at partially audible material.
::	Colons indicate the stretching or prolonging of the sound that immediately precedes them.
word	Underlining indicates stress or emphasis either through increased loudness or higher pitch.
WORD	Upper case indicates especially loud talk.
↓	An arrow indicates a strong fall or rise in pitch in accordance with the direction of the arrow.
°	Degree signs indicate that the talk enclosed by the signs is markedly quiet or soft.
Yes:	If the letters preceding a colon are underlined, this indicates that there is a falling intonation contour; you can hear the pitch turn downward.
Yes:	If the colon itself is underlined, this indicates a rising intonation contour; you can hear the pitch turn upward.
hhh	Hearable aspiration is shown where it occurs in the talk by the letter "h," the more "h"s the more aspiration is heard.
(hh)	Aspiration representing breathing or laughter may occur within a word. It may be enclosed in parenthesis to set it apart from the letters of the word.
$	$ represents a voice quality that betrays that the speaker is smiling while speaking.
#	A creaky voice quality that betrays that the speaker is close to tears.

(( ))   Double parentheses are used to mark descriptions of events, for
             example, ((telephone rings)).
> <   The combination of "more than" and "less than" symbols
< >   indicates that the talk between them is compressed or rushed.
             Used in the reverse order, these symbols indicate that the talk
             between them is markedly slowed down or drawn out.

PART II
QUALIFICATIONS AND COMPETENCIES

CHAPTER FOUR

EVALUATING THE SPOKEN ENGLISH PROFICIENCY OF INTERNATIONAL MEDICAL GRADUATES FOR CERTIFICATION AND LICENSURE IN THE UNITED STATES

Marta van Zanten

ABSTRACT

International medical graduates seeking to practice in the United States must pass the United States Medical Licensing Examination® (USMLE®) Step 2 Clinical Skills (CS), a seven-hour performance test which incorporates an assessment of an examinee's spoken English proficiency evaluated by trained lay raters who are simulating patients in a mock medical environment. This chapter focuses on issues associated with that assessment, including scale development, rater training, standard setting, and ongoing reliability and validity data. Aggregate IMG performance statistics are provided. While overall reliability for the spoken English proficiency measure in the Step 2 CS is high, future studies are needed to better understand nonnative English-speaking IMGs' performance in the medical workplace.

English Language and the Medical Profession: Instructing and Assessing the Communication Skills of International Physicians
Innovation and Leadership in English Language Teaching, Volume 5, 75–90
Copyright © 2011 by Emerald Group Publishing Limited
All rights of reproduction in any form reserved
ISSN: 2041-272X/doi:10.1108/S2041-272X(2011)0000005010

INTRODUCTION

Verbal communication skills are essential elements of physician competence. In providing patient care, doctors must be able to ask precise and unambiguous questions to accurately solicit descriptions of their patients' current symptoms, past medical histories, and pertinent family disease information. Physicians must possess the language skills necessary to express empathy and compassion as well as to counsel their patients with tact and clarity. In addition, it is essential that patients fully understand diagnosis and treatment regimens. While the patient–physician dialog can be impeded for numerous reasons, including the complexity of the information being exchanged and the emotional responses often associated with illnesses, it is essential that health-care providers communicate effectively with patients, family members, and other associates in the health-care team.

Successful communication between doctors and their patients has been shown to lead to more efficient health-care delivery and more desirable patient outcomes (Stewart, 1995). Patients express greater satisfaction with care, better compliance with treatment regimes, and enhanced recall and understanding of the information received when they perceive that their doctors communicated effectively.

Conversely, deficiencies in communication skills inhibit a physician's ability to effectively interview patients, to understand their narratives and concerns, and to interact with patients' family members and other medical staff. Some malpractice claims have been shown to be the result of a physician's poor communication skills and a lack of understanding between the doctor and patient (Levinson, Roter, Mullooly, Dull, & Frankel, 1997). A lack of precise and effective communication among medical team members has also been demonstrated to contribute to adverse patient events (Reader, Flin, & Cuthbertson, 2007).

Communicating in English in the medical environment may be more challenging for nonnative English-speaking physicians as compared to their native speaker peers, due to both potentially lower language proficiency and/or cultural differences in health-care expectations. Yet poor communication skills are not solely a problem of nonnative speakers. Most studies documenting breakdowns in communication in the medical setting include a sample of health-care providers without regard to language background. The literature on communication skills of physicians usually encompasses communication in the broadest sense, including the speaker's topic and word choice, tone, demeanor, body language, and interpersonal behaviors, in addition to language accuracy. Therefore, although issues associated with the assessment of spoken English proficiency of nonnative English-speaking physicians practicing in the United States is the focus of this chapter, the topic of ensuring adequate communication skills of physicians is applicable to all health-care providers.

NONNATIVE ENGLISH-SPEAKING PHYSICIANS IN THE UNITED STATES

Due to workforce needs and training opportunities, many physicians who do not speak English as their first language choose to practice medicine in English-speaking countries such as the United States, the United Kingdom, and Australia. Currently, approximately 25% of physicians in training and in practice in the United States are graduates of international medical schools (IMGs) (Brotherton & Etzel, 2009), and approximately 75% of these internationally trained physicians self-report a native language other than English (van Zanten, Boulet, McKinley, De Champlain, & Jobe, 2007).

IMGs seeking to enter accredited graduate training programs in the United States must first be certified by the Educational Commission for Foreign Medical Graduates® (ECFMG®). The purpose of ECFMG certification is to ensure that IMGs possess knowledge and skills at a level comparable to graduates of United States medical schools. While the specific ECFMG certification requirements have been modified over the years, current requirements include verification of a medical diploma, graduation from a medical school listed in the International Medical Education Directory (IMED), and passing scores on the United States Medical Licensing Examination® (USMLE®) Step 1 Basic Science, Step 2 Clinical Knowledge (CK), and Step 2 Clinical Skills (CS) exams. Step 1 is a multiple-choice exam that assesses an examinee's ability to understand and apply important concepts of the sciences basic to the practice of medicine, with special emphasis on principles and mechanisms underlying health, disease, and modes of therapy. Step 2 CK is a multiple-choice exam that assesses an examinee's ability to apply medical knowledge, skills, and understanding of clinical science essential for the provision of patient care under supervision. Step 2 CS is a performance exam that tests a physician's ability to gather information from patients, perform physical examinations, and communicate the findings to patients and colleagues. Step 1, Step 2 CK, and Step 2 CS may be completed in any order.

While passing Step 1, Step 2 CK, and Step 2 CS are the prerequisite exams for ECFMG certification, IMGs usually take an additional exam, Step 3, during residency. Step 3 assesses whether physicians can apply medical knowledge and understanding of biomedical and clinical science essential for the unsupervised practice of medicine, with emphasis on patient management in ambulatory settings. Step 3 provides a final assessment of physicians who will be assuming independent responsibility for delivering general medical care and is required by most state medical boards for licensure (Federation of State Medical Boards, Inc., & National Board of Medical Examiners, 2011).

THE STEP 2 CLINICAL SKILLS (CS) EXAM

Clinical performance evaluations such as the Step 2 CS have been widely used around the world to assess a physician's ability to communicate with patients. Certification and licensure examinations in Australia, Canada, the Netherlands, the United States, and other countries all include a measure of physicians' spoken language proficiency (Boulet, Smee, Dillon, & Gimpel, 2009; Boulet, van Zanten, McKinley, & Gary, 2001; Chur-Hansen, Elliott, Klein, & Howell, 2007; Chur-Hansen & Vernon-Roberts, 1999; Chur-Hansen, Vernon-Roberts, & Clark, 1997; Hawkins et al., 2005; Rothman & Cusimano, 2000, 2001; Sonderen, Denessen, Ten Cate, & Splinter, 2009). While the spoken language proficiency of physicians is assessed in numerous countries, in the United States the ECFMG has included a spoken English proficiency requirement as part of a performance examination of clinical skills for IMGs since 1998. From 1998 until 2004, the ECFMG Clinical Skills Assessment® (CSA®) fulfilled this requirement. Beginning in 2004, all allopathic (physicians who receive an M.D. degree) graduates, including both graduates of U.S. medical schools (USMGs) and IMGs, have been required to demonstrate appropriate clinical skills in a simulated medical environment. The ECFMG CSA was replaced by the USMLE Step 2 Clinical Skills (CS), a comprehensive exam with three evaluated dimensions: Integrated Clinical Encounter, Communication and Interpersonal Skills, and Spoken English Proficiency. The CS is currently required for all physicians who seek graduate training positions in the United States, including graduates from medical schools located in the United States and all other countries. Therefore, the primary focus of this chapter will be on the CS exam, and specifically the spoken English proficiency component of the assessment.

In the Step 2 CS (Hawkins et al., 2005), physician test-takers rotate through a series of 12 stations, encountering a different standardized patient

(SP) in each room. The SPs are lay persons who are extensively trained to portray a particular patient, memorizing details of the present complaint, past medical history, social history, etc., and learning affective mannerisms and the appropriate responses to various physical examination maneuvers. The physician test-takers are aware that the SPs are actors simulating their complaints, not actual patients. Nevertheless, physicians are instructed to interact with the SPs as they would with actual patients, gathering relevant data through questioning the patients about their illnesses, performing physical exams, counseling patients on risky behaviors, and providing SPs with information about possible diagnosis and follow-up plans.

The CS exam is approximately seven hours in duration. After arriving at the test center, physician test-takers view a short video that provides orientation information regarding expectations and exam logistics. Physicians are also instructed on all exam policies, such as the prohibition of recording devices and the sharing of exam information with other test-takers. Each of the 12 cases is 25 minutes in duration—15 minutes for the patient interview and 10 minutes for the written patient note. Because the exam is modeled on a first-time ambulatory care visit and physicians are instructed to take a focused history based on the patient's chief complaint, 15 minutes is considered adequate time for a patient interview. The physicians are not expected to take a complete history, and invasive physical exam procedures are prohibited. Immediately following the patient encounter, the physician exits the room and is given a minimum of 10 minutes to sit at a designated station and complete a written documentation of the encounter. (If a physician exits the patient's room prior to the 15-minute warning, the physician may begin writing the patient note immediately. The physician is not permitted to re-enter the examination room after leaving.) Currently, test-takers are given a choice to either type using a computer provided at each station or handwrite their patient notes on paper provided by the exam proctors. As of July 17, 2011, physicians will be required to type all patient notes. Test-takers are given one 30-minute break and one 15-minute break during the day.

Before entering each room, physicians are instructed to read a short description of the patient they are about to examine. This printed information includes the patient's name, age, gender, vital signs, and a brief reason for the visit. In most encounters, the SP is wearing a hospital gown and is sitting or lying on the examination table when the physician enters the room. In some special cases, the SP is wearing street clothes and the physician is informed that the focus of the case is on counseling skills and that no physical exam is required. In other special cases, the physician does not meet the SP face-to-face but instead is instructed to use a telephone in the exam room to call the patient and conduct the encounter. The SP is sitting in another room waiting to answer the calls, and because the physician and the patient do not meet face-to-face, no physical exam of the patient is required.

The entire pool of potential cases is comprised of various clinical problems and types of patients that are typically encountered by a doctor in the United States. The 12 cases that make up each specific CS exam are selected based on a blueprint designed to ensure that each physician encounters an equivalent but not identical sample of different complaints, conditions, and patient demographics (i.e., age, gender, and acuity of the illness). The presentation categories include, but are not limited to, cardiovascular, constitutional, gastrointestinal, genitourinary, musculoskeletal, neurological, psychiatric, respiratory, and women's health. While physician test-takers may not see a patient in each of the defined categories, the exam blueprint ensures that physicians encounter a reasonable mix of cases and patients.

SCORING THE EXAMINATION

Immediately following each encounter, the SPs document the clinical skills of the physician test-taker by completing a case-specific checklist indicating which history items were asked and which physical exam maneuvers were performed correctly according to predetermined protocols. Scores for this checklist comprise the data-gathering (DG) component of the exam.

As part of the CS, physicians are instructed to establish rapport with the patients, elicit pertinent historical information from them, perform focused physical examinations, answer questions, and provide counseling when appropriate. The SPs provide ratings of physicians' communication and interpersonal skills (CIS) along three dimensions, questioning skills, information-sharing skills, and professional manner and rapport. These ratings are provided on a scale from 1 (needs significant improvement) to 9 (very good).

The first CIS dimension, questioning skills, includes assessment of various abilities, such as a physician's use of open-ended questions, transitional statements, facilitating remarks, and summarization, and avoidance of leading or multiple questions, medical terms/jargon unless immediately defined, and interruptions when the patient is talking. For the second dimension, examples of information-sharing skills include an evaluation of a physician's ability to acknowledge patient issues and concerns and to then clearly respond with information. Physicians are also evaluated on their ability to provide counseling when appropriate and to close the encounter with statements about what happens next. The final subcomponent, professional manner and rapport, includes criteria such as asking about the patient's expectations, feelings, concerns, support systems, and impact of illness, with attempts to explore these areas. Other examples of rated behaviors include the physician's ability to provide opportunities for the patient to express feelings and concerns, to encourage additional questions or discussion, to make empathetic remarks, and to show consideration for patient comfort during the physical examination.

The spoken English proficiency (SEP) rating is based on how effectively a physician test-taker is able to communicate with the SPs in English. Mispronunciations, incorrect word choice, or other language deficiencies that may have caused a breakdown in communication between the patient and doctor are all considered by the SPs when providing their rating. The SPs are instructed to make a holistic judgment of their overall listener effort and how effectively the physician communicated, not simply whether or not the physician had a foreign accent. The SEP rating tool is a holistic rating scale, and the rating descriptors range from 1 (needs significant improvement) to 9 (very good).

Patient notes (PN), completed by physician test-takers after the patient encounters, are scored holistically by trained physician raters. The PN exercise is used to assess the physician's ability to summarize and synthesize the history-taking and physical examination data collected in the patient encounter.

To pass the CS, physician test-takers are required to pass all three conjunctive components (Integrated Clinical Encounter, a combination of DG and PN scores; CIS; and SEP) in the same administration. Physicians who fail one or more of the three components must retake the entire exam; there is currently no limit on the number of times a physician can take the CS.

HISTORICAL DEVELOPMENT OF ENGLISH LANGUAGE PROFICIENCY REQUIREMENT

Before the currently administered CS exam, the preceding exam, the Clinical Skills Assessment (CSA), was the requirement for ECFMG certification from 1998 to 2004. Prior to the CSA implementation in 1998, numerous needs assessments, validation studies, etc., were conducted to justify and plan for all aspects of the assessment, including the spoken English proficiency component. Since IMG physicians are seeking ECFMG certification for admission into supervised training programs, the spoken English proficiency rating tool needs to measure entry-level skills. Staff first reviewed the literature available at that time (prior to 1998) (i.e., Arthur, Brooks, & Long, 1979; Chur-Hansen et al., 1997; Eggly et al., 1999; Sutnick, Kelley, & Knapp, 1972; Sutnick et al., 1993) and solicited expert opinions concerning the specific English proficiency competencies required of first-year residents. A similar development process was undertaken in 2002–2003 prior to the implementation of the revised spoken English proficiency tool used in the CS exam. While nonnative physician test-takers are not required to sound like a native speaker, they are expected to be able to communicate effectively with patients. A rating instrument and associated training protocols were developed and piloted that could be used by lay raters (the SPs) in a high-stakes simulated medical testing environment. Because the SPs represent a sample of potential patients that a doctor would be likely to encounter in a typical hospital or clinic setting in the United States, the raters are a heterogeneous group of people. The SPs frequently do not have a linguistic or teaching background, range widely in age and education level, and sometimes do not have significant previous exposure to individuals who speak English as a second or other language. Additionally, the SPs' tasks in each encounter are quite complex. They are required to accurately portray their cases, which often include simulation of symptoms such as pain or emotional affect; to remember which history items are asked and physical exam maneuvers are completed by the physicians; to assess three separate communication and interpersonal skills competencies; and also to evaluate spoken English proficiency. Due to the realistic nature of the examination format, the SPs are not able to view any of the rating instruments or take notes during the encounters. All scoring and documentations are completed from memory immediately following each interaction. Therefore, the rating instruments need to be relatively basic and easy to use. While the encounters are recorded, these recordings are used for security and training purposes only. No rescoring of physician test-takers is conducted using recordings.

THE STEP 2 CS (CLINICAL SKILLS) EXAM

Rater Training

As part of the CS exam, the SPs are trained to evaluate the spoken English proficiency of physicians in a half-day workshop using a variety of techniques, including an explanation of the rating process, presentation of the rating tool, review of benchmarked recorded encounters, individual rating of additional recorded encounters, and group discussion. Following training, SPs are required to show competence in portraying their particular case, accurate documentation of the history and physical exam checklist items, and justifiable CIS and spoken English proficiency ratings. Also, to ensure that their SEP ratings did not drift over time, SPs are subject to various quality assurance procedures. All ratings are monitored for outliers, and a small percentage of each SP's ratings are double scored by trainers. SPs with inconsistent ratings are retrained as necessary, or terminated if their ratings do not conform to acceptable standards.

Language Testing Environment

A fundamental difference between the CS and other measures of oral language proficiency is the high-fidelity simulated clinical environment in which the communication assessment takes place. The CS centers were built to resemble medical clinics, with standard size evaluation rooms equipped with authentic examination tables and equipment, such as ophthalmo-scopes, reflex hammers, tongue depressors, etc. The physician test-takers wear lab coats and carry stethoscopes. Except for a small number of SPs portraying patients in special cases, the SPs are dressed in authentic hospital gowns. The SPs do not come out of role as a patient to score the physician until after the physician has completed the encounter and left the room. Physicians and SPs enter the rooms from separate hallways and do not come in contact with each other except in the clinical encounters.

While the physicians are aware that the patients are simulating their roles, this high-verisimilitude testing environment provides an advantage over other spoken language tests such as oral interviews between an interlocutor and examinee. Guided role-plays, such as the CS, have been shown to be more effective than nonscripted interview tests at compelling examinees to exhibit their true conversational competence (Kormos, 1999). Even though each rater in the CS has a role of a particular patient that they portray in every encounter, the speech produced by the physician test-taker is not directly dictated by the evaluator. The realistic clinical setting encourages examinees to "buy in" to the role-play scenarios and produce authentic language.

Additionally, while it is possible for test-takers to prepare for the exam by memorizing certain high frequency key phrases such as "Tell me about your complaint" or "Now I will listen to your heart," the assessment is designed so that physicians will also be required to produce a large quantity of unrehearsed speech. Each exam administration consists of 12 out of a pool of over 100 possible cases which change daily. It is therefore highly unlikely that a test-taker can memorize all needed history items and diagnostic explanations for every possible clinical scenario and simulate a language proficiency level that he or she does not control.

Allowing the physician test-taker instead of the rater (SP) to lead most of the communication in the encounters lessens potential interviewer effects. Brown (2003) demonstrated the impact of various interlocutors on examinee performances and raters' perceptions of examinee ability. When interviewers differ in the way they structure the conversations, their questioning techniques and feedback provided to examinees in the form of ratings will be less reliable. In the CS, the communication between the patient and the doctor unfolds with the examinee (as the doctor) leading almost all communication in each encounter. The doctor asks questions and the patient responds with memorized scripted responses, standardizing inter-locutor effects on the communication elicited in the encounters.

While the large majority of the communication that takes place in the encounters is physician-led, there are occasions built into the exam structure where the SP initiates the topic. Most SP roles incorporate a communication challenge statement which is designed to deliberately elicit a physician's response. Communication challenge statements often include emotional assertions by the patient such as "I'm really frightened I may have AIDS," "I really don't like doctors," or "No one in this clinic is listening to me!" Other communication probes by the SP, such as "If I can't lose weight I'm going to start smoking again" or "I am taking my boyfriend's prescription pills," are scripted to be deliberately provocative. These challenges not only provide an opportunity for the physician to respond (or not respond) and thus demonstrate his or her guidance, advisory, and interpersonal skills, but the probes also provide a forum for the physician to produce additional spontaneous language that can be evaluated by the SPs.

Standard Setting

The standard setting process used to determine pass/fail thresholds for the CS involves the medical education and practice communities. Individuals from these groups review data from live administrations of the exam and provide opinions on the minimal standard of performance in the areas tested. Medical school administrators, undergraduate and graduate medical educators, clinicians, state medical board members, and physician test-takers themselves complete surveys aimed at identifying the prevalence of substandard clinical and communication skills. The USMLE Step 2 CS committee, which is made up of leaders in medical education and licensing, review these data and make a decision regarding the minimal acceptable performance for all of the CS components. These pass/fail cutoff points are periodically reviewed to ensure that they remain relevant and appropriate.

Exam Administration

The CS exam is offered at five testing sites in the United States: Atlanta, Chicago, Houston, Los Angeles, and Philadelphia. Test-takers are permitted to take the exam at any of the five locations. These test centers operate year round and up to seven days per week, with as many as three test administrations (12 examinees per administration) per day, depending on test-taker volume. An additional testing site in Philadelphia was opened in 2010 to accommodate extra exams at peak periods and to provide a venue for testing new methods and populations. From June 30, 2008 to July 1, 2009, there were 17,034 administrations for IMGs of the CS exam, of which 13,162 were for first-time exam takers, and 3,872 were repeat attempts.

VALIDITY AND RELIABILITY OF THE SPOKEN ENGLISH PROFICIENCY (SEP) RATING IN THE STEP 2 CS

The Step 2 CS was first administered in 2004, and numerous studies have been conducted demonstrating the validity and reliability of the SEP rating. Harik et al. (2006), investigated the relationship among subcomponents (including SEP) of the Step 2 CS exam, the Step 2 Clinical Knowledge (CK) exam, and the Step 1 exam for all physicians who tested between June 2004 and July 2005. For the 12,300 IMGs in the sample, the overall reliability for spoken English proficiency (SEP) was 0.94. The reliabilities for the data-gathering checklist (DG), communication and interpersonal skills (CIS), and the patient note (PN) components were 0.73, 0.80, and 0.74, respectively.

As expected, spoken language ability has some influence on physicians' performance on other CS components. The correlation between the SEP ratings and the communication CIS ratings was 0.55, indicating a moderate relationship. This finding was anticipated because in the CIS rating, SPs evaluate aspects of communication that certainly would be influenced by language ability. Physicians who lack sufficient spoken English skills would likely have some difficulty gathering and sharing information with the patients. Nonproficient physicians may also struggle in their attempts to build rapport, and in counseling patients with tact and clarity. Stronger associations were not, however, anticipated, as the CIS rating tool also includes nonverbal measures, such as appropriate eye contact, body language, and actions taken to make the patient feel at ease during the physical exam. The moderate correlation between SEP and CIS, albeit scored by the same person, demonstrates that the two instruments measure somewhat related, but not identical, competencies.

The correlation between SEP and the data gathering (DG) component of the exam (the score on the checklists completed by the SPs indicating the number of correct history items asked and the physical exam maneuvers performed) was 0.11, indicating almost no relationship. Although one would expect that physicians who spoke English well may also have the ability to conduct a more thorough interview, the DG measure is designed to assess a physician's application of clinical knowledge and reasoning, not language ability. Physicians receive credit for all appropriate questions that are asked, whether or not the questions contain mispronunciations or are awkwardly phrased. In addition, the total DG score consists of both history-taking and physical exam scores. The ability to conduct an appropriate physical exam is a skill that, for the most part, is unrelated to spoken language proficiency.

Spoken English proficiency scores and patient note (PN) ratings were modestly correlated, at 0.35. A physician who speaks English well is also likely to be better able to document his or her findings. However, since the patient note was designed to evaluate clinical judgment, not written language ability, the nominal shared variance between the two measures yields some evidence for the discriminant validity of the SEP ratings.

Physician performance on the two multiple-choice examinations that measure basic and clinical science proficiency (Step 1 and Step 2 CK) was not related to SEP ability. The correlations between SEP and Step 1 and Step 2 CK were 0.00 and 0.05, respectively, indicating that the competencies required for these multiple-choice tests do not appear to be related to a physician's spoken English ability (Harik et al., 2006).

Raymond, Clauser, Swygert, and van Zanten (2009), used generalizability theory to obtain reliability indices for the SEP rating separately for native and nonnative speakers of English, and at various points along the nine-point rating scale. The total sample consisted of 29,084 physician test-takers, of which 11,283 self-reported that English was not their native language. The mean SEP score for this nonnative group was 7.20 (scored on a 1 to 9 scale) and the standard deviation was 1.13. In contrast, the mean SEP score for the native speakers was 8.80 (with standard deviation of 0.43). Although overall reliability indices for native and nonnative speakers combined were very high (0.95), the authors also examined measurement error for SEP ratings along the score continuum and reported that measurement error increases toward the middle and bottom of the scale. These findings could be due to a number of factors, including a ceiling effect (the SPs cannot rate very proficient physicians higher than a 9), whereas for less proficient physicians, SPs have more scale points from which to choose when assigning a rating. Rater leniency or stringency tendencies could also vary across the scale continuum and examinees. In addition, the spoken English ability of physicians could fluctuate throughout the testing day and across cases. Some physicians' speech may improve as they become comfortable with the test, whereas in contrast, some physicians may become fatigued during the seven-hour testing day and experience a decline in spoken language ability. Specific cases may also impact SEP performance. A highly emotional patient, a complicated case, or an unfamiliar clinical problem might cause a nonnative speaker to become anxious and suffer a temporary deterioration in spoken English proficiency (Raymond et al., 2009).

VALIDITY AND RELIABILITY OF THE SPOKEN ENGLISH PROFICIENCY RATING IN THE PREVIOUSLY REQUIRED CLINICAL SKILLS ASSESSMENT (CSA)

In addition to the above Step 2 CS research, many studies were also conducted to support the use of spoken English proficiency ratings for the very similar previous ECFMG certification requirement, the Clinical Skills Assessment (CSA). The CSA was operational from 1998 to 2004 and was only required for IMGs, not graduates of U.S. medical schools. The CSA included a measure of physicians' spoken English skills based on a four-point scale from 1 (needs significant improvement) to 4 (excellent). Prior to CSA implementation, pilot studies of volunteer physicians supported the psychometric adequacy of the English proficiency rating instrument (Friedman et al., 1991; Friedman, Sutnick, Stillman, Regan, & Norcini, 1993). In terms of potential sources of score invalidity, differences in English ratings as a function of physician and SP gender and native language (English versus all other languages) were explored. Controlling for ability, no significant SP gender by physician gender effect was found (van Zanten, Boulet, McKinley, & Whelan, 2003). As would be expected, native English-speaking physicians received significantly higher spoken English proficiency ratings from the SPs, regardless of the SPs' native language. Other physician characteristics in addition to gender and native language—that is, age and years since graduation from medical school, and performance on qualifying examinations, including the Test of English as a Foreign Language (TOEFL) (which was discontinued in 2004 as a certification requirement) and USMLE step exams—were studied to determine their relationship, if any, to CSA outcomes. Passing the doctor–patient communication component of CSA was associated with female gender, recent graduation, higher Step 2 CK and TOEFL scores, and was more likely for native English language speakers (van Zanten, Boulet, & McKinley, 2003). Evidence was also gathered using the ratings of external observers, further supporting the validity of communication ratings provided by the SPs (Whelan, McKinley, Boulet, Macrae, & Kamholz, 2001).

IMG PERFORMANCE ON THE STEP 2 CS

Table 4.1 provides information on the number of IMG USMLE Step 2 CS test-takers and pass rates for the one-year period June 30, 2008 through

Table 4.1. IMG USMLE Step 2 CS Performance (June 30, 2008–July 1, 2009).

	Number of Administrations	Number Passing	Percent Passing
Total	17,034	12,045	71
First-attempt takers	13,162	9,595	73
Repeaters[a]	3,872	2,450	63
U.S. citizens[b]	3,738	2,959	79
First-attempt takers	3,176	2,608	82
Repeaters[a]	562	351	62
Foreign citizens[b]	13,296	9,086	68
First-attempt takers	9,986	6,987	70
Repeaters[a]	3,310	2,099	63

Source: <www.ecfmg.org>.
[a]The data for repeaters represent examinations given, not number of examinees.
[b]Citizenship is at the time of medical school.

Table 4.2. IMG and USMG First-Attempt Passing Rates on USMLE Step 2 CS Exam Components (July 1, 2008–June 30, 2009).

	Percent Passing the Integrated Clinical Encounter (ICE) Component	Percent Passing the Communication and Interpersonal Skills (CIS) Component	Percent Passing the Spoken English Proficiency (SEP) Component
International medical graduates[a]	84	84	94
United States medical graduates	98	99	>99[b]

Source: <www.usmle.org>.
[a]Includes both U.S. citizen and foreign citizen IMGs.
[b]>99 signifies that the passing rate would round up to 100%.

July 1, 2009. Seventy-one percent of the total number of IMGs who took CS during the study period passed the exam. Passing rates were somewhat higher for United States citizen IMGs (79%) as compared to foreign citizens (68%).

Table 4.2 provides information on CS exam components first-attempt passing percentages for IMGs for the one-year period July 1, 2008 to June 30, 2009. For comparison, this information is also provided for United States Medical Graduates (USMGs). Overall 94% of IMGs taking the CS for the first time passed the SEP component. USMGs outperformed IMGs on all components. Because failing one (or more) of any component of the CS (ICE, CIS, or SEP) results in a failure of the entire exam, Table 4.2 does not show the overall pass/fail rates for the exam.

CONCLUSIONS AND FUTURE RESEARCH

Internationally trained physicians for whom English is not a native language will likely continue to seek opportunities to practice medicine in the United States for many years to come. Because IMGs are more likely than graduates of U.S. medical schools to practice primary care and serve underserved populations, this group of physicians plays a significant role in the provision of health care in this country.

Due to the importance of IMGs in providing care in the United States, the heterogeneity of their educational settings, and the fact that currently approximately 75% do not speak English as a native language, the quality of the care provided by IMGs has been the subject of ongoing concern. The goal of high-stakes performance tests, such as the USMLE Step 2 CS, is to ensure that these IMG physicians possess the adequate skills to provide appropriate patient care, yet little research has been conducted that provides validity evidence that the exam appropriately screens out inadequate physicians. Norcini et al. (2010) recently investigated the quality of care provided by IMGs. The authors studied 244,153 hospitalizations in Pennsylvania of patients with congestive heart failure or acute myocardial infarction. Patients of non-U.S. citizen IMGs had significantly lower mortality rates than patients cared for by USMG doctors or IMG doctors who were U.S. citizens and received their degrees abroad. The authors found no significant mortality difference when comparing all IMGs with all USMGs. In addition to country of a physician's medical school as a factor influencing patient outcomes, the number of years since graduation from medical school was positively related to mortality, and specialty board certification was associated with a decrease in mortality.

While studies such as the Norcini et al. (2010) investigation provide some important validity evidence that supports the use of ECFMG certification requirements, including the Step 2 CS and the associated English proficiency measure, additional research focused on the real-world performance of nonnative English-speaking IMGs in the workforce is warranted. For example, investigations of IMGs' specific communication skills, including the adequacy of their spoken English proficiency, from the multiple perspectives of patients, patients' families, supervising physicians, and other members of the health-care team, are needed to further validate decisions made in the Step 2 CS. Additional measures of physicians' ability and skills, such as residency directors' ratings and specialty board certification rates could also be compared to spoken English proficiency ratings to determine the relationship, if any, to these scores. These types of validity studies will lend continued evidence supporting the use of the spoken English proficiency measure in the Step 2 CS.

CHAPTER FIVE

THE CLINICAL SKILLS (CS) TEST: IMG PREPARATION AND PERCEPTION

Sara M. Tipton

ABSTRACT

Prospective international medical graduates (IMGs) approach the United States Medical Licensing Examination® (USMLE®) Clinical Skills (Step 2 CS) test from vastly different backgrounds. This chapter discusses the variety of challenges examinees face in preparing for the exam. It further describes assessment activities and tools as well as methods and materials consulted in designing individualized preparation programs to hone the skills needed to pass the exam. Finally, it presents how the communication skills examined in the CS are linked to those required for success in a residency program.

INTRODUCTION

Since 1989, I have coordinated the International Teaching Assistant (ITA) program and taught in the English Language Institute (ELI), an intensive English program, at Wayne State University in Detroit, Michigan. ITA

English Language and the Medical Profession: Instructing and Assessing
the Communication Skills of International Physicians
Innovation and Leadership in English Language Teaching, Volume 5, 91–110
Copyright © 2011 by Emerald Group Publishing Limited
All rights of reproduction in any form reserved
ISSN: 2041-272X/doi:10.1108/S2041-272X(2011)0000005011

testing and training involves assessing the communicative competence of all prospective graduate teaching assistants whose native language is not English and then providing linguistic and cultural training to those who do not pass the assessment before they enter the classroom. It also involves delivering orientation workshops and ongoing programs to all ITAs on campus. IMGs and ITAs are similar in many ways: they are entering professional training with advanced degrees and preparing to work with the American population. (For more on the frameworks of ITA education and their applications for IMG education, see Hoekje, this volume).

I began conducting individual tutoring sessions for IMGs at metro-Detroit hospitals in 1997, with the focus on supporting their communication skills to enable them to interact more confidently and effectively with patients and families as well as attending physicians and other health-care professionals. This began through personal references as well as via calls to our ELI from medical directors at metro-Detroit hospitals asking for "English help" for first-year residents, known as interns, who were experiencing difficulty in their residency programs.

In 2000, I widened my instructional practice to include preparing IMGs to take the Clinical Skills Assessment® (CSA®), now the Clinical Skills (CS) exam. The CS exam (Step 2 of the United States Medical Licensing Examination®, USMLE®) tests applicants' communication skills in the context of twelve clinical scenarios using standardized patients. (See van Zanten, this volume, for a thorough description of the CS exam, including the history of the exam, its rubrics and scoring, the feedback examinees receive with their scores, and data on passing rates.) While I continue to tutor currently employed intern and resident physicians at their workplace, I tend to meet CS examinees through word of mouth via their language communities. Usually an intern or resident whom I have previously tutored will refer a friend to me for CS test preparation; that CS examinee will then refer future friends. At the time of this writing (2011), I have prepared 19 candidates for the CS or CSA exams.

In this chapter, I discuss my encounters with these examinees, the skills they bring, and the perceptions they have of the task. I discuss (1) how I assess the strengths and weaknesses of their communication skills as well as those required specifically by the CS; (2) how I design an individualized tutoring program that meets their needs in the time period remaining before their exam date; and (3) what resources, methods, and materials I use to deliver the training. Finally, I present examinees' comments and feedback collected at three points: after the training concludes, after they have taken the exam, and after they have begun residency.

Work with an ESP communication specialist can benefit the IMG in many important ways. For IMGs preparing for residency, such support can boost confidence, cultural knowledge, and language skills in a nonthreatening environment, allowing the IMG to practice, make mistakes and receive tips and feedback before the first few months of rotations and the resulting feared evaluations from senior residents and attending physicians. For IMGs identified as having communication problems in their residencies, the ESP consultant can be all of the above and more: a trusted confidante from outside the program and medical community who serves as a cultural informant and coach to overcome difficulties and help them regain status in the program. Thus, at various points in their education, IMGs will find value in working with an ESP communication specialist in addition to focusing on clinical skills and medical knowledge.

MY ENCOUNTERS WITH CS EXAMINEES AND THEIR RANGE OF SKILLS AND EXPERIENCE

Prospective CS examinees come to the task from a wide variety of backgrounds. Based on my experience in preparing 19 candidates for the exam, I can categorize them into two groups in terms of their background. The first group (10 out of 19) comprises those who have come to the United States on a short-term visitor's visa to take the CS exam, perhaps do observerships or externships in a local hospital or clinic (i.e., they shadow physicians in a medical setting such as a clinic or private practice without having direct patient contact), and stay long enough for the residency match period, the fall and winter interview season leading up to March each year when prospective residents are matched to a residency program based on rankings submitted by all involved. In my experience, these CS examinees have all been in their mid-to-late twenties and from the Middle East. They have strong family ties or friendships in the Detroit area, so they come months before the exam to prepare. They have graduated from medical school one to two years prior to taking the exam, with little or no residency training in their home countries. Thus, while their medical knowledge seems fresh, their clinical skills appear rather weak due to lack of experience.

The other group (9 out of 19) comprises experienced physicians who have been working in the United States at hospital research labs or other related tasks for 7 to 15 years while raising families; in most cases, a research opportunity or a spouse's employment brought them to the United States.

Prior to that, they had many years of medical practice in their respective countries in specialized fields such as obstetrics, cardiology, pathology, or radiology. They plan to take the test in hopes of beginning an internal medicine residency program so they can be licensed to practice medicine and remain in the United States. Their ages have ranged from the mid-thirties to early fifties. In my experience, those in this general group have been from China (5), South Korea (2), and Russia (2). While their experience before coming to the United States has been rich in terms of dealing with patients and doing clinical procedures related to their respective specialties, they admit that their medical knowledge is outdated, especially in the wider realm of internal medicine, which is the focus of the CS test. In several cases, their expertise in specific fields such as pathology or radiology never prepared them for the clinical encounters with standardized patients that they must face in the CS test. In those cases, the CS test proves especially challenging.

In both groups, familiarity with the culture as well as proficiency and level of confidence with spoken American English also varies widely but does not necessarily relate to the number of years they have lived in the United States. Understandably, those in the first group of recent arrivals from the Middle East have had very little opportunity to interact with Americans. Most have had recent English instruction in private schools in their home countries as well as some medical school education in English but little opportunity to speak the language or experience the culture. Despite that, their colloquial English and knowledge of current cultural references can be effective due to their exposure to English through travel, Internet use, and the growing dependency on English texts in medical training abroad. (See Olmstead-Wang, this volume, for global trends in the use of English in medical education.) By comparison, those in the second group who have lived in the United States for decades often reside in isolated language communities, speaking their native language at home and in a neighborhood with others of their native culture, so that shopping, worshipping, and socializing revolve around the native community. They often admit to not interacting much in their labs with colleagues from the United States or other language groups and cultures, but rather they report focusing on their work, eating lunch with colleagues from their native culture, and avoiding interacting more widely.

These factors greatly affect the type of preparation required for success on the test and, ultimately, in a residency program. I find that both groups struggle with managing the clinical encounter required by the CS test comfortably in every facet, from establishing rapport, opening and closing the encounter, and understanding patients' direct and implied comments, to taking patients' histories and offering appropriate counseling. With each prospective CS examinee, my goal is to identify strengths and weaknesses and then provide information, feedback, and practice to help them achieve the confidence and skills they need for success on the exam and beyond.

As mentioned above, those in the first group who have participated in observerships may be more familiar with the many aspects of the clinical encounter: the greeting, opening and closure; the order and grammar of questions to ask; expected active listening skills and empathic responses; effective body language and eye contact while interacting and taking notes; commands and explanations during the physical exam; and typing or handwriting legible, organized notes after the encounter. However, despite their familiarity with these points, they do not, in my experience, exhibit ease and confidence in their delivery, a critical part of the CS exam. These candidates may be more likely to have greater familiarity with pronouncing patient names (and knowing what is a first name rather than a family name or whether to call the patient Ms., Miss, or Mrs., etc.) and the names of common over-the-counter medications. While some have more comprehensible pronunciation, grammar, or fluency, most need work on colloquial vocabulary, speaking rate, fluency, volume, stress, and emphasis—not to mention cultural orientation.

In comparison, examinees with years of clinical experience in their home countries may demonstrate greater ease and professional confidence in the entire encounter compared with recent graduates. For example, they appear familiar with the order of questions in taking the history, comfortable doing the physical exam, and less shaken by being in the role of the physician; however, they may have spent a decade or more away from clinical medicine doing research. I have found that in those cases, even if they had clinical experience in the past, the practice of medicine varies greatly among cultures; thus, many aspects of the standardized patient encounter appear alien to them, especially in cases that involve culturally specific issues related to sexual health and practice, mental health and depression, domestic violence, or social issues, such as referring the elderly to a social worker for help in finding suitable housing.

Finally, prospective examinees come to me with varying degrees of experience with the exam. Three had failed the test once and realized that their preparation had not been sufficient. Others had completed a preparation or a practice test with a private company such as Kaplan (www.kaptest.com/Medical_Licensing/Step-2-CS/index.html) and felt they needed to polish their skills or work on weaknesses identified in those practices. Other types of preparation courses abound. One examinee described a physician in Philadelphia who offers individual training for the CS exam as well as room and board in his home for three days, one week, or two weeks for "a high fee." My informant attended one such session for three days and reported appreciating the expertise provided from a clinician although feedback on language was minimal. Others have come to me because they found it difficult to find a partner other than their own family members with whom to practice the cases. One examinee stated that it is possible to find informed partners over the Internet who will practice using Skype; he reported, however, that they are no longer interested if they find that his English skills are weak or learn that he failed the exam in his first attempt. Thus, I have found that when setting up a training program for the CS exam, it is important to take into account the background knowledge and experience of the examinee; there is no such thing as "one size fits all."

ADDITIONAL BARRIERS FACING PROSPECTIVE CS EXAMINEES

CS examinees frequently discuss the high anxiety they experience regarding the test due to many factors. First are the costs involved, including the test fee ($1,355, as of March 2011; see www.ecfmg.org/fees.html), the travel expenses required to get to one of the five test sites in North America, and any costs involved in taking preparation courses. In addition to the financial burden, those CS examinees who are already in the country are usually working at full-time jobs and need to use vacation time to prepare and travel, while as mentioned above, others travel to the United States just to take the test, apply to residency programs, and go to interviews. Thus, some have months or years to prepare for the test, whereas others have much less time, leading to the time pressure that many describe.

A further hurdle is they must pass both the Step 1 and Step 2 written licensing exams before they can take the CS exam; all three exams must be passed to be able to then interview in that year's residency match process in March. That interview season is generally from October to January. If they fail the first time, their goals will be postponed; some report that they only have one chance due to external circumstances such as financial support. Therefore, the stakes are high for applicants; in some cases the inability to get a medical license in the United States can mean loss of visa status and hope of becoming a permanent resident. In other cases, it means the end of a goal to seek training in the United States and further a career. Thus, this fear of failure and loss of face in their families and communities can lead to an overall problem with performance anxiety as described anecdotally by examinees I have tutored over the years.

Finally, despite the vast and thorough information on the official Web sites (www.usmle.org; www.ecfmg.org) and in textbooks, I have found many test-takers may not have read that information carefully beyond what is necessary for registration. Rumors abound in the examinees' language or cultural communities and on the Internet. One such recent rumor was that it is better for Asians to take the test in Los Angeles because standardized patients in other centers are not accustomed to Asians. Thus, it has been my experience that examinees can be poorly informed about the test objectives and not take advantage of all that the official Web sites have to offer, including videos of patient encounters, models of notetaking, tips for how to manage time, explanations of how the examination will be rated, etc. Instead, they spend valuable time memorizing rote phrases. One examinee showed me a notebook of test preparation materials that he had gotten from blogs and Web sites developed by other examinees from his native country; fellow nationals had taken the test, typed up descriptions of the twelve encounters they had faced on the test, and listed set phrases and questions to memorize for each case. In spending time memorizing these points, this examinee had neglected to review the official Web site and thus lacked a true understanding the purpose of the test and how he was expected to react to the scenarios. More specifically, he did not know how to respond when our practice sessions did not follow a prepared script exactly as is true of authentic communication.

Taking all these factors into account, I set out to identify where IMGs are at the time of our first meeting, how far they need to go to be successful on the exam, and what type of instructional activities will best help them achieve their goals.

DESIGNING AN INDIVIDUALIZED TUTORING PROGRAM

Introduction

An individualized program to prepare for the CS exam must not only target the test and the examinee's needs, but it also needs to be grounded in sound ESP research, including developing a needs analysis, creating instructional activities, providing feedback, and tracking progress. In the chapter

"English for Medical Purposes," Shi (2009) reviews the different types of needs analyses employed in designing training programs that target the distinct needs of various groups of medical English learners. Following Bruce (1992) and Maher (1986), Shi explains that EMP (English for medical purposes) on the macro level is either professional or educational, the former referring to the English required of those already using the language on the job, and the latter to that of those entering educational programs to prepare for medical and health professions careers. On the micro level, EMP can be subcategorized into specializations or different communication tasks that the physician performs in the workplace. The CS test, with its focus on the patient interview and brief physical examination, aims to evaluate the ability to perform such micro tasks.

Among the various types of needs analyses that EMP instructors employ, Shi (2009) describes a *deficiency needs analysis* as one in which gaps are identified between the proficiency required to be successful at the targeted task and current student performance. Shi, Corcos, and Storey (2001) used this approach to design individualized courses to meet student needs, incorporating "episodes of videotapes and transcripts of student performance data in teaching and learning tasks to illustrate and provide practice in the relevant linguistic repertoire" (p. 217). Such elements can be applied in preparing students for a micro task such as the CS test.

As in all ESP situations, the EMP instructor must first gain expertise about the test: how it is rated, what is considered a passing performance, and what preparation materials are available. In addition, the instructor must then gain familiarity with the genre of the doctor–patient interview. Finally, the EMP professional must assess the skill level of each prospective CS examinee at the beginning of the practice and measure how much progress must be made to reach acceptable performance. This assessment shifts throughout the practice, with ongoing data collection informing the original findings. Using these principles as a guide, I have developed the following needs analysis.

Conducting a Needs Analysis

When I first meet any prospective CS examinee, I conduct an initial needs analysis via a 60- to 90-minute interview covering the following points:

• Background of the examinee, including nationality, education, experience, length of time in the United States, familiarity with the American medical system, current status, and future goals;

- Scheduled test date and number of times taken;
- Steps already taken to prepare and become familiar with official preparation materials and a review of what the examinee has already acquired, assembled, and studied;
- Current status of the Step 1 and Step 2 exams;
- Nonverbal communication and overall professional demeanor, such as eye contact, gestures, handshake, poise, and confidence;
- Overall assessment of pronunciation, grammar, vocabulary, fluency, rate, intonation, and comprehensibility.

During this initial interview, I take notes on all of the above using the CS Test Assessment Sheet (see Appendix 5.1) I developed. The initial interview is an informal, conversational encounter and generally does not cover much medical terminology. I do not videotape this portion of the assessment. I bring my laptop if necessary to review the USMLE Web site as well as recommended materials together with the examinee. To conclude this initial session, we discuss my general findings, how much time remains until the exam, how frequently we plan to meet, my fees, and a proposed plan of work.

Based on this analysis, the candidate and I decide whether we agree to further sessions. In one case, I declined because the examinee had failed the Step 2 Clinical Knowledge (CK) exam and thus had to cancel his scheduled CS date indefinitely. I counseled him to work on Step 2 CK and then contact me in the future. I feel it is important to be realistic about what I can do as an ESP practitioner in helping the client set priorities and experience success in our work together.

Likewise, two candidates did not choose to continue with me; one said he wanted to work with a physician, and the other said she wanted a guarantee she would get her money back if she did not pass the exam. Again, while I do everything possible to support my clients, some requests are impossible. Whether or not we decide on further sessions, I always send my findings in a follow-up email, detailing strengths, weaknesses, and suggestions.

If we agree to work together, I decide on whether a more comprehensive assessment of spoken English is necessary; if so, I use the excellent diagnostic tools found in Grant (2009) and Wilner and Whittaker (2008). However, in most cases, the initial needs analysis provides enough information to discern the candidate's language skills as they relate to the SEP (Spoken English Proficiency) component on the CS exam, such as question word order, verb tense, or frequent and consistent errors with consonants, vowels, and syllable stress, as well as nonverbal skills, professional demeanor, poise, and confidence. Based on my findings in the needs analysis, gaps in the examinee's language and test-related skills are identified and compared to the skills needed to succeed in the CS exam. I then prioritize what needs work and use this as the basis of course design. However, before beginning our sessions, there is still one more piece of the needs analysis puzzle: ascertaining how the IMG perceives the exam.

IMG PERCEPTIONS OF THE EXAM

Many CS examinees have misperceptions of the goals of the CS exam, perhaps as a result of the frustration they face in preparing for such an exam; while they are all seasoned test-takers of standardized exams, the CS is quite different and has such a critical impact on their future. Below are some of the comments I have encountered anecdotally through the years that demonstrate misunderstandings of the purpose of the exam.

- "My Step 1 and 2 scores are high; why do I need to do this? It is just a formality."
- "There isn't time to let patients talk in the exam, so I will just memorize what to say and do all the talking."
- "The most important point is clinical knowledge, right?"
- "We don't learn or do this in my country, so how can I be expected to know it? Won't they train me in a residency program?"
- "Patients in my country do whatever the doctor says. They never argue with or challenge the doctor. How can I be expected to handle that?"

Clearly, successful examinees must demonstrate that they can get the information they need in the time allotted while employing effective communication skills. They cannot memorize what to say; they must be flexible and confident in their clinical skills while being good listeners. Further, while clinical and medical knowledge is indeed important, the CS exam evaluates the ability to communicate with patients in a clinical encounter, different from the Step exams. Step scores and performance on the CS test are not necessarily related; the first is knowledge, and the second is application of that knowledge in a clinical setting. It is not just a formality; people do fail. (See van Zanten, this volume, for statistics on the pass/fail rate.) Finally, when assuming a residency position, interns will be expected to perform as confidently as American medical graduates and be familiar with how to conduct interviews, perform physical exams, and write notes on the clinical encounter on their first day of residency.

Therefore, while focusing on individual skills, it is also important to dispel any myths such as those recounted above. The CS test is in fact a threshold for success in any medical residency program. The skills examined by the CS test must be demonstrated with cultural appropriateness and sincere empathy, effective verbal and nonverbal communication, medical accuracy, and professional demeanor. It is ineffective to memorize a list of phrases and questions to run through; rather, it is essential to listen to the standardized patient, be flexible in the path that the questioning takes, and manage the entire encounter with confidence. This is the goal we set out to achieve together in preparing for the CS exam.

COURSE DESIGN AND INSTRUCTIONAL METHODS

Courses are designed around practice of the standardized patient encounter since that is the concern of most examinees. Based on how many sessions we have planned, my initial findings, and the examinee's previous preparation and assembly of materials, we begin our sessions. The examinee prepares by reviewing the USMLE Web site and other materials (such as Le, Bhushan, Sheikh-Ali, & Abu Shahin, 2010) for cases likely to be encountered, choosing one or two to practice together per session and then reading relevant medical textbooks to prepare the content and order of interview questions. I generally ask that one case be prepared for each one-hour session at first, leading to two per hour later; the CS test has twelve encounters, with fifteen minutes allotted for the patient interview and targeted physical exam and 10 minutes for notetaking, so it is important to begin slowly to focus on details and then recreate the quicker pace in later practice. The examinee chooses the cases to be reviewed in the next session and emails me the numbers of those cases from texts such as Le et al. (2010), which offers 41 complete cases. We both then independently review the cases and prepare our roles. In preparing to be the standardized patient, I read the entire case and focus on the patient description, notes to the patient on how to act, challenging questions to ask, and sample responses to deliver. The Le et al. (2010) text also offers a checklist for what the examinee should remember to do; other textbooks likely offer similar materials. What comes next is based on the number of weeks before the test date or the number of sessions to be arranged. With the 19 candidates I have prepared, the number of sessions has varied from three to twelve, at the rate of one to two sessions each week.

When the test date is weeks away, there is only time to practice a few cases and suggest ways to help the candidate communicate more clearly. I have found that in those cases, providing exhaustive comments and feedback only serves to make the candidate more nervous and befuddled and less confident. Instead, I prioritize what is most important, based on the needs analysis and the most frequent or troublesome problems that require the greatest listener effort. For example, there may not be enough time to realize improvement in language issues such as verb tense or syllable stress, but it is possible to practice greeting the patient and opening the encounter confidently, taking a patient history on a few cases with clear question word order, maintaining effective eye contact, and managing time effectively.

If the exam date is more distant, exam preparation can be divided into four segments:

(1) The clinical encounter, part 1: taking information at the door, greeting the patient, washing hands, asking questions about the chief complaint and taking the relevant patient history.
(2) The clinical encounter, part 2: summarizing the findings, counseling the patient, and concluding the encounter.
(3) The physical examination: while I reserve the right to decline practicing the actual physical examination, we hone the key commands needed, such as imperatives ("Breathe in, hold it, breathe out" and "Push back on my hand") as well as directive language ("Now I'm going to listen to your heart"). Tips for this section include remembering to wash hands before beginning, listen to breath sounds with the stethoscope on the skin by first untying the gown, and offer the drape provided for privacy.
(4) Notetaking: practicing the format, managing the 10-minute time frame, and communicating the required information.

In my experience, most of our time is spent on the clinical encounter, parts 1 and 2 above. Tips, checklists, models, and formats for all four areas can be found at www.usmle.org and www.usmleworld.com, as well as in Le et al. (2010). Occasionally, some practice sessions are recorded via my Flip video camera, with an opportunity for playback and feedback either at that moment or sent via a large file sharing Web site such as www.yousendit.com. Improvement is discussed and assignments are set for the next session.

For every case practiced, I complete a feedback sheet (see Appendix 5.2, CS Practice Feedback Sheet) based on the subcomponents that are evaluated in the CS exam: Integrated Clinical Encounter (ICE), Communication and Interpersonal Skills (CIS), and Spoken English Proficiency

(SEP). We discuss improvement from the previous practice as well as weaknesses encountered, such as unclear terminology, pronunciation, and grammar; inappropriate nonverbal communication; insincere, robotic pseudoempathic remarks; unorganized flow of questions in the patient interview; and missing or inadequate counseling at the end. Homework for each session is to review the weak points for the cases practiced that day so that we can practice them by either repeating that case or transferring that skill to the next case. Near the end of the practice sessions and the looming test date, we usually practice two cases per hour to become accustomed to the rigor of the exam without stopping for comment or feedback; a stopwatch is used for accuracy. At that point, I tend to focus my comments on the overall performance rather than detailed feedback on each grammar or pronunciation problem; I generally record these final practices for individual or shared feedback sessions.

On occasion, an examinee demonstrates particular skill and expertise in one or more parts of our practice. For example, experienced physicians may do well in the physical exam but not in taking the history, so we may only briefly practice the stronger points to focus our resources on what needs work. In one case, we practiced only the greeting and opening of the encounter for weeks so that the examinee could be more comfortable communicating with correct vocabulary, grammar, nonverbal communication, and pronunciation as well as developing rapport with the standardized patient. Thus, it is common that one aspect of the CS test remains a barrier throughout the practice, requiring that we return to it time and again for special focus.

AREAS OF FOCUS AND SUGGESTED RESOURCES

The four segments listed above can be broken down into the following specific areas the ESP consultant may need to focus on in greater detail, with suggested resources for further research and support.

Taking the Patient's History

In taking the patient's history, there are many commonly used statements, transitions, rituals, and questions that must be repeatedly practiced in different scenarios to achieve effective communication. Areas that are essential to include are those reviewed below.

(1) Entering the room, greeting the patient by name while making eye contact, shaking the patient's hand, stating name and role, offering the drape to the patient, sitting down, and explaining what is going to happen (see www.usmle.org, www.virtualmentor.org, and www.ecfm g.org for tips, checklists, and videos, as well as Le et al., 2010). Problems in these areas need to be mastered for greater confidence and to make a good first impression.

(2) Asking questions that are relevant to the chief complaint as explained on the chart outside the door, with clear grammar, vocabulary, and intonation as well as in the proper order (see Bickley, 1999; Cohen-Cole, 1991; Glendinning & Holmström, 2005; Le et al., 2010; Maher, 1992). This is a complex task due to the time constraint. It takes much practice and familiarity with forty or more practice cases to know which questions need to be asked and in what order and with what language.

(3) Using verb tenses appropriately, especially present perfect, as in "How long have you had this pain?" versus past, as in "When did it start?" (see Glendinning & Howard, 2007; Le et al., 2010; Maher, 1992; McCullagh & Wright, 2008).

(4) Employing active listening strategies (Candlin, Bruton, Leather, & Woods, 1981) and appropriate turn-taking in the genre of doctor-patient communication, not just firing off questions as though moving through a list. It is important for the candidate to be flexible and to know which question to ask next based on the flow and nature of the patient's response.

(5) Responding to rather than avoiding issues described earlier regarding culture and lifestyle (such as depression, sexuality, substance abuse, etc.) as well as calmly handling unexpected tears, outbursts, or silence. The candidate must avoid judging the patient or reacting surprised or shocked by anything the patient says (i.e., "I am an exotic dancer").

(6) Asking for clarification if anything is unclear rather than pretending to understand.

(7) Transitioning into and conducting the physical examination (see Bickley, 1999; Cohen-Cole, 1991; Le et al., 2010; Maher, 1992).

(8) Summarizing the relevant findings from the patient interview and physical exam (see Le et al., 2010).

(9) Offering future counseling as well as support from social workers, nutritionists, and programs on smoking cessation, substance abuse, nutrition, and weight loss as needed (see Le et al., 2010).

(10) Bringing closure to the encounter by discussing tests to be ordered and future appointments (see Le et al., 2010).

As mentioned above, it is essential to practice all of these skills numerous times, with a variety of cases, using a stopwatch set for 15 minutes. In this section, pronunciation and grammar errors are identified and corrected either immediately or upon review of the recording. The goal is to identify patterns of high frequency pronunciation and grammar errors that can be prioritized, and then to locate support material and exercises for practice, rather than to itemize and correct every incidence of error.

Responding to the Patient and Expressing Empathy

In this area, the examinee must demonstrate the ability to respond appropriately to what patients say. Common inappropriate responses to a standardized patient's explanation of pain or distress range from a blank, emotionless stare that comes from learned but insincere empathy, to mumbling the following while scribbling notes: "God will take care of you," "I'm sorry," or even "Good" or "OK."

A more appropriate response to such disclosures from a patient, accompanied by effective eye contact, could be "That sounds difficult/painful," "That must be tough," "I see," or "Uh-huh. Go on. Tell me more about the pain" (see Le et al., 2010, and O'Grady, this volume, for more on expressing empathy).

Using Effective Nonverbal Communication

The third area is in using effective nonverbal communication to demonstrate self-confidence and professionalism. This includes working toward the goal of erect but relaxed posture, direct eye contact, and a range of facial expressions as well as practicing the handshake, taking notes while talking and listening, and knowing when to stand or sit, when to touch or not, and what gestures are appropriate compared to those that reveal nervousness. These features can be noted in the practice videos provided at www.usm le.org and then later reviewed in recordings of practice sessions. In my experience, the greatest hurdle to overcome in this area is the lack of eye contact while taking the patient's history. Instead of looking at the patient, ineffective behavior includes asking questions while looking at notes or looking up in the air while imagining the checklists of questions needed to ask. In many cases, this nonverbal behavior at the least makes it difficult to develop rapport, but in the worst case the physician misses important clues as to the diagnosis; for example, if the physician asks the patient to point to the pain or to show where the pain radiates, he or she could miss that gesture. It is common that we reverse roles in practicing nonverbal communication so that I can model appropriate body language.

Notetaking

The final area is in writing notes in a timely, organized, legible fashion upon exiting the encounter. The examinee is given the opportunity to choose whether to type or handwrite the notes as well as to use a narrative style or bullets, but all must follow a particular order, use conventional abbreviations, and be grammatically correct (as of July, 2011, all notes must be typed, see www.usmle.org). The notetaking form and conventions identified on the USMLE Web site must be followed; a stopwatch set for 10 minutes is recommended. We compare the completed notes to the examples provided in the USMLE practice Web site and in Le et al. (2010) to identify strengths and weaknesses. I then ask the candidate to rewrite the notes for homework.

COMMENTS FROM EXAMINEES AFTER COMPLETING THE CS

Over the past decade, I have polled all of the IMGs I have trained for the CS exam via email at three intervals: after the training concludes, after they have taken the exam, and after they have begun residency. All 19 report having passed the exam and matching in a residency program; recall that at the time I met them, some were taking the test for the first time, but others were repeating the test. In addition, some had attended other forms of test preparation programs before we began working together.

All 19 responded regarding the immediate effectiveness of the training program. Many report that even though they could always study for the test alone or with their friends or family, those methods did not allow them to have any feedback on language; further, they rarely if ever would have had the opportunity to practice with a native speaker or experienced instructor of communication skills. They report finding that watching recordings of their practice was a shock at first but a good learning experience; in some cases, they found they did not have a realistic understanding of their ability but rather over- or underestimated their language, nonverbal, or clinical skills.

Further, they often express that they did not realize they were not thinking of the patient in the practice encounters but were rather just thinking about what to say next, visualizing the notes they needed to write and imagining checklists from memory. Finally, all felt they could not have prepared as effectively by themselves; they appreciated having a professional educator to encourage them and help them practice, someone who was "not just another scared guy with bad English like me," as one IMG wrote in an email message.

Examinees polled via email again soon after they had taken the CS exam were asked what advice they had for future test-takers; 16 responded. While all said they had been extremely anxious for the first few of the 12 encounters in the test, most (14 of 16) reported feeling that they overcame their nervousness and found a rhythm by their third encounter. They felt there had been no surprises: the materials that had been provided and our sessions prepared them as well as possible for what to expect.

Finally, IMGs were polled once they passed the CS, matched in a program, and began working as a resident. While it is difficult to maintain communication after time has passed, I have remained in contact with 6 of 19; I have continued working with three into their internship year and beyond. Two reported that studying for and taking the CS test helped them greatly in preparing for their residency. Three wrote that the CS test was easier than real work on the hospital floors. In contrast, one wrote that the CS test was harder than her real work as a resident because "real patients are nicer and more cooperative than actors."

FINAL NOTES TO THE ESP CONSULTANT

Although I have been working with CS exam preparation materials for more than a decade, I continue to be current with official Web sites regarding the CS test as well as test preparation texts and trends, carefully reviewing the main tasks, goals, and instructions as well as training material provided. It is also important to review the abundant material, blogs, and support services available on the Internet, from USMLE as well as other sources, to discern what may or may not be accurate or helpful and to encourage prospective examinees to do the same. Further, it is helpful to stay abreast of new medical English and ESP texts, journal articles, and research in related fields as well as newspaper articles (see the Health section of the *New York Times*, for example) on doctor–patient communication that can lend insight and provide information to share and discuss. Finally, it is key that when training for the CS test, examinees must realize that they are also training for the residency to follow; therefore, it is important to build the confidence of IMGs by enhancing their ability to communicate clearly and professionally. Their sessions with communication and English language specialists may be their only chance for individual feedback and support from an ESP professional, leading to improved confidence, clearer communication skills, and more effective interactions with patients and other health-care professionals.

APPENDIX 5.1

CS Exam Assessment Sheet: Initial Interview

Name _____   Date _____

Email _____   Phone _____

Background and goals:

CS test date, test history and preparation; status of Steps 1 and 2:

Nonverbal communication, professional demeanor and confidence:

Oral communication skills: 3 (strong)   2 (acceptable)   1 (weak)

Pronunciation ____   Grammar ____   Vocabulary ____

Fluency/rate ____   Volume/projection____   Intonation/stress ____

APPENDIX 5.2

CS Exam Practice Feedback Sheet

Name _____   Date _____

Case _____

Rating Key: 3 (effective)   2 (acceptable)   1 (needs work)

Subcomponents of Clinical Skills

1. Integrated Clinical Encounters (ICE)
____ Data gathering: order, flow, accuracy, effectiveness, completeness

____ Documentation: format, accuracy and clarity in notes

Comments:

2. Communication and Interpersonal Skills (CIS)

____ Questioning skills: verb tense, clarity, word order, accuracy

____ Information sharing skills: counseling, transitions,

____ Professional manner and rapport: nonverbal communication and empathy

Comments:

3. Spoken English Proficiency (SEP)

____ Pronunciation of consonants and vowels

____ Intonation/prosody and syllable stress

____ Voice projection (volume)

____ Word choice, expressions

____ Grammar/syntax

Comments:

CHAPTER SIX

ASSESSING CULTURAL KNOWLEDGE AMONG INTERNATIONAL MEDICAL GRADUATES IN THE UNITED STATES

William Rozycki, Ulla M. Connor, Laurie Lipsig Pylitt and Lia Logio

ABSTRACT

This chapter describes how an English for specific purposes unit at an American university formed a team with medical professionals at a major Midwestern medical center to jointly produce an assessment tool for family medicine residency training. The assessment is designed to identify knowledge gaps regarding clinical and residency norms, especially among international medical residents, and therefore allow proactive training during the first year of residency.

English Language and the Medical Profession: Instructing and Assessing
the Communication Skills of International Physicians
Innovation and Leadership in English Language Teaching, Volume 5, 111–132
Copyright © 2011 by Emerald Group Publishing Limited
All rights of reproduction in any form reserved
ISSN: 2041-272X/doi:10.1108/S2041-272X(2011)0000005012

INTRODUCTION

In the United States since the 1980s, a rapid increase in international medical graduates who enter residencies for medical specialization has created a pressing need for linguistic and cultural education. On many university campuses with medical complexes and residency training programs in the United States, there exists some type of English for specific purposes (ESP) resource that offers education and remediation to international residents, often through departments such as applied linguistics or English. These ESP personnel and resources are generally well equipped to handle the linguistic issues of international residents. However, when it comes to cultural training, there are few resources available to language teachers, perhaps because disciplinary knowledge (i.e., knowledge of clinical practice and routines) is required to identify and address divergence from cultural norms in the clinical and residency medical setting. This often leaves disciplinary/professional training solely to the medical educators, creating an unnecessary division between specialized language teaching and cultural training. This chapter describes how one ESP center on a university campus responded to the needs of a particular residency program, and how that led to the joint (ESP and medical residency trainers) development of a cultural knowledge assessment tool that is grounded in and validated by the practices of a local clinical environment. At the end of the chapter, the lasting benefits of this collaboration, both to the ESP trainers and to the medical educators, are also briefly examined.

BACKGROUND

In recent decades, calls for better interpersonal communication skills on the part of physicians have led to inclusion of assessment of communication skills as part of the United States Medical Licensing Examination® (USMLE®), and to inclusion by the Accreditation Council for Graduate Medical Education (ACGME) of Interpersonal and Communication Skills as one of six general competencies (see ACGME General Competencies). While the attainment of communication skills can be challenging for any physician, since it appears to be facilitated by a combination of attitude and knowledge (Zoppi & Epstein, 2002), the challenge is greater for medical graduates trained outside the United States.

These graduates enter U.S. residence programs—a type of clinical apprenticeship typically leading to specialist certification in a period of three years—in a cultural setting that is often unfamiliar, and in which the norms of clinical practice and communication may be different from those in which they trained.

In the United States, international medical graduates (IMGs)—graduates of medical schools outside the United States, Puerto Rico, and Canada—are increasingly entering specializations that have a shortage of domestically trained physicians. Among these specializations is family medicine (previously also called family practice). At the Indiana University family medicine residency program, the number of IMGs in residence has risen dramatically in the past decade, and in some years IMGs now make up 100% of the first-year residents. The program, situated in a large university medical center located in Indianapolis, began the decade with lower rates of IMG representation than nationally. However, from 2001, the numbers accelerated to well past the national average (see Fig. 6.1, national data from Pugno, McGaha, Schmittling, DeVilbiss, & Kahn, 2007). As the numbers of IMGs rose, so did the number of miscommunication incidents in clinical settings. Local program administrators came to recognize that some IMGs required enhanced training in communication skills.

In 2004, educator-administrators in Indiana University (IU) Family Medicine began referring IMGs with recognized communication difficulties to the Indiana Center for Intercultural Communication (ICIC), a campus unit specializing in ESP and discourse analysis research. The center already had experienced in assessing and training referred residents from other

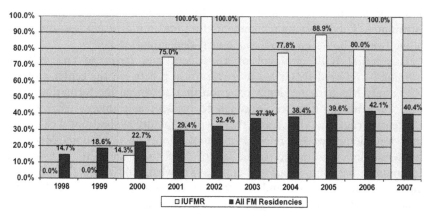

Fig. 6.1. Ten Years of First-Year IMG Residents in IU Family Medicine (Light Bars) and Nationally (Dark Bars).

medical residency programs and had established a protocol for assessment and training. Once referral was made, ICIC staff typically administered a set of instruments to each referred resident with the view of assessing the full range of linguistic and sociolinguistic competencies:

- Standard test of grammar, vocabulary, and reading (75 minutes).
- Standard listening test (20 minutes)
- Oral proficiency test (audiotaped, modified SPEAK test, 5 minutes)
- Elicited writing sample (written on the theme of professional goals, 20 minutes)
- Personal interview (audiotaped with interviewer notes, on origin, education, family situation, goals and aspirations, perceived communication competency, approximately 20 minutes)
- Examination of the resident's Objective Standardized Clinical Exam (a videotaped assessment of clinical rounds with simulated patients, an instrument given to all incoming residents by IU Family Medicine, approximately 50 minutes)

In addition, a supervisor of each referred resident was interviewed to identify the incidents that caused referral, and to discuss the goals to set for training.

Following analysis of test results and interviews, ICIC linguists then produced an individual assessment report and a training recommendation. One-on-one training could then be contracted with the center, and typically addressed such problems as pronunciation, grammar, and pragmatics. Training sessions were tailored to the resident's schedule and lasted 90 minutes. Total training recommendation for an individual resident could range from 3 hours up to 30-plus hours, depending on need.

This initial ICIC protocol of assessment and language and cultural training of referred IMGs led to a relationship between the center and the IU Family Medicine residency program that advanced the formation, over time, of a more proactive approach to resident assessment. After seeing residents struggle in clinics and receive poor faculty evaluations well *before* they were identified for referral and mediation, the IU Family Medicine residency director decided in the fall of 2005 to utilize ICIC in assessing communicative competence and cultural knowledge differences[1] for incoming first-year residents, and to provide training and resources to new residents before problems arose in the clinics. This broad vision for assessment meant that *all* residents, whether domestically trained or IMGs, were to be assessed.

As part of this plan, ICIC and the IU Family Medicine curriculum developer were asked by the residency director of IU Family Medicine to undertake joint development of a novel instrument to identify each incoming resident's degree of knowledge of clinical norms and of practices in the residency program. The development of this instrument was motivated by a number of critical incidents, of which the following are illustrative but not exhaustive:

- Low-income, minority patients at a community clinic complain about a lack of respect from a first-year resident;
- Attending and chief residents evaluate a first-year resident as "aloof, arrogant, untrustworthy" after resident claimed competence with a procedure but then failed to perform it stating "lack of practice";
- Two second-year residents are written up by faculty for arguing about round assignments within the hearing of patients and staff.

It became clear that such incidents did not arise from language differences alone, and that much of the discrepancy between expectations and actual performance was due to extralinguistic factors involving understanding of the role of a medical resident and appropriate behavior in that role (including being an active participant in team activity, acting appropriately within a hierarchy, proactively asking questions to facilitate learning, etc.). In other words, some IMGs were coming into the program without knowledge of disciplinary/professional culture in the local context.

Thus, for ICIC, what began as language assessment and training soon evolved into cultural assessment and training as well. This expansion was inevitable; pragmatic linguistic skills such as requests, complaints, commands, and polite hedges cannot be taught without understanding of context (and therefore, for these residents, of local and disciplinary culture). Hymes (1972) lists sociolinguistic competence (using language appropriate to context) and grammatical competence (language proficiency) as two factors in communicative competence. Canale and Swain (1980), in their expanded conceptualization of communicative competency, confirm sociolinguistic competence as a factor among the required competencies that make up communicative competence. Knowledge of local and disciplinary culture can be fit into the construct of sociolinguistic competence within the wider frame of communicative competence.

Stern (1992) offers the most specific theorization of the relation of cultural knowledge to communicative competence. He considers cultural knowledge and communicative competence to be linked through the intermediate stage of cultural competence.

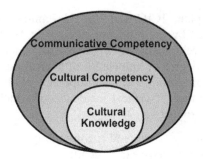

Fig. 6.2.   The Communicative Competency Spheres.

Stern identifies cultural knowledge as "systematic conceptual knowledge about the culture and society" and states that cultural competence "implies the ability to recognize culturally significant facts, and a knowledge of the parameters within which conduct is acceptable or unacceptable" (Stern, 1992, p. 82). Stern considers cultural competence to be distinct from communicative competence in that it points to "social and cultural behavior and less to linguistic manifestations" (Stern, 1992, p. 82). Cultural competence, according to Stern, is a necessary component of communicative competence. The conceptualization can best be understood through a Venn diagram, as in Fig. 6.2.

Cultural knowledge for the purposes of the IMG training means knowledge of the norms of the clinical practice and the residency program. In other words, the most vital cultural knowledge for these residents is knowledge of disciplinary culture. Disciplinary culture has been theorized under different names by various scholars. For our purposes here, perhaps the best descriptions are offered independently by James Gee and John Swales. Gee (1999) calls the concept big "D" Discourse—to distinguish from the broader term *discourse* of linguistics and rhetoric—and in his view this Discourse involves "acting-interacting-thinking-valuing-talking (sometimes writing-reading) in the 'appropriate way' with the 'appropriate' props at the 'appropriate times' in the 'appropriate' places" (p. 17). Years before Gee (1999), Swales (1985) had described a shared disciplinary community as having "institutional attitudes and expectations ... the belief-systems, initiation ceremonies, rites of passage, rituals, taboos, value judgments of excellence or otherwise, codes of practice, etc. of doctors, lawyers, navigators, geologists, and so on ..." (p. 212). In both of these descriptions, values, norms, and appropriate behavior are central to the concept, and language plays only a supporting role. It is precisely this construct of disciplinary/professional culture that ICIC and IU Family Medicine residency trainers were tasked to assess by developing a novel instrument.

Joint development of the instrument by the ESP practitioners of the center and the medical educators of IU Family Medicine would assure that both sociolinguistic considerations and medical certification criteria were brought to the table. To have face validity in the arena of medical residency training, the instrument had to fit within the framework of the six competencies—(1) Patient Care, (2) Medical Knowledge, (3) Interpersonal and Communication Skills, (4) Professionalism, (5) Practice-Based Learning and Improvement, and (6) System-Based Practice—established by the ACGME for resident training and certification (Accreditation Council for Graduate Medical Education, 2007b, see ACGME General Competencies). Additionally, all developers had to be familiar with trends in the social, ethical, and legal environments impacting clinical care—the adoption of patient-centered care as the working model for health-care systems; the ramifications of the 1996 Health Insurance Portability and Accountability Act (HIPAA) on patient privacy and patient autonomy requirements; and the increasing effect of third-party payers on health-care systems, resources, and delivery. For the ICIC team, this meant research of the literature and then discussion with the medical faculty and administrators who already were deeply immersed in these issues and their impact on practice.

DEVELOPMENT OF THE INSTRUMENT

The first step in development of the instrument was to search the literature on assessment instruments in regard to physicians. Assessment and training instruments are already available to test physician interpersonal communication skills (e.g., Common Ground, see Lang, McCord, Harvill, & Anderson, 2004) and cultural adaptability (e.g., the Cross-Cultural Adaptability Inventory (CCAI), see Majumdar, Keystone, & Cuttress, 1999). However, these tools measure general abilities (Common Ground: rapport building, active listening, addressing feelings, etc.) or attitudes (CCAI: flexibility, emotional resilience, autonomy, etc.) with the aim of predicting success in communication. Another instrument, the Cultural Competence Assessment (CCA, see Schim, Doorenbos, Miller, & Benkert, 2003) has been developed to measure components (fact, attitude, knowledge, and behavior) of hospice workers with a broad range of education and professional levels. None of the above assessment tools, nor other available cultural and communication instruments, met the exact needs of ICIC for evaluating incoming residents to IU Family Medicine.

In line with the English for specific purposes approach of ICIC, and following Crespi (1977), who indicates that the more specific the survey, the more useful its prediction of specific behavior, ICIC and the IU Family Medicine residency program jointly developed an assessment tool specific to residency clinical practice, named the Interpersonal Communication Assessment (ICA). The ICA name was given to the instrument for reasons of face validity, as the name aligns with the ACGME general competency of Interpersonal and Communication Skills.

Our original goal in developing the instrument was to identify attitudes that hampered effective communication in the clinical setting. In focus meetings with IU Family Medicine behavioral and epidemiologic researchers in late 2005 and early 2006, it became clear that measuring attitudes was not as useful as measuring knowledge—in part due to social desirability bias when surveying attitudes. Since the institutional aim of the assessment was to aid in the (proactive) training of the residents, and because knowledge can be measured more effectively than attitudes, the decision was made to assess knowledge of norms in the Indianapolis clinical and residency training setting.

With this change in direction, we set about identifying knowledge differences that might hamper effective performance by medical residents in their work and training (including doctor–patient, resident–supervisor, resident–nurse, resident–colleague, and resident–staff interactions). We used three sources to identify knowledge variability that might lead to critical incidents, low evaluations, or other problems in the resident's clinical setting. The sources for these were:

(1) literature on cultural misunderstandings in clinical encounters and medical education (e.g., Desai, 2003; Gropper, 1996; Roberts & Sarangi, 2005);
(2) observations of, and action research gained from, training of international medical residents in the past years by staff at ICIC;
(3) input of educators and behavioral scientists at IU Family Medicine, drawing on their years of experience in training both international and domestically trained residents.

From this information, the team made a list of specific norms, beliefs, and behaviors, the presence or absence of which led to critical incidents or low performance evaluations, and found that these included nonprofessional behavior and ethical questions as well as communication difficulties. When these were identified, two focus groups, using chief residents and former residents now on faculty, looked over the list and suggested additional topics. The most common themes of this input involved the patient-centered care of American clinics, patient autonomy and privacy rights established by HIPAA, and different patient and doctor expectations for pain alleviation.

Working from this list, the development team then composed 30 statements, each to be eventually linked to a Likert scale for agreement or disagreement. The team mapped these 30 items to the ACGME general competencies (see ACGME General Competencies). We found that while one main construct was in the area of interpersonal communication, two other competencies were also represented. Thus, three competencies became fields in the instrument: the above-mentioned Interpersonal and Communication Skills; Patient Care; and Professionalism. These three ACGME general competencies are listed in detail in Table 6.1, and underneath each competency are listed items from the original ICA corresponding to that competency.

Table 6.1. ACGME Interpersonal and Communication Skills, Patient Care, and Professionalism and Corresponding ICA Item.

Residents must be able to demonstrate interpersonal and communication skills that result in effective information exchange and teaming with patients, their patients families, and professional associates. Residents are expected to:

Create and sustain a therapeutic and ethically sound relationship with patients

Use effective listening skills and elicit and provide information using effective nonverbal, explanatory, questioning, and writing skills

Work effectively with others as a member or leader of a health-care team or other professional group

ICA items corresponding to the Interpersonal and Communication Skills competency:

- Doctors work with nurses and other medical staff to encourage patients and people in their communities to maintain good health practices.
- Nurses and assistants follow the doctor's orders without question.
- Smiles are appropriate only between equals during social occasions.
- A nurse, staff member, patient, or patient's family member should never question a doctor's diagnosis.

- Raising your voice or speaking very loudly is a sign of anger.
- Maintaining eye contact is polite only with one's peers of the same gender.
- Smiling indicates lack of seriousness in a person.
- It makes no difference which hand is used to receive or give an item.
- The doctor has the responsibility to deliver all information (including bad news) directly to the patient.

PATIENT CARE

Residents must be able to provide patient care that is compassionate, appropriate, and effective for the treatment of health problems and the promotion of health. Residents are expected to:

Communicate effectively and demonstrate caring and respectful behaviors when interacting with patients and their families

Gather essential and accurate information about their patients

Make informed decisions about diagnostic and therapeutic interventions based on patient information and preferences, up-to-date scientific evidence, and clinical judgment

Develop and carry out patient management plans

Counsel and educate patients and their families

Use information technology to support patient care decisions and patient education

Perform competently all medical and invasive procedures considered essential for the area of practice

Provide health-care services aimed at preventing health problems or maintaining health

Work with health-care professionals, including those from other disciplines, to provide patient-focused care

ICA items corresponding to the Patient Care competency:

- Most doctors and patients share the same religion and same culture.
- The doctor is responsible for making the ultimate decision about a patient's treatment.
- Doctors work with patients, their families, and nursing staff to decide on the best care and treatment.
- The patient has the final decision in his or her own medical care.
- Doctors speak openly to patients about terminal illnesses and the patient's approaching death.

- Patients will follow the doctor's orders.
- Patients expect doctors to address them formally (e.g., "Mr. -," "Mrs. -").
- Preventive health-care is an important part of a doctor's work.
- The husband is responsible for deciding if his wife should be operated on.
- A "pregnancy" refers only to conditions that result in a live birth.
- The man is acknowledged as head of his family at all times.
- The birth mother is not allowed to make decisions for the baby.
- A health-care provider must include the decision maker of the family in the consultation process.

PROFESSIONALISM

Residents must demonstrate a commitment to carrying out professional responsibilities, adherence to ethical principles, and sensitivity to a diverse patient population. Residents are expected to:

Demonstrate respect, compassion, and integrity; a responsiveness to the needs of patients and society that supersedes self-interest; accountability to patients, society, and the profession; and a commitment to excellence and ongoing professional development

Demonstrate a commitment to ethical principles pertaining to provision or withholding of clinical care, confidentiality of patient information, informed consent, and business practices

Demonstrate sensitivity and responsiveness to patients' culture, age, gender, and disabilities

ICA items corresponding to the Professionalism competency:

- Patients believe it is okay if a doctor interrupts an examination to take a personal, nonemergency phone call.
- Doctors decide which patients receive treatment when resources are scarce.
- A doctor should not accept any gifts from a patient or the patient's family.
- It is considered unprofessional for a doctor to share a laugh or joke with a patient while treating that patient.

The process also produced some items not mapped to a specific competency, but related to the environment of the residency. Some of these items were motivated by specific critical incidents mentioned earlier, and like the preceding also are relevant to non-IMG residents:

- A student or resident should never question what a faculty member says is the correct diagnosis or treatment plan.
- Both parents often work, so children are frequently left in a day-care facility until parents finish work.
- As a student or resident, it is acceptable to answer a faculty member's question with "I don't know."
- Childcare is supervised closely by the husband's mother.

Pilot Version

Once the construct had been mapped to individual items, the team prepared a pilot version of the ICA. Test-takers were asked to rate their agreement or disagreement with each statement in two environments: the environment in which they received their medical education and their expectation of the environment they were entering into as clinical residents in Indianapolis. To avoid pattern bias, we phrased some statements to elicit positive (agree) response and others to elicit a negative (disagree) response. This initial design, with examples of the first two items presented in each of the two environments, is given below.

Part I

Answer the following questions based on your experience during your previous medical school or residency training. Place an X in the box corresponding to your answer.

1. Most doctors and patients share a common religion and culture.
   Strongly Agree ☐   Agree ☐   Disagree ☐   Strongly Disagree ☐
2. The doctor is responsible for making ultimate decisions about a patient's treatment.
   Strongly Agree ☐   Agree ☐   Disagree ☐   Strongly Disagree ☐
   etc.

Part II

Answer the following questions based on what you believe will be the situation during the next three years of your training as an IU Family Medicine resident.

---

1. Most doctors and patients share the same religion and same culture.
   Strongly Agree □   Agree □   Disagree □   Strongly Disagree □
2. The doctor is responsible for making ultimate decisions about a patient's treatment.
   Strongly Agree □   Agree □   Disagree □   Strongly Disagree □
   etc.

We piloted the assessment with a focus group of residents (made up of third-year IMGs in IU Family Medicine), and again with a group of behavioral scientists associated with the IU Family Medicine at the Bowen Research Center in the IU School of Medicine. From the feedback of those focus groups we ultimately reduced the item number to 28, dropping two of the original items. One of these was "Most doctors and patients share the same religion and culture," meant to identify expectations of a monoculture for residents from such environments, yet problematic because the majority of patients in Indianapolis clinics are nominally Christian, and some in the focus group argued that a shared culture did indeed exist in local clinics. The other was "Doctors decide which treatment patients receive when resources are scare," meant to test understanding of operating protocols that are systematized in health-care organizations. However, the focus group argued that system protocols differ from health-care organization to health-care organization, and in some circumstances the doctor may be assigned such a role, in others not. Incoming residents could not, it was argued, have knowledge of the system in place locally.

The focus group's recommendations also influenced a decision to change the format of the instrument. It was decided to eliminate the half of the ICA that tested cultural knowledge in the test-taker's earlier medical education. The focus group suggested that a two-part instrument was too long, and information about a previous experience was irrelevant to knowledge about the current residency environment.

Alpha Version

The ICA then took shape in its 28-item alpha version, with each item a statement with a Likert scale for agreement, with "Don't know" added as a possible answer. An additional development was the creation of a cover sheet to go with the instrument. The cover sheet explained the purpose of the instrument and attempted to ease the stress that incoming residents felt during the orientation period, when they took many tests and filled out many documents. The cover sheet assured test-takers that the purpose of the assessment was solely to improve training for the residents, and that scores would not be used to in any way punish the test-taker. Because some residents looked for hidden meaning or "trick" questions in the instrument, wording was also added requesting test-takers to mark their exams according to first impressions, and assuring them that there were no hidden meanings or trick questions in the items. The original cover sheet for IU Family Medicine use is reproduced in Appendix 6.1, along with the first page (the first 12 items only) of the 28-item alpha version of the ICA.

The 28-item instrument was trialed with a group of experienced IU Family Medicine faculty ($n = 6$) in the spring of 2006 to determine a baseline "expert" score. A decision was made to set a threshold of 80% agreement among faculty before an "expert" answer was determined. This had two effects: (1) it was necessary to collapse "strongly agree" with "agree" and to collapse "strongly disagree" with "disagree" in order to obtain sufficient expert concordance to meet our criteria; and (2) the 80% concordance standard meant that in regard to faculty (i.e., expert) scores, we were operating in a criterion-referenced domain while keeping a norm-referenced domain for residents. Considering the purpose of the instrument, we deemed this acceptable. In the summer of 2006, the alpha version of the ICA was administered to the incoming IU Family Medicine first-year residents ($n = 10$).

Beta Version

After studying the expert and resident scores from the alpha version, the development team analyzed differentiation in expert scores and identified one item as problematic ("Raising your voice or speaking very loudly is a sign of anger") because faculty scores failed to meet an 80% concordance level. The item was meant to identify those from cultures in which loud voices were considered invariably as signs of aggression. However, since loud voices can *sometimes* be a sign of aggression, the faculty diverged widely in their answers. The solution was to drop this item from the instrument.

The team then reworded four other items in hopes of producing a minimum of 80% agreement by faculty in establishing an "expert" score for the instrument. The four items that required revision were (1) "Doctors speak openly to patients about terminal illnesses and the patient's approaching death," rewritten so it was less descriptive and more prescriptive as "Doctors *should* speak openly to patients about terminal illnesses and the patient's approaching death"; (2) using the same approach, "Patients will follow the doctor's orders" became "Patients *must* follow the doctor's orders without question"; (3) the item "Doctors speak openly to patients about terminal illnesses and the patient's approaching death" became "Doctors *must* speak openly to patients about terminal illnesses and the patient's approaching death"; and (4) "It makes no difference which hand is used to receive or give an item," which was rewritten as "You *must* use your right hand to receive or give an item."

The result was a 27-item beta version used in 2007 for incoming residents in IU Family Medicine and IU Internal Medicine. It was taken by IU Family Medicine residents ($n = 12$) and IU Internal Medicine residents ($n = 40$). A separate cover sheet, similar to the IU Family Medicine cover, but appropriate to IU Internal Medicine's needs, was developed by IU Internal Medicine trainers. The results were analyzed for item distinction and differentiation. Four items were still problematic.

One item, "Patients believe it is okay if a doctor interrupts an examination to take a personal, nonemergency phone call," failed to gain more than 60% agreement of faculty in this round of testing. Meant to stress the requirement to deliver patient-centered care, the actual culture of the clinics apparently did not recognize a clear-cut case in that context. The item was dropped. Two other items, "Preventive health-care is an important part of a doctor's work" and "Maintaining eye contact is polite only with one's peers of the same gender," failed to differentiate test-takers in any way, as all test-takers scored identically with the faculty score (in agreement with the former item, in disagreement with the latter). These two items were also dropped from the instrument. A fourth problematic item, "A doctor should not accept any gifts from a patient or the patient's family," was rewritten to elicit better agreement from faculty in the "expert" score. For the gamma version of the ICA, the item became, "A doctor should not accept *even small* gifts from a patient or the patient's family." These revisions brought about the 24-item gamma version.

Gamma Version

Before its release, the 24-item gamma version underwent a change in format and in cover sheet. This came about through consultation with Srikant Sarangi, the director of the Health Communication Research Centre, Cardiff University, who is the founding editor of the journal *Communication and Medicine.* Sarangi, an associate research fellow of ICIC, consulted on the ICA project and recommended the cover and the instrument be presented in a way that residents could draw on their previous experience and provide their answers within a salient context. Thus, the revised cover sheet asks residents to draw on their previous knowledge and experience in answering the items on the instrument (see Appendix 6.2 for gamma version cover sheet). The ICA items in the gamma version instrument itself are presented in the labeled contexts of the clinic, the residency, and the general environment, providing clearer orientation to the context for test-takers.

Reliability Testing

To date, 69 residents have taken the gamma version, a number which limits the statistical significance of reliability analysis. As described below, the instrument has its immediate uses, even though the development process ahead is still long and iterative. When we have gathered data from 150 test-takers, we plan to run internal consistency analyses of the entire instrument and its subsections (clinic, residency, and community), domains (interpersonal and communication skills, patient care, and professionalism), and subjects (IMG and American-trained). These coefficient alphas will guide further revision to increase internal reliability.

Current Use

The ICA is now in use for all resident assessment in IU Family Medicine and in limited use by IU Internal Medicine, and is also used in assessment of residents in other departments (e.g., oncology, obstetrics-gynecology, and psychiatry) when individuals are referred to ICIC by those departments.

The instrument can be used in two ways, either as a small-scale instrument for use by hand, or, in future, as a large-scale differentiation instrument. In the small-scale approach, as used at our center, each resident's ICA is analyzed as one data set among many that inform the assessment report. If, for example, a resident answers "Agree" to the item "A student or resident should never question the diagnosis or treatment plan that a faculty member has made"—as happened recently—then the training recommendation will suggest explicit training on the norms of the residency and the value of speaking up and sharing opinions during the clinical practice period.

In future, when sufficient numbers of test-takers have provided a basis for establishing reliability of the instrument, residents' answers on the ICA will be compared to the preestablished expert answers. For each answer that diverges from the expert score, one point is assigned to the score of the test-taker. The higher the total score of the individual, the greater the difference in knowledge concerning the local clinical and residency environment. The highest scoring quartile or third can then be assigned to either individual or group education and remediation regarding the norms of the residency environment.

LESSONS LEARNED AND BENEFITS GAINED

This team development of an assessment instrument meant an opportunity for specialists to learn from counterparts across disciplines. For the medical educators, this created a deeper understanding of the language and cultural challenges facing international medical graduates; for the linguists of ICIC, this meant immersion in the discipline of medicine, including literature studies, interaction with medical doctors and educators, and presentation at medical communication conferences nationally and internationally (Connor, Goering, Hamilton, & MacNeill, 2007; Connor & Rozycki, 2007; Connor, Rozycki, & Ruiz-Garrido, 2006). Dudley-Evans and St John (1998) call on ESP practitioners to learn the conceptual and discoursal framework of the specialized subject, and this collaborative effort led to exactly that end. As a result, ICIC strengthened its standing as a provider of ESP training to the medical profession. The center has since responded to requests for cross-cultural communication workshops at the university medical center and now has clients from other residency programs in the urban area.

Additionally, having established this base in medical discourse, ICIC embarked full-scale on health discourse research. This led to the establishment of an interdisciplinary team at the center consisting of applied linguists, discourse analysts, physicians, pharmacologists, sociologists, intercultural specialists, and communication theorists. Results to date include a transnational study of patient information leaflets (Connor, Ruiz-Garrido, Fortanet, & Palmer, 2006; Connor et al., 2008), and funding from the Eli Lilly and Company Foundation for a three-year research project on the relationship of health literacy to medication adherence (the degree to which patients take the medication prescribed to them, including at the directed times and in the directed dosage). That project produced in-depth interviews and survey data of type-2 diabetes patients (Connor, Goering, Matthias, & MacNeill, 2009).

In sum, the joint development of the ICA instrument produced several beneficial results. First, the interdisciplinary team produced a useful tool for residency assessment that is now undergoing long-term reliability testing. Second, the residency trainers gained a better understanding of the linguistic challenges and the resources available to meet them; the ESP trainers at ICIC have gained face validity within the medical community in Indianapolis, and the center is now in demand for assessment and training in the areas of cross-cultural medical communication and health discourse. Finally, the Indiana Center for Intercultural Communication has through its research, training, and assessment become a leader in health discourse and health communication training.

NOTE

1. We adopt the view of Belz (2002) that there are differences but not "deficiencies" in communicative competence. These differences do affect evaluations by faculty of the residents, and so are addressed in a manner that involves negotiation and accommodation (Connor, 1999) with a view to making residents successful in the program.

APPENDIX 6.1: INDIANA CENTER FOR INTERCULTURAL COMMUNICATION AND IU FAMILY MEDICINE

The Interpersonal Communication Assessment Survey
(Cover Sheet to Alpha Version)

Goals of the Introduction to IU Family Medicine month include (1) assessing new learners' baseline knowledge and skills, (2) acclimation of new learners to the environment in which they will be working, and (3) identification of both group and individual learning needs so that learning can be directed toward shoring up any deficiencies, and all learners can be brought to a minimum entry level within a short time of starting residency training. All of the above goals are guided by the ACGME's Six Competencies: (1) Patient Care, (2) Medical Knowledge, (3) Interpersonal and Communication Skills, (4) Professionalism, (5) Practice-Based Learning and Improvement, and (6) System-Based Practice (see ACGME General Competencies).

Many of the activities in which you have already participated, or in which you will participate in coming days and weeks are aimed at assessing your entry-level status relative to these competencies. The attached survey is but one more tool used in this process.

You should answer the survey questions based on your expectation of the environment you will be training in for the next three years as an IU Family Medicine resident. Please read each question, and choose a response based on your first impression. The questions are meant to reflect general statements, not specific incidents, and are *not* meant to trick you.

Your responses to this questionnaire will be incorporated into the overall report you will receive from the Indiana Center for Intercultural Communication. The Residency and your Advisor will also receive this report, and together you will use it to direct learning toward shoring up any identified deficiencies. There will be no adverse or punitive actions taken as a result of responses, so please answer openly and honestly.

When directed to begin, please turn the page. Put a check mark in the box below each question that indicates your answer. Check only one answer for each question. Remember, answer each question is based NOT on your previous experience, but on your understanding of the Indiana University School of Medicine environment you are entering here in Indianapolis.

Indiana Center for Intercultural Communication and IU Family Medicine.

NAME _____

1. The doctor is responsible for making the ultimate decision on what treatment the patient receives.
☐ Strongly Agree ☐ Agree ☐ Disagree ☐ Strongly Disagree
☐ Don't Know

2. Doctors work with nurses and other medical staff to encourage patients and people in their communities to maintain good health.
☐ Strongly Agree ☐ Agree ☐ Disagree ☐ Strongly Disagree
☐ Don't Know

3. Nurses and assistants follow the doctor's orders without question.
☐ Strongly Agree ☐ Agree ☐ Disagree ☐ Strongly Disagree
☐ Don't Know

4. Doctors work with patients, their families, and nursing staff to decide on the best care and treatment.
☐ Strongly Agree ☐ Agree ☐ Disagree ☐ Strongly Disagree
☐ Don't Know

5. The patient has the final decision in his or her own medical care.
☐ Strongly Agree ☐ Agree ☐ Disagree ☐ Strongly Disagree
☐ Don't Know

6. Doctors speak openly to patients about terminal illnesses and the patient's approaching death.
☐ Strongly Agree ☐ Agree ☐ Disagree ☐ Strongly Disagree
☐ Don't Know

7. Patients will follow the doctor's orders.
☐ Strongly Agree ☐ Agree ☐ Disagree ☐ Strongly Disagree
☐ Don't Know

8. Patients believe it is okay if a doctor interrupts an examination to make a phone call.
☐ Strongly Agree ☐ Agree ☐ Disagree ☐ Strongly Disagree
☐ Don't Know

9. It is considered unprofessional for a doctor to share a joke or laugh with a patient while treating that patient.
☐ Strongly Agree ☐ Agree ☐ Disagree ☐ Strongly Disagree
☐ Don't Know

10. A student or resident should never question the diagnosis or treatment plan that a faculty member has made.
    ☐ Strongly Agree ☐ Agree ☐ Disagree ☐ Strongly Disagree
    ☐ Don't Know

11. Patients expect doctors to address them formally (e.g., "Mr. -," "Mrs. -").
    ☐ Strongly Agree ☐ Agree ☐ Disagree ☐ Strongly Disagree
    ☐ Don't Know

12. Preventive healthcare is an important part of a doctor's work.
    ☐ Strongly Agree ☐ Agree ☐ Disagree ☐ Strongly Disagree
    ☐ Don't Know

APPENDIX 6.2: THE INTERPERSONAL COMMUNICATION ASSESSMENT SURVEY (REVISED COVER SHEET FOR USE WITH GAMMA VERSION)

Many of the activities in which you have already participated, or in which you will participate in coming days and weeks, are aimed at assessing your entry-level status relative to competencies of the Accreditation Council for Graduate Medical Education (ACGME). The attached survey is but one more tool used in this process.

Based on your prior experience and/or what you may have read or heard about clinical work in the United States, please answer the questions in the survey according to your expectations of clinical work and the residency program in Indianapolis. Please read each question, and choose a response based on your first impression. The questions are meant to reflect general statements, not specific incidents, and are *not* meant to trick you.

Please complete the questionnaire in 10 minutes or less. There will be no adverse or punitive actions taken as a result of responses, so please answer openly and honestly.

When directed to begin, please turn the page. Put a check mark in the box below each question that indicates your answer. Check only one answer for each question. Remember, each question is about the medical environment you will be working in here in Indianapolis.

© 2008 The Trustees of Indiana University.

CHAPTER SEVEN

BY THE BEDSIDE: LESSONS ABOUT COMMUNICATION FROM AN INTERNAL MEDICINE PROGRAM DIRECTOR

MaryGrace Zetkulic

ABSTRACT

In the course of a rapid transition from a program in internal medicine staffed by U.S.-trained residents to one staffed by internationally trained doctors, the program director created a one-station Objective Structured Clinical Examination (OSCE) test for all residents to serve as a diagnostic for clinical and communication skills. The OSCE proved useful as an ongoing tool for formative assessment and instruction for all residents working in this urban hospital clinical setting. This chapter is a narrative of the overall transition and focuses on the lessons on communication gleaned from that transition.

INTRODUCTION

The bedside to a physician is hallowed ground. Here practitioner and patient meet in a unique moment and begin a relationship infused with trust

English Language and the Medical Profession: Instructing and Assessing
the Communication Skills of International Physicians
Innovation and Leadership in English Language Teaching, Volume 5, 133–146
ISSN: 2041-272X/doi:10.1108/S2041-272X(2011)0000005013
133

or mistrust. Here at the bedside, communication, the natural currency of all human interaction, gains even greater power—the power to diagnose, to heal, to comfort, or to do irreparable harm. As such, communication, verbal and nonverbal, is the most fundamental and necessary tool of the physician. Its diagnostic value supersedes that of any MRI. The initial medical history taken and recorded is used by teams of clinicians to determine diagnosis and care through a course of illness. Information that is overlooked or inaccurate in the initial history of illness may never be asked again. Only more recently have U.S. medical schools focused more extensively on communication. The international medical graduate for whom English is a second language or who is trained at an institute that does not commit time to developing this skill is at a notable disadvantage.

Given its importance, one would believe evaluation and education in communication would be a priority for residency directors and educators of international medical graduates (IMGs); however, it remains an after-thought. This is significant as data from the National Resident Matching Program for 2010 indicate that 40% to 60% of residency slots are filled by IMGs, depending on the specialty. Some of this oversight is the culture of U.S. graduate medical education. Having completed medical school, physicians complete three to six years of training in an accredited residency program directly caring for patients in a system of graduated supervision. Residents learn by watching and doing and are expected to learn and perform simultaneously and quickly. Training in communication is time-intensive. The rapid pace of hospital medicine is not conducive to the necessary observation and feedback which communication training requires. Faculty are often not comfortable with this area of education and have little training in assessment of communication. Moreover, the supervision of residents varies. Most often the highly technical skills such as placing a central line or performing a lumbar puncture have the most supervision. But the taking of a medical history or the reviewing of a therapeutic plan with a patient or family is rarely observed. It is fair to say that most assessments of communication in residencies across the country more accurately reflect how a resident communicates with his attending physician, not from objective evaluation but direct observation. Due to these reasons combined with the significant momentum of residency training, it is often six months before deficits in communication are fully realized.

This is a narrative of my experience as Internal Medicine Associate Program Director at an urban hospital in the northeast United States as we transitioned the program from one with 100% U.S. medical graduates to one that consisted of 70% international medical graduates (IMGs).

Implementing this transition required reflection and analysis of the limitations of current practices in residency training. The transition provided a vantage point to observe the communication challenges of the IMG. It demanded novel solutions to these challenges to ensure success of the new residents and the safety of the patients under their care.

THE STRUCTURE OF U.S. GRADUATE MEDICAL EDUCATION

A Program in Transition

A U.S. residency program must be accredited through the American College of Graduate Medical Education (ACGME). The ACGME has worked hard to ensure uniformity of standards in American Graduate Education. Having considerable influence over funding of graduate medical education, their standards have transformed educational practice. The vocabulary of graduates of medical education is taken from the ACGME's program requirements. Regardless of the field of medicine, residents must be evaluated in six general competencies: (1) Patient Care, (2) Medical Knowledge, (3) Interpersonal and Communication Skills, (4) Professionalism, (5) Practice-Based Learning and Improvement, and (6) System-Based Practice (see ACGME General Competencies). The program director must administer and maintain an educational environment conducive to educating the residents in each of the ACGME general competency areas. The program director must oversee and ensure the quality of didactic and clinical education in all institutions that participate in our program. In addition, the program director is responsible for the selection and evaluation of the residents in the program. It is the program director who must certify at the end of training that a physician is competent to practice independently.

In 2005, as a result of irreconcilable differences among participating institutions and our sponsoring university, our long-standing multiinstitution residency had to be restructured as a new residency with a single institution and a new university affiliation. This meant that until June 30, 2005, we ran a 110-resident program, with 100% U.S. medical graduates (USMGs). On July 1, 2005, the new smaller residency began with 36 brand new residents, 70% of whom were international medical graduates (IMGs). Our hospital resides in a smaller urban center in the northeast United States, with 450 beds, a 30-bed intensive care unit (ICU), and a 40-bed neonatal ICU. We serve as a tertiary care center for high-risk deliveries, in addition to caring for medical conditions from sepsis to renal failure. Our residents provide medical consultations for our high-risk pregnant patients. We also provide medical school training for a large U.S. medical school, having approximately 60 medical students per month integrated into the medical services. The Herculean transformation of the residency did not occur in a classroom but in the context of this busy hospital, filled with patients—at the bedside. On July 1, the doctors, nurses, and patients saw all new faces. Thirty-six residents saw a whole new world. The information offered here is drawn from this experience and the continued experience of training IMGs (and USMGs) in caring for patients.

Initial Assessment

With concern over the response of patients and staff to our program filled with "foreign" medical graduates, all with different accents and cultures, the first great challenge was to assess with confidence the baseline medical knowledge and clinical competency of the new group, given their diverse educational backgrounds. We understood that communication skills would be integral to both perceived competence and actual effectiveness. Normally, in a residency, only the first-year residents (the "interns") are new whereas one can rely on the second- and third-year residents, who are acclimated to the institution and whose strengths and weaknesses are well known. These more experienced residents buffer the transition of the interns and ensure competent care of patients, while faculty learn the baseline abilities of the new interns. In this system of graduated supervision, second- and third-year residents provide much of that supervision. Moreover, much of the teaching third- and fourth-year medical students receive comes from upper level residents. In our case, everyone was new and the level of the clinical competence, medical knowledge, and communication skills for all residents was unknown. We needed a tool to directly observe residents and take stock of basic knowledge, communication and interpersonal skills with patients, staff, and physicians in a safe way. It was understood that in the first few months the attending physicians would have to provide intensive levels of supervision extending to a level of detail to which they were not accustomed. Such an inventory of basic knowledge, communication, and interpersonal skills would provide these attending physicians with reference points on which they could focus.

What evaluations of competency were available to us and, indeed, all program directors?

All new residents are required to be certified by the Educational Commission for Foreign Medical Graduates® (ECFMG®) prior to applying to residency training. Of the many ECFMG requirements, physicians must take a language proficiency test. They must pass the initial Step 1 and 2 exams necessary for all U.S. medical graduates. Then they must pass the Clinical Skills (CS) exam also required of all U.S. medical graduates. The CS exam is an objective skills evaluation with standardized patients in multiple simulated medical scenarios. Physicians are evaluated by both the standardized patients and multiple physician evaluators. The purpose is to ensure the physician has the minimum necessary clinical skills, communication correctly categorized as a clinical skill, to proceed further in training. This exam is pass/fail. The residency program directors are only assured the new residents meet minimum requirements.[1] While this evaluation is valuable, it does not provide actionable information that a supervising physician would desire when working with a new physician by the bedside, especially when the senior resident's abilities are equally unknown. Though the recruited second-year residents had completed a year of training in the United States or United Kingdom prior to beginning, the available assessment of their ability was disappointingly superficial. It is important to note that all major accrediting bodies in the United States, the National Board of Medical Examiners® (NBME®), the ACGME, and the ECFMG, identify communication as a fundamental competency, both as an independent skill and as a component of the other five identified necessary competencies (see ACGME General Competencies for a complete description of the six competencies). Guidance in evaluating and certifying competency after entering a residency program, however, is left up to educators and institutions, leading to very variable and subjective implementation.

Development of the One-Station OSCE

To meet the need for objective observation and evaluation of communication and clinical skills, a clinical skills evaluation tool to provide the necessary baseline inventory needed to be developed and implemented. The clinical skills evaluation was performed for all residents, both international and domestic, during orientation in the last week of June. The clinical skills evaluation was a "single station simulation"—that is, a roleplay, or simulation of a patient, played by an actor, or "standardized patient." It was a modification on the multistation Clinical Skills (CS) exam administered as part of the United States Medical Licensing Examination® (USMLE®). In this standardized simulated encounter, referred to as an "OSCE" in medical education (Objective Structured Clinical Examination), the resident evaluates a standardized patient having chest pain. There is a nurse in the room, available to provide any additional information or assistance. The resident has 20 minutes to evaluate the patient. A physician observer (myself) is positioned behind a two-way mirror evaluating each resident's communication skills with the patient and the nurse as well as the competency in the approach to the clinical task. The resident is then required to present the case over the phone to the physician observer. In this way the resident's phone communication skills can be assessed, as well as the essential ability to identify the most salient elements of a patient's condition and communicate them succinctly.

Though the anxiety provoked by the exercise affected performance, the inventory was helpful. USMGs had more familiarity with the exercise due to U.S. medical schools practicing similar yet longer exercises to prepare their students for the CS exam. However, salient aspects of interpersonal interactions, such as response to nonverbal cues, were elicited for all residents. As residents presented the case over the phone—an essential skill—how they responded to questioning was reflective of future performance. Sometimes residents would provide information that was not actually asked. Often medical jargon was substituted when a physician had less ability in colloquial language. This was a problem for USMG as well as IMG residents. Some residents who performed poorly on the OSCE were fine when observed by the bedside, but the evaluation highlighted the need to facilitate direct bedside observation in the area of communication. Supervising attending physicians could tailor their approach and super-vision based on more specific information; moreover, they would not be surprised by deficiencies.

Ongoing Use of OSCE

Though this was not originally planned, the program training team opted to continue this one-station OSCE, which we modified to perform monthly or every other month. Each month we changed the scenario to evaluate the residents' knowledge on clinical topics like headaches, memory loss, and musculoskeletal conditions while continuing to assess the development of their communication skills. We could give immediate feedback to the residents on the areas of weakness and question them to find out if poor performers lacked medical knowledge or communication skills. We expanded the number of faculty evaluators to four, but intentionally kept this group small. This way our objectives, evaluations, and feedback became uniform within the group.

Five years later, this one-station OSCE has remained a powerful tool to evaluate and educate. It continues to provide a routine opportunity for our best educators to observe and teach each resident one-on-one. It gives me an instrument to later teach and evaluate the ability of residents in communication tasks that are especially complex, such as identifying sexual abuse, receiving consent for procedures, or discussing end-of-life issues. Keeping the exercise to one station maintains the procedure's simplicity, flexibility, and routine. While a multistation exercise can touch on multiple areas of medical knowledge, the communication skills are reviewed in each station repeatedly, making the more cumbersome multistation approach redundant when evaluating communication. Furthermore, being able to perform the exercise with increased frequency allows evaluation of progress in communication which would be lost in another approach.

Having to rethink our residency and being unable to assume the adequacy of our residents' communication skills offered a new opportunity to advance our teaching methods. Having recognized the need for objective observation and evaluation of communication skills, we found that the standardized simulated OSCE, though invaluable, also had limitations. It is formalized and structured, and it does not simulate with high fidelity the subtleties of patient–doctor interactions. Also, even a single OSCE takes time and resources that limit the frequency with which it can be performed. For these reasons, we adopted the "mini Clinical Exercise" (mini-CEX) for ongoing evaluation of residents' skills in real encounters with patients as an additional tool.

Adopting the Mini-CEX

The mini-CEX (Clinical Exercise) is a tool validated by the American Board of Internal Medicine. This is a brief evaluation form that a physician can utilize when observing a resident during a *real* patient encounter. The tool facilitates observation and feedback to the resident. The form itself is deliberately nonspecific so educators can tailor it to meet their educational objectives. This Mini-Clinical Evaluation Exercise is available at the

American Board of Internal Medicine Web site (see www.abim.org), and is reproduced in Appendix A.1. (For details regarding the use of this form, see Norcini, Blank, Arnold, & Kimball, 1995).

The mini-CEX can be woven in the daily routine of caring for patients and supervision of residents. Because this is done in relation to patients directly under the care of the resident being evaluated, it gains the power of relevance. A small group of physicians who work side by side with residents can be trained to observe with a critical eye the data-gathering, medical interviewing, and counseling skills of residents. From there, the physician can diagnosis communication difficulties with residents and plan the means of remedy. For example, an attending physician can supervise a resident in delivering difficult news on a diagnosis and analyze how the resident responds to questions. As new patients are admitted from the ER, the attending physician can directly observe and later evaluate and provide feedback on how a resident gathers sensitive history such as sexual history or alcohol use.

When using the mini-CEX as an evaluation and education tool for communication, faculty education and training is important. In most residency programs, the strongest educators are supervising residents in July, when the residency year and the new interns begin. The supervising faculty should be instructed to perform mini-CEX evaluations in essential communication areas as described below.

(1)   The taking of an initial patient history
      As stated earlier, the initial history taken and recorded by an intern or resident will be used by attending physicians and consultants to determine the patient's care. Some questions may never be asked again. Inaccurate information will be repeated ad infinitum. Therefore, the downstream effects of a poor initial patient's history may be disastrous. New interns should be deemed competent in this skill within the first few weeks through direct observation. Their weaknesses here need to be identified early.

(2)   Counseling
      Counseling can be as simple as explaining the side effects of a medication to the complexity of delivering difficult news. There are some basic competency requirements for this, but one never stops improving this skill. Treatment may require a patient to understand complex tasks such as self-administering insulin or responding to changes in blood sugar. If this is done poorly, such as if a resident cannot sense when a patient does not understand or cannot respond

empathetically to their distress, he or she will irreversibly lose the trust of the patient. A vulnerable patient may be hurt deeply by information delivered incorrectly and insensitively. The patient may leave an encounter without the information necessary to make educated medical choices.

(3) Clinical reasoning

Precision in science and medicine begins with precision in language. Conversely, sloppy language both reflects and enables sloppy reasoning. Both USMGs and IMGs may obfuscate clear and thorough understanding of diagnosis and management with medical jargon. Moreover, the area of clinical reasoning involves synthesizing information from patients, other physicians, and laboratory data, and ultimately formulating a diagnosis. Physicians with communication difficulties often omit or minimize the input of the patient's history and rely on technical input or the written records of others because it is easier for them. Yet it has long been recognized that difficulties in the effective delivery of healthcare can arise from problems in communication between patient and provider rather than from any failing in the technical aspects of medical care.

COMMUNICATION AND CLINICAL SKILLS IN MEDICAL PRACTICE

Communication Issues and Resident Evaluation

It should be clear from the previous paragraphs that safe, effective medical practice is impossible without competent communication. It also defines the prerequisite for all other clinical skills. We recognized this early in the transition of the program. We learned in the crucible of the transition that no educator can assess and ameliorate communication skills without effective direct observation early in training. The OSCE and mini-CEX are precisely that: tools utilized to facilitate direct observation. These tools were of particular importance with regard to communication skills because in a busy residency, communication skills are the least likely skills to be observed.

Observations need to be frequent, focused, and resulting in feedback. Medical educators need to identify high-risk communication areas and ensure there are multiple observations of residents enacting these scenarios,

preferably through both OSCE and mini-CEX observations early in
training, in the first one to two months.

The Role of a Communication Consultant

Our program faced a particular challenge that made early evaluation
imperative, but as is the case in most residencies, a particularly important
time in new resident evaluation is the six-month mark. This six-month mark
is the program director's mid-year evaluation mandated by the Accreditation Council of Graduate Medical Education (ACGME). At this time,
communication deficits may be misdiagnosed as lack of medical knowledge
or professionalism. If communication deficits are correctly identified,
professional consultation may be initiated.

With all the above information, how does the communication consultant
integrate his or her expertise in the graduate medical education process
when a program director has identified a problem. To be effective, the
communication consultant should identify a physician partner who will
have the most opportunity for direct observation. This person may not be
the program director who calls for the consultation.

In internal medicine, family medicine, psychiatry, and pediatrics, the
ACGME governing regulations require a continuity clinic. This is an
outpatient setting where residents practice at least one day a week. In this
setting, the residents will interact with the same attending physicians,
nursing staff, and patients weekly over a three-year period. This is the place
where a communication consultant can best integrate into the resident
educational process, identify the resident's continuity clinic supervising
physician, and interview him or her and other staff for the deficits that are
perceived. The ancillary staff in the facility will also have valuable input.
The consultant can arrange to be present for a mini-CEX observation with
the attending physician and resident during a real outpatient encounter. As
long as the patient gives consent, a communication consultant can be
present in an encounter. Patients who attend resident-run clinics are aware
that their physicians are in training. They are used to having observers and
are rarely reluctant to consent. This will give the consultant the best insight
in to the resident's deficits. After the encounter, the consultant should
debrief the attending physician and the patient for their impressions of the
resident's deficits. The different perspectives will be illuminating and give the
consultant a key to collaboration.

As a communication consultant works with a resident, frequent meetings
with the supervising attending physician can give a feedback loop where

effort and progress can be observed at the bedside on a weekly basis. The consultant should be aware that by the time a consultant has been called, the resident—without exception—will have lost the trust of his supervisors and colleagues. Indeed, consultations are driven more by complaints than evaluations. Tools for rebuilding this trust must be part of any practice improvement intervention. Often this may require that the resident reiterate what a patient or colleague has said to demonstrate understanding.

Summary of Experience and Lessons Learned

Communication problems in international medical graduates are in fact not so different from those of U.S. medical graduates, but IMGs are less likely to be forgiven for them. Our experience with early direct observation demonstrated that we had taken for granted communication skills in our U.S. graduates without cause.

Nonverbal communication skills are most essential. This should be encouraging to physicians with strong accents or language difficulties. Responding to patient nonverbal cues about discomfort, suffering, or confusion builds essential trust with the patients. Having worked side by side with IMGs by the bedside, I have seen residents with poor verbal skills become beloved by their patients. Since patients often come with their own communication difficulties, a physician who communicates well using all aspects of communication succeeds.

The physician needs to listen, listen, listen. Patients decide to trust a physician early in their interaction. This decision is based largely on their perception of being listened to and far less by how well their doctor speaks. The physician's nonverbal and verbal communication should unequivocally demonstrate that he or she is listening to the patient.

It is essential that when a resident misunderstands information from a colleague, supervisor, or patient, this must be acknowledged. The resident must stop and clarify points, even if it is embarrassing or if the resident feels it may make him or her appear incompetent. Expressing understanding when points are unclear starts a cycle that will cause the loss of the trust of patients and colleagues.

CONCLUSION

This transition provided a great professional challenge. Working with our new IMGs proved a great privilege. The challenge opened an opportunity to reflect upon and readdress our approach to graduate medical education. Working by the bedside with our new physicians threw into relief the importance of communication—in all its aspects. The exigencies of recreating a residency in a high-stakes environment where failures would result in poor patient care forced us to address the complacency that graduate medical education often has with regard to communication. Turning that sense of urgency into routine practice and habits of good training has become our new challenge.

NOTE

1. An interesting historical note: While U.S. graduates are also required to pass the clinical skills exam, this was required of IMGs through the ECFMG many years earlier. See van Zanten, and Whelan (both this volume) for a discussion of the development of the Clinical Skills Assessment® (CSA®) and the Clinical Skills (CS) Exam.

APPENDIX 7.1 MINI-CLINICAL EVALUATION
EXERCISE (CEX)

Evaluator: Date

Resident: O R-1OR-2OR-3

Patient Problem/DX

Setting	Ambulatory	In-patient	ED	Other
Patient	Age:	Sex:	New	Follow-up
Complexity	Low	Moderate	High	
Focus	Date Gathering	Diagnosis	Therapy	Counseling

Medical Interviewing Skills:	1	2	3	4	5	6	7	8	9
Physical Examination Skills:	1	2	3	4	5	6	7	8	9
Professionalism:	1	2	3	4	5	6	7	8	9
Clinical Judgment:	1	2	3	4	5	6	7	8	9
Counseling Skills:	1	2	3	4	5	6	7	8	9
Organizational/Efficient:	1	2	3	4	5	6	7	8	9

7. Overall Clinical Competence (O Not Observed)

1   2   3   4   5   6   7   8   9

UNSATISFACTORY   SATISFACTORY   SUPERIOR

Mini-CEX Time: Observing   Mins.   Providing Feedback:

Mins

Evaluator Satisfaction with Mini-CEX

LOW   1   2   3   4   5   6   7   8   9   HIGH

Resident Satisfaction with Mini-CEX

LOW   1   2   3   4   5   6   7   8   9   HIGH

Comments:

Resident Signature   Evaluator Signature

DESCRIPTORS OF COMPETENCIES
DEMONSTRATED DURING THE MINI-CEX

Medical Interviewing Skills: Facilitates patient's telling of story; effectively uses questions/directions to obtain accurate, adequate information needed; responds appropriately to affect, nonverbal cues.

Physical Examination Skills: Follows efficient, logical sequence; balances screening/diagnostic steps for problem; informs patient; sensitive to patient's comfort, modesty.

Humanistic Qualities/Professionalism: Shows respect, compassion, empathy, establishes trust; attends to patient's needs of comfort, modesty, confidentiality, information.

Clinical Judgment: Selectively orders/performs appropriate diagnostic studies, considers risks, benefits.

Counseling Skills: Explains rationale for test/treatment, obtains patient's consent, educates/counsels regarding management.

Organization/Efficiency: Prioritizes; is timely; succinct.

Overall Clinical Competence: Demonstrates judgment, synthesis, caring, effectiveness, efficiency.

Reprinted from the American Board of Internal Medicine (www.abim.org).

PART III
COURSES AND CURRICULA

CHAPTER EIGHT

DEVELOPING CURRICULUM AND STRATEGIES FOR A CHINESE-LANGUAGE MEDICAL UNIVERSITY IN TAIWAN ADOPTING ENGLISH AS A MEDIUM OF INSTRUCTION

Susan Olmstead-Wang

ABSTRACT

This chapter describes efforts by a faculty development center at a medical university in Taiwan to provide workshops, lectures, and practice sessions to assess and address current English language and teaching pedagogy needs. The focus in this chapter is on helping physicians and biomedical instructors transition from using Chinese to using English by building their oral English language skills and confidence. Suggestions are given for improving English language training curricula in international medical universities, especially in those already using interactive problem-based learning (PBL) as a teaching technique.

English Language and the Medical Profession: Instructing and Assessing
the Communication Skills of International Physicians
Innovation and Leadership in English Language Teaching, Volume 5, 149–174
ISSN: 2041-272X/doi:10.1108/S2041-272X(2011)0000005014

INTRODUCTION

With the globalization of education (Friedman, 2005; Gaston, 2010; Likic, Dusek, & Horvat, 2005), there is increased use of English as a medium of tertiary instruction and as a "language ... of wider communication" (Graddol, 2000, p. 58), and of English for specific purposes (ESP), including English for medical purposes (EMP). Purposes include increasing international exchange at international conferences, assisting international students who choose to study in formerly non-English-speaking institutions or in English-speaking countries, and developing medical tourism.

Some international medical universities in India and China (www.chi naenglishmedium.com/Medical_Council_India_China) and a few in Taiwan (www.english.moe.tw.edu) have adopted English as a medium of instruction as part of their curriculum. Medical university administrators seek to adopt and transition to English textbooks and to English as a medium of instruction in order to raise the prestige of their institution (Graddol, 2006, p. 74), to attract international students to campus (Harden, 2006, pp. S25–S26), and to link the medical university more closely to the international medical community of practice (Harden, 2006, p. S23).

Improved English not only facilitates these institutional goals, but also strengthens the communication skills of these schools' graduates who may later take up residencies or fellowships as international medical graduates (IMGs), including in the United Kingdom or the United States, where they constitute 25.3% of the physician workforce (www.ama-assn.org). In order to "track the global pipeline of medical education" and to "better understand the global capacity to educate physicians" (Boulet, Bede, & McKinely, 2007, p. 20), more studies are needed which focus on English language training in the medical universities from which IMGs come. To link language training programs, improve the flow between segments of this global pipeline, and reduce the negative impact of "additional hurdles" (Hoekje, 2007, p. 328) which IMGs encounter in English-speaking countries and culturally diverse environments, coordinated efforts are needed to prepare IMGs in professional medical communication in English before they receive any additional medical training in English-speaking environments.

"Global flows" (Burns & Roberts, 2010, p. 409) of medical doctors and patients are changing; in addition to international medical graduates seeking residencies in English-speaking countries or wealthy international patients seeking high-end medical treatment in the United States, there are now many medical students traveling as international students to countries which offer medical education in English and many medical tourists who seek reasonably priced medical care outside the United States (Turner, 2007, p. 307). With the rise in countries actively recruiting international students MESDCs (major English-speaking destination countries) and in global medical tourism, there are changed global dynamics and increased demand for English language skills.

In addition to the positive aspects of countries developing English-language programs to attract new students and to link more closely to the global learning community, there are many challenges to such undertakings. This chapter raises complex issues of language and educational policy on the national level in Taiwan as well as medical university curricular reform at a global level and at one medical university in the southern part of the island. It focuses on some challenges encountered and opportunities realized as this university transitioned from using Mandarin to English as its medium of instruction in its Post-Graduate (post-baccalaureate) Medical Department. In response to a challenge from the university president for volunteers to come to campus to contribute in various areas of expertise and endeavor, I organized specific English language training in a series of four intensive workshops over a two-year period. Because this medical university (then, college) is the place where I began my EFL/ESL career decades ago, it was interesting on a number of levels to return and teach. In the 1970s, a medical English course consisted of long lists of English words to be memorized but not necessarily pronounced. Now, English use is ubiquitous and central to all campus efforts to publish and present internationally.

Kaohsiung Medical University's efforts to attract international students to study and to "better position its graduates in the international medical community" (www.kmu.edu.tw/~spbm/eng-web/programs/overview.html) requires concerted, coordinated effort on the levels of planning, assessing, implementing, and providing ongoing support, especially for middle-aged and older professors who have been teaching in Mandarin or Taiwanese their whole careers and who did not possess high levels of skill or confidence in speaking English at the beginning of the transition.

To provide background on the current language situation in Taiwan, this chapter first reviews the complex language history of the island and of its educational system. It then discusses recent government policies that promote English language development and medical tourism and addresses medical university English language policy decisions that impact local curriculum development. The chapter focuses on several practical aspects of implementing the policy decisions and describes the four workshops developed to improve Chinese biomedical professors' own English language skills, confidence, and interactive teaching techniques. PBL is considered as an example of an interactive learning environment and as a prototype for introducing other interactive teaching techniques into institutions that wish to improve English language proficiency.

The chapter concludes by advocating student-centered learning techniques like problem-based learning where possible for material formerly presented in teacher-centered, lecture-based formats and offers practical suggestions for assisting a university department as it transitions to English as a medium of instruction.[1]

TRENDS TOWARD ADOPTING ENGLISH AS A MEDIUM OF INSTRUCTION FOR HIGHER EDUCATION

English in International Higher Education

The internationalization of higher education around the globe is closely linked in a concurrent, if not cause–effect, pattern of adopting English as a medium of instruction around the world. Internationalization of English in global higher education can aid in the clear exchange of scientific information at international conferences, attract international students to institutions of higher education, including medical universities, assist medical scholars and graduates who want to immigrate to English-speaking countries or to new English-using programs in countries where English is not an official language for further study or training, and promote medical tourism.

Graddol (2000) notes that "[o]ne of the most significant educational trends worldwide is the teaching of a growing number of courses in universities through the medium of English" (p. 45). In the short term and midterm, the use and promotion of English allows access to the most current science information (textbooks, research articles, online sources). In the long term, the trend has major effects on increasing the reach, influence, and prestige of English and making possible "rapid internationalization of education ... [that] allows developing countries to reposition themselves as exporters of education services" (p. 45) and thus "become major competitors to native-speaking countries in English-medium education" (p. 54).

Graddol (2006) identifies a strong link between English language use as a medium of instruction and the global prestige of an institution. Because "around two-thirds of the world's top 100 universities are in English-speaking countries" (p. 74), English is seen as a driver for improving an institution's reputation and draw. Graddol concludes that if a university "wishes to become a centre of international excellence, it needs both to attract teachers and researchers from around the world, and to encourage international students to enroll on its courses, enriching the university's prestige, revenue, and intellectual climate" (p. 74). Using English as a medium of instruction facilitates "entrepreneurial universities," further establishing a country as a major English-speaking destination (p. 76).

Teacher training is a challenge in "English-medium education … where teachers are not fully proficient in the English language and where there is little use of English in the community … " (Graddol, 2000, p. 38). In some environments this sets up "the development of an elite group" (Graddol, 2000, p. 38) of those with access to English language skills who continue to garner more educational advantages. In an environment where rapid, poorly planned languages or curricula changes are forced, some medical professors may be challenged by having to teach before being well trained or by having to use English that is inferior to that of their international students. In addition, students may come from countries where English is an official language but speak a form or variant of English that is different from the target English of the professors.

English in International Medical Institutions and for International Scholarly Exchange

International medical universities may decide to instigate use of English in order to attract English-speaking international students to their campuses for economic reasons or to strengthen international links to overseas universities. Because most major medical journals have shifted to publishing in English (Gibbs, 1995, p. 77), English has become the medium for "an enormous amount of intellectual property" (Graddol, 2000, p. 9).

Many of the medical universities now using English are in countries where English is not an official language. As Boulet et al. (2007) note, "Of the 1,771 medical schools located outside the United States or Canada, 664 (37.5%) offer instruction in English. However, only 22% of the countries where these schools are located list English as an official language" (pp. 22–23). Additionally, Boulet et al. (2007) observe rapid growth of medical schools in Asia where English is being adopted as one of the tools for modernization and internationalization (p. 23).

Where English is not an official language of a country and where all business is conducted in a two-tier, bilingual environment, a basic step in standardizing language use involves developing standard medical terminology equivalents in all languages used for medical purposes. By carefully instituting the clearest equivalents and most accurate translations for medical terms, and by eliminating use of inaccurate or imprecise terminology, bilingual medical universities can clarify meaning and improve communication. Medical institutions that use native languages together with English medical terminology in a side-by-side model need to respond to modest international goals such as developing usage of "common medical education vocabulary or terminology ... recognized by the International Institute of Medical Education (IIME)" (Harden, 2006, p. S23). A well-known example of idiosyncratic naming is Mandarin's sound transliteration for AIDS: 愛滋病 or 艾滋病, both pronounced *ai dzu bing*. Although the first character in each sequence reflects a difference between usage in Taiwan and China, respectively (Hornby & Wehmeier, 2004), each produces a rough sound equivalent of the term "AIDS" and reflects a folklore explanation of a cause of the disease (especially the first, "love proliferation disease"). These variations create an unscientific terminology "equivalent" for the English term HIV/AIDS. Such nonstandard or multiple terminologies must be standardized for clear English medical usage.

Medical institutions that use English as a medium of instruction must develop appropriate language policy responses and English training initiatives. In addition to needs for English inside international medical universities, momentum for adopting the use of English in medical education is driven by needs for English in the broader international medical community. Adequate English skills are necessary for precision and clarity in medical presentations (spoken and written) for international conferences and journals and for medical graduates who migrate to English-speaking countries for advanced medical training. For those who migrate to the United States for these purposes, the need is perhaps more immediate and specific: they need to pass English language qualifying tests and to perform in a high-stress English-speaking environment. More fortunate international medical graduates (IMGs) taking up residencies in English-speaking countries have had excellent English-language training at home and/or benefit from institutional training resources designed to facilitate their transitions and to maximize their success at their new institution (Tipton, 2005, p. 396). Others less fortunate may struggle to bring their English language skills up to the high levels of communication required and may experience significant stress while trying to do so.

English Language Development in Medical Tourism

Due to the high expense of medical care in the United States and elsewhere, seekers of affordable medical care are traveling to other countries aided by a "new global industry" that has brokered international trade agreements (e.g., the General Agreement on Trade in Services (GATS)) and other services to support "this cross-border traffic" (Turner, 2007, p. 307). In general, the international medical tourism industry was worth about US$40 billion in 2010 and served 40 million medical travelers in a trend to "outsourcing health-care" (Turner, 2007, p. 305). One projection suggests that 1.6 million Americans will travel abroad for medical care in 2012 (Sun, shopping, and surgery, 2010, p. 78).

Singapore, a leader in "'exporting' healthcare by 'importing' patients," has found that medical tourists bring in big profits (Turner, 2007, p. 314). In a new global economy in which international medical travel is becoming "normal," there is increased justification for using "portable, borderless health insurance" from any country in any country (p. 317). "Medical tourism" has created a global health services marketplace in which patients fly to wherever they can afford the treatments they need, and usually, to where English is the language of communication (p. 323).

In Taiwan, new government and industry initiatives seek to transform Taiwan into a major medical tourism location by 2015 (www.imtj.com/news/?EntryId82 = 172651). In 2007, Taiwan's Department of Health began to plan links between tourism and medical services, including construction of whole health-care villages, beginning with the first one conveniently located near the large international airport that serves the capital of Taipei. Up eightfold from 5,000 people in 2008 to 40,000 medical travelers in 2009, the numbers are expected to increase rapidly. To date most medical tourists have been overseas Chinese returning for care, mostly focused on medical check-ups and cosmetic surgery. In 2011, the Taiwan government began to offer changes in visa applications to allow potential medical tourists a check box for "medical care." This change will make it easier for mainland Chinese to travel individually, separate from organized (and supervised) tour groups and will facilitate travel and medical tourism. Although Taiwan is currently behind neighboring countries (e.g., Singapore, Thailand, and Japan) in medical tourism, Taiwan's medical care is highly ranked in the world and poised to adapt to this emerging opportunity. To date, Taiwan has attracted mostly overseas Chinese and those of Chinese descent (www.imtj.com/news/?EntryId82 = 172651). Nonetheless, Asian countries "feel confident that large numbers of Americans are going to be forced to look abroad for affordable healthcare" (Turner, 2007, p. 316). Taiwan touts itself as an "English friendly country" where bilingual signage and "no social shock" will attract a broad range of medical tourists (see www.tmtda.org/en/index2.php?option = com_content&task = vie).

By looking at global trends in medical English education, and by integrating communicative approaches and language skills development early in the training framework, it is possible to improve use of English as a medium of international medical communication and to coordinate efforts on behalf of IMGs flowing to English-speaking countries through the global pipeline. Furthermore, better English training may also have an effect on the English development of major English-speaking destination countries and of medical tourism. Although opportunities and challenges will vary according to differences in specific situations, ranging from historical and philosophical orientations to financial considerations, more research on needs and better implementation of best educational practices can improve training in using English as an international language of medicine.

THE SITUATED NATURE OF LANGUAGE USE IN TAIWAN'S MEDICAL COMMUNITY AND CURRICULAR CHANGE

Local language history and politics as well as global language trends interact in specific ways to create unique language profiles that must be taken into account in assessing an institution's language background and in accounting for policy choices. A brief review of the complicated language histories of Taiwan and of medical higher education in Taiwan provides insight into attitudes about language in that educational setting. Colonization and historical events motivated radical changes in the languages used in Taiwan, and international trends in the dominant languages of medicine affected the medical higher education community.

Taiwan has used a number of languages over its history, including aboriginal Austronesian languages, Fukienese/Taiwanese, Hakka, Japanese, and Mandarin, with most people being bilingual. During the Japanese occupation of Taiwan from 1895 to 1945, Japanese was used as the language of government, business, and higher education. After the end of World War II, Japan returned Taiwan to Chinese control, and the new government instigated the use of Mandarin. As a result of these historic events, the Austronesian and Taiwanese-speaking population had to learn new languages, Japanese and Mandarin, to attend university (Wu, Chen, & Wu, 1989, p. 124).

Changes within medical education in Taiwan have included shifts in the dominant language of medicine from Latin, Japanese, and German to English. The governmental and educational leaders established a side-by-side model of language use, including Chinese plus Latin and Chinese plus German (Mainland China also used Chinese plus Russian). From 1943 to 1950, mainland China used language textbooks that gave English equivalents to science terminology (Haas, 1988, p. 46). These changes in the preferred foreign language for medical purposes over decades meant that some medical students had to learn a smattering of Latin, German, Japanese, and English for reading, grammar, or technical medical terminology as well as Mandarin for their mainstream training. With English stabilizing as the dominant language of science now (and most likely for some time to come), there is a demand for more thorough language training. Although English language textbooks in natural science paired with Chinese language oral instruction have long been used (Wu et al., 1989, p. 132), the trend is now to use English language texts *and* English language instruction. The growing use of English in Taiwan higher education may be seen as a "foreign impact" (Wu et al., 1989, p. 129) or as a strategic choice within the new global environment that differs from the language colonization of the past.

Although more studies of English use in higher education and medical university classrooms around the globe and in Chinese-speaking environments are needed, some immediate challenges are how to provide effective English language training and support for busy medical professionals. In one of the few studies on faculty levels of English competence in medical universities in Taiwan, Chia, Johnson, Chia, and Olive (1999) reported that all (100%) of the 20 biomedical faculty members surveyed at a major medical university said they taught course content in Chinese, but provided medical terms in English (p. 111). Faculty and students did not agree on the need for English or on priorities for English instruction: faculty perceived English as "more important for the students than the students did" (p. 111) and emphasized medical research reading and writing while students emphasized developing medical terminology. However, all agreed in desiring more than the one-year required English course for first-year students.

When teachers are asked to change from teaching in Mandarin to teaching in English, they may experience stress (Penner, 1995, p. 2) and may wish to continue using teacher-fronted lecture formats under the presumption that they will need *less* English than if they use other formats. However, they often need to develop English-speaking skills and teaching approaches (situational and problem-based) in order to communicate well with the international students the university has attracted. To assist in building speaker skill and confidence in English and to bring in best classroom practices, newer problem-based or student-centered formats can be used to supplement traditional teacher-fronted lecture formats in another version of the side-by-side model. Teacher education begins with assessment of existing language practices, educational resources, and needs. Assessment is ongoing and formative, as well as summative, and involves learners, staff, and administration. By learning about a university's current approaches and near- and long-term goals, language facilitators can build upon current program proficiencies while helping to shape specific desired changes.

Penner (1995) reports on early use of Communicative Language Teaching (CLT) approaches for teaching English in China and addresses cultural and pedagogical issues related to introducing change in educational institutions. Cultural preferences, traditional educational goals, and ingrained expectations affect language policy and classroom interaction and must be carefully considered when initiating radical curricular, language, or pedagogical changes (Penner, 1995, p. 3). Educational and curricular reform may involve first-order changes that seek only to modify current practices slightly or second-order changes that seek to modify the basic structure of organizations. Changing the medium of instruction to English may seem to be simple, but it may prove to be a second-order change that carries new expectations and teaching approaches with it. Successful educational reform must understand both first- and second-order kinds of change, undertake change with appropriate steps so it is experienced as "evolution, not revolution" (Penner, 1995, p. 7), and involve connections among methodology training, language proficiency, and properly designed materials (p. 3).

Chinese traditional approaches focused on transmission of a body of knowledge; whether for learning medicine or foreign language, memorization and lecture formats were preferred over other methods such as case studies or interactive approaches (Penner, 1995, p. 4). While traditional approaches were seen as "a knowledge receiving process" with the teacher as the sole authority, communicative approaches may be seen as "skill development" with the teacher acting as "helper" rather than "knower" (Penner, 1995, p. 5). Implementing curricular change can be threatening and disruptive. For the many teachers who were "teaching to the limits of their knowledge of English ... it was very threatening to use methods that allowed for unpredictability, such as student questions" (p. 6). Agents of change must understand "which aspects of the communicative approach can be adapted or adopted to suit their teaching and learning culture" (p. 14).

In order to attract international students who had earned bachelor's degrees outside of Taiwan to study medicine at its institution, the Kaohsiung Medical University (KMU) decided to use English rather than Mandarin as the medium of instruction in its Post-Graduate Medical Department. The next section of this chapter describes four English workshops designed to assist KMU biomedical professors and physicians transition to using English to teach, and discusses the key language and pedagogy issues that arose.

DEVELOPING ENGLISH WORKSHOPS FOR CHINESE PHYSICIANS AND BIOMEDICAL PROFESSORS

Background

The original project for the Kaohsiung Medical University (KMU) was conceived in response to the university president's call for alumnae/alumni and interested parties practicing or teaching medicine in North America to return to campus to contribute to the medical university's development as volunteers in their various areas of expertise. Because my husband is a graduate of this university and because my first English as a Foreign Language (EFL) job was teaching there in the mid-1970s, we were very interested in exploring the opportunity. I was teaching advanced second language writing full time at a major US university, so I decided to focus on medical writing and arranged to conduct a week-long workshop to assist physicians, biomedical researchers, and medical university professors.

The Team

The Kaohsiung Medical University Center for Faculty Development administrators and staff publicized the workshops, registered all participants, issued continuing education units, and provided audiovisual support, meeting space, and a hot lunch for participants daily. Two biomedical professors who had earned their doctorate degrees in the United States were particularly helpful and perceptive about the challenges of transitioning from Mandarin to English and of changing to newer teaching approaches that would be familiar to the international students arriving on campus to pursue medical degrees. These professors and my husband, a native of Kaohsiung and a graduate of KMU, were tireless in interviewing administrators, physicians, faculty, and students about their perceived needs and in facilitating workshop sessions. I did all of the teaching and peer reviewing. Although one never has the whole language picture until arrival (Pilcher, 2006, p. 83), we were fortunate to have good support and guidance from the Center for Faculty Development (CFD), to encounter enthusiastic and motivated participants, and to be fluent in local languages (Mandarin and Taiwanese) so that we could refine our sense of the needs through informal conversation before and after class.

Overview of English Camps

The First Workshop (January 2007)
The original plan for the first English workshop was a writing workshop for medical researchers who had research papers in process. When we arrived on campus, however, we learned that the medical university had decided to introduce English as the medium of instruction in July of that year for its Post-Graduate Medical Department and that many professors were experiencing stress at the prospect of having to switch from teaching in Mandarin or Taiwanese to teaching in English. In response, I rewrote the curriculum to include developing English-speaking skills and to introduce several student-centered, interactive teaching techniques that teachers could use in our English classes (and perhaps adapt to their biomedical science classes).

During the eight-day workshop, we alternated four full days of reviewing research papers with four afternoons of explicit instruction on how to put research papers together. Writers with manuscripts in process signed up at the Center for Faculty Development for one-hour long appointments with me. We met one-on-one in a conference room where we talked about their goals for our sessions and discussed their questions about their papers, and I read their papers for structural and organizational issues. While consultations were a one-time only event for a few of the writers, 8–10 of the writers established successful drafting cycles with me in face-to-face sessions, continued in online consulting after my return to the States, and polished their prose. Forty-three writers started in the first workshop; many finished at least one paper, and three writers finished two papers while in drafting cycles with me over two years.

Four afternoon sessions offered explicit instruction on how to construct research papers. Topics included how to write a scientific paper in general and how to write the introduction, discussion, and conclusion sections, in particular. I built on participants' confidence in their reading ability in English and their familiarity with information structure in science genres, using slide presentations I developed while teaching advanced academic writing at Johns Hopkins School of Advanced International Studies. Although English for medical purposes (EMP) is sometimes described as teaching in English as a second language (ESL) rather than English as a foreign language (EFL) environments, or as verbal interaction in English between medical staff and patients, I used the definition of EMP as "genre-informed pedagogy based on needs assessment of specific groups of learners" (Shi, 2009, p. 205) and extended its application to the EFL (or English as an International Language, EIL) context of our workshops and our participants' needs. Participants learned to notice and employ sentence stems commonly used in science writing and other key, repeated features of genre-based science formats (Zeiger, 2000). Following each lecture, we conducted hour-long discussions in a small group with interaction, writing advice, feedback, and examples. There were 30–40 attendees at the lectures and 10–12 who stayed for the less formal interactive sessions afterwards.

A small retrospective survey at the end of this workshop provided key information on how to shape the next workshop. Less than a third (31%) reported having adequate English training, 26.6% felt they had adequate speaker training in English, and only 18% felt they had "adequate, specific instruction" for how to teach in any language (see Appendix 8.1).

The Second Workshop (July 2007)
With a clearer grasp of the needs and a sense of urgency to help the teachers who would soon begin to teach in English, I used two-hour blocks of time each of the first three mornings to focus on key "how to" topics: How to teach in English, how to build up self-confidence in teaching, and how to make smooth transitions in oral presentations. Because of a strong Taiwanese preference for teacher-fronted lecture and the large number of attendees, I presented these topics in lecture format, although I did try to make the presentation somewhat relaxed and interactive by talking informally and directly with the audience. To make the experience as authentic as possible under the circumstances, I spoke in English and I modeled conventional transition phrases between slides in presentation (Olmstead-Wang, 2009).

During the 90-minute lunch period, many participants and I ate together and chatted in English or Mandarin about the medical university's upcoming transition to using English in its postgraduate medical department and about participants' goals for their own English development. Afternoon sessions were four hours long and allowed for nine participants (professors or medical doctors) each day to practice delivery of conference papers or classroom lectures. We requested that all participants remain to listen to their colleagues' presentations, and this request was largely honored in spite of the participants' very busy teaching and clinical schedules. I provided immediate feedback and I offered one-to-one playback sessions by appointment. Although many Taiwanese may traditionally seek only negative feedback on their performance deficiencies, I chose to offer them encouragement about the proficiencies I noticed as well as to give specific information about patterns of error. The Center for Faculty Development made video-ecordings and uploaded them to the CFD Web site for faculty to review at their convenience.

The Third Workshop (January 2008) and the Fourth Workshop (June 2008)
The third and fourth workshops used similar formats developed from and built on needs that were identified in earlier workshops and fine-tuned by e-mail in the weeks and months prior to the workshops. Workshops were five full days and featured a focus on oral skills development. For three hours each morning, we worked in six to eight small groups with selected chapters from published materials (Duncan & Parker, 2007) in order to practice language skills and model interactive teaching techniques. As with other workshops, these five-day workshops had participants from all parts of campus and the hospital, some of whom took vacation days to attend.

Participants wanted to have a variety of kinds of speaking practice and writing assistance, including speaking practice to include pronunciation help, extemporaneous speech training, and conference paper preparation and presentation assistance. In addition to their requests, I added many opportunities for interactive, communicative, and authentic use of language in small groups. Although the typical Taiwanese medical university classroom is not using these kinds of interactive teaching techniques and student-centered learning activities, I included these features to decenter the teacher and to take pressure off the teacher's developing but not yet excellent English; to prepare student problem-solving skills and to allow them to develop their speaking and negotiating skills; and to align

Taiwanese medical training to the expectations of incoming international students.

On Thursday and Friday mornings in a large auditorium, I presented three-hour writing modules on writing skills, including prioritizing and organizing, editing, using writing tools, responding to reviewers, drafting and refining, and improving rhetorical and self-editing skills. We highlighted two kinds of medical information structure: Introduction, Methods and Materials, Results, Discussion (IMRD) for research faculty, and History and Physical (H&P) for clinical faculty. Each afternoon, I met individually with 12 writers who had biomedical papers in middle or late stages of drafting for publication. There were 6 hours of individual peer reviewing, which allowed only about 15 minutes for each of 24 writers. Depending on the writers' levels of comfort with me and with spoken English, I used Mandarin or English to ask about their wishes for the writing session and their focal questions about the paper. Some came with the expectation that we would do line-by-line editing, but many understood the process of drafting and editing in broader ways. Many continued to discuss their drafts with me through an e-mail account dedicated to this project.

On Monday, Tuesday, and Wednesday mornings, I presented three-hour writing modules on using information structure to organize lectures, building academic vocabulary, managing question and answer sessions, participating in meetings, and negotiating meaning.

I conducted three-hour morning sessions using *Open Forum* Book 3 (Duncan & Parker, 2007) with a CD for interactive teaching techniques and language practice. The medical university purchased a class set of these materials, and some individuals purchased copies for their own use at home.

After lunch, we focused on pronunciation for 30 minutes, an inadequate amount of time for any real improvement in sentence intonation or general pronunciation. Given the limitations, I asked participants to bring a list of the top 25 English terms in their areas of expertise that they need to pronounce properly in order to "sound like" the experts they are when discussing those topics in international settings (following Braasch, 2009). Participants knew exactly what words they wanted to pronounce accurately and came prepared with lists and recording devices. I recorded for them and with them, then provided some tips for them to listen independently to the two samples and to improve their pronunciation of these most important technical terms.

In the second part of the afternoon, students practiced short extemporaneous speaking tasks to help them operationalize their "passive" English and to produce speech more actively and spontaneously. Several participants were members of the Kaohsiung Toastmasters'[®] Club and were very enthusiastic about this type of activity for developing more fluency and skills-based confidence. In the last part of the afternoon, individuals practiced 15-minute segments of speeches with technical slides that they were preparing for international conferences. The audience (all of the presenters) and I listened and prepared comments on language and delivery (including projection and posture). Technical support staff videotaped the presentations and made them available on the CFD Web site so that participants could see their videos at will and improve from observation.

While planning the fourth workshop, the CFD and I clarified the question of whether we wanted to repeat some of the core material for a new audience or to build on and extend the skills presented to our existing audience, a core of repeat attendees from the previous three English workshops. In terms of curriculum development, the issue was whether to develop more breadth or more depth. Offering the fourth workshop to new audiences would introduce more teachers to strategies for approaching the new medical university demands for increased use of English in the classrooms but would not be able to significantly help them develop their actual language skills. Offering the workshop to former participants would help a smaller group develop their language and classroom management skills more fully. We compromised and decided to offer some of the basic materials to new medical university populations and to offer core group skills development opportunities to help them practice at the next levels of complexity in their language development. Those who had attended in the past received e-mail notification of the new workshop and many knew about it because I was working with them on their writing on an ongoing basis through a dedicated e-mail address. New participants heard about the workshop by word of mouth or saw colorful posters announcing the workshops in Chinese and English around campus.

LEVERAGING INSTITUTIONAL FAMILIARITY WITH PROBLEM-BASED LEARNING

PBL in Taiwan Medical Universities

In addition to its strong tradition of teacher-fronted lectures, the Kaohsiung Medical University is actively developing a more interactive model of teaching, problem-based learning (www.kmu.edu.tw/~spbm/eng-web/pro grams/overview.html). Problem-based learning (PBL) is especially interest-ing as a recent curriculum innovation in many medical universities in general and at this medical institution, in particular. PBL was initiated at Kaohsiung Medical University (KMU) in 2002 and now is an integral and successful part of the medical curriculum. In PBL, medical professors move from the center of the knowledge exchange (or knowledge generation) process and function from the periphery of the learning space as coaches. Students engage in case studies or problems to solve, and they work together to discuss diagnoses, negotiate and clarify meaning, determine solutions, and persuade a group to follow a course of action, all critical functions of language. Whether conducted in the students' first language or in English, the interactive quality of the process increases student participation and learning (Spencer & Jordan, 1999, p. 1280). Due to KMU's institutional familiarity with and affinity for PBL, the approach may prove to be a pathway for other forms of interactive learning to inform curricular and pedagogical development, including how English will be used at KMU as a medium of instruction.

Variously defined, PBL is "an instructional strategy" used by students to identify problems, solutions, or foundational "phenomena that need explanation" (Spencer & Jordan, 1999, p. 1281). PBL began at McMaster Medical School (Canada) in the 1960s and is now used in 150 medical universities around the world (Spencer & Jordan, 1999, p. 1282).

Hwang (2006) reports that there were few changes in the Taiwan medical education between the end of World War II and 1993, when PBL was first adopted in Taiwan's premier medical university (Taiwan National University) in order to "improve learning processes and overcome the limits of lecture-based education" (Hwang, 2006, p. 812). Taiwan's other 10 medical universities, including the Kaohsiung Medical University, followed with various combinations of PBL and traditional teaching approaches in basic medical education or clerkship courses. By 2002, PBL was well-established and respected throughout the Taiwan medical curriculum (Hwang, 2006, p. 813). Soon after, the Taiwan Association of Medical Education extended curricular development by adding medical humanities coursework and instigating Objective Structured Clinical Examinations (OCSEs) (p. 814).

KMU's enthusiasm for the PBL approach is demonstrated by the fact that it hosted a large international PBL conference in July 2008 and annually thereafter. PBL coaches and medical student participants came from Taiwan, Hong Kong, the United States, England, Australia, and

KMU's sister institution, Posnan Medical University in Poland. Medical and dental students discussed integrating PBL into the curriculum and practiced the techniques on detailed case studies with comments from process coaches. Because the conference overlapped the end of our cycle of English training workshops, I was able to attend and observe how the interactive approach worked with English as the lingua franca.

As an approach to self-directed and life-long learning, PBL represents a major curricular innovation. KMU's decision to use English as a medium of instruction for its international students in the Post-Graduate Medical Department is also a major innovation requiring careful planning, skills development, and observation.

PBL and English

There is limited literature addressing how PBL and English language use in problem-solving interact in Taiwan and global contexts (Chen et al., 2009; Hutchinson & Waters, 1987; Kashani, Soheili, & Hatmi, 2006). There is little information on how English is used *inside* PBL groups in international settings, in part because use of English "has largely been treated as a given" (Wilkinson, 2008), is taken for granted, or is otherwise rendered invisible. Belcher (2009) addresses the development of PBL in the context of medical and nursing education, notes the function of language in the method, and supports PBL as an approach for teaching English for specific purposes (ESP).

One of the few studies looking at PBL, English for academic purposes (EAP), and English for medical purposes (EMP) demonstrates that interactive learning techniques like PBL put the focus on student interaction and practice opportunity. Students work in groups, analyze posed problems, discuss options, develop a variety of suggestions, seek additional information, research possibilities, reflect on the problem-solving process, evaluate themselves and others in terms of quality of participation, and sometimes persuade their group members to adopt one of the generated solutions. PBL is a "context-based approach which treats learning in a contextual, holistic fashion" that is interactive and student-centered (Wood & Head, 2004, p. 5). Learning is contextualized by the immediate "problem to be solved" (Wood & Head, 2004, p. 9) and "combine(s) a considerable degree of student-centeredness with a concentration on EAP needs which is as focused as any traditional needs analysis on the target situation" (p. 9). Question posing, clarification, and feedback keep group and potential audience members communicating in focused ways (p. 12). Learning to notice communication breakdowns and to repair them is key to "communicative effectiveness" (p. 15). The PBL approach engages student motivation, links present and future needs for interactive problem-solving, and *depends on* good language skills, here English (p. 10, my emphasis).

In a study conducted at the University of Brunei Darussalam (UBD), undergraduates who are in a joint premedical program with the University of Queensland, Australia (UQ), prepare English language and PBL skills in their home university (UBD) before transferring to UQ (Wood & Head, 2004). UQ teachers sought to "determine how they could prepare students for their future studies, maximize their motivation" (p. 4). Teachers looked ahead to the use of PBL and English in Australia, the destination country of most of their premed students.

Tiwari, Lai, So, and Yuen (2006) studied the relationship between using PBL and the development of critical thinking skills over time and in comparison to lecture-based approaches in first-year undergraduate nursing students at a general university in Hong Kong. In the study, PBL groups, which were comprised of 10 students and a PBL tutor, met for 3–6 hours per week for 28 weeks. Students honed the skills of defining, analyzing, prioritizing, synthesizing, and others while tutors helped prepare, facilitate, and evaluate both process and outcomes (p. 549). Students in the lecture-based control group attended lectures 3–6 hours per week for 28 weeks. Both groups studied nursing therapeutics and had similar course objectives. The study showed that PBL "provide[d] students with a statistically reliable advantage in the development of critical thinking disposition over students who are taught using a lecturing format" (Tiwari et al., 2006, p. 552.) Although there was no information on whether and how English per se functioned in these groups, the study does indicate that Chinese students from teacher-centered backgrounds can "sustain self-competence and to acquire a critical approach during the PBL process" (Tiwari et al., 2006, p. 552).

PBL is an example of interactive instruction that can inform KMU's developing English language training program as well as an approach for teaching English for specific purposes. While KMU teachers still need help with the English language skills necessary for teacher-fronted lectures and for conference paper presentations (e.g., the ability to introduce content slides in a one-way delivery format), they also need practice in the English language skills required in interactive classrooms and PBL (e.g., the ability to manage two-way give and take and to negotiate meaning in problem-solving situations).

DISCUSSION

This chapter has reviewed the content of four week-long English workshops given over a two-year period at a major medical university in southern Taiwan, the Kaohsiung Medical University. Although the first workshop was planned to address writing science research articles in English, the focus shifted to include speaking skills in order to support the university's decision to transition to English as the medium of instruction in the Post-Graduate Medical Department, a department poised to attract international students to Taiwan. The workshops focused on improving participants' English through explicit lecturer-fronted instruction, one-to-one reviewing sessions, small groups, and interactive practice.

Throughout the workshops, we engaged principles of adult learning by providing material that is relevant, focused, immediately applicable, and "designed so they can take responsibility for their own learning" (Spencer & Jordan, 1999, p. 1231). With respect for the proficiencies that adult professionals bring to language study, we were aware that affective concerns can cause "crippling anxiety" (Tipton, 2005, p. 395), and we engaged in face-sensitive approaches to error correction (Maynard & Heritage, 2005, p. 431). Because international students in the postgraduate medical program may have higher levels of English than their Taiwanese instructors, professors may experience anxiety about how to convey the material in which they are experts without possible "loss of face" due to inadequate English (Hu, 1944). Dedicated biomedical scientists and professors, many had published journal articles in Chinese and some had published in English. However, only some had been outside of Taiwan to study in an English-language environment. Because their English practice heavily depended on reading and grammar translation, they tended to have a static notion of what English proficiency is and what English teaching should "look like" but not to have confidence in their listening comprehension or speaking abilities. Our workshops and interactive approaches may have increased the "confidence required to overcome hurdles and be comfortable working in English" (Tipton, 2005, p. 396). The stimulating activities and problem-based approaches used in our workshops helped develop professors' English and provide a variety of ways to convey medical content information during the period of transition from Mandarin to English as the medium of teaching and from teacher-fronted lectures to a broader repertoire of teaching techniques that incorporates interactive approaches, including PBL.

English is used strategically as a shared language of international medical communication and has developed significant gatekeeper functions

(Graddol, 2000). Curriculum and language needs must be assessed accurately, and training must be planned and executed well. The process of developing curriculum is complex and nonlinear, involving the interconnected processes of "conceptualizing content, assessing needs, formulating goals and objectives, developing materials, and organizing the course" (Hoekje, 2007, p. 336).

The chapter notes that two key challenges include the dearth of qualified teachers and a tendency to underestimate the complexities of learning and using English well enough to communicate clearly. It suggests that interactive language teaching helps teachers improve their own English and models new, effective approaches to content learning.

By taking advantage of the medical university's recent adoption of PBL, English language training and pedagogy development have a model for decentering learning from teacher-fronted classroom lecture to student-centered interactive problem-solving (Hwang, 2006). This chapter has argued that increased use of interactive and communicative teaching approaches for English language skills can add to these stepwise improvements in Taiwan's medical education curriculum.

CONCLUSION

Taiwan has turned to English to aid in "its modernization and economic growth" (Tsao, 2000, p. 82), to rapidly increase internationalization, and to attract international students to Taiwan. Taiwan's methods of teaching English may need to move beyond "attempting to create equivalent terms lists of vocabulary equivalents in scientific and technical fields, including various specialties in medicine" (Tsao, 2000, p. 69) and to integrate and "standardize scientific terminology" (p. 69). Teachers need more in-service training to develop their own English language abilities, familiarity with current pedagogy, and use of audiovisual aids (p. 85). In a non-English language environment, learners need more opportunities to use English in authentic ways. Inside the classrooms, teachers need to shift from pedagogies that emphasize grammar, translation, reading, and writing (p. 85). In addition to more research on best practices for English for medical purposes in English as a foreign or international language setting, more information is needed on best practices in language policy development and on integrating innovations across the curriculum. Just as the Taiwan Association of Medical Education skillfully instigated medical humanities coursework, OSCEs, and PBL innovations, Taiwan medical universities can carefully plan change and sequence transition to English as a medium of instruction and to interactive teaching approaches that support language and the development of critical thinking.

NOTE

1. In this department (the Post-Graduate Medical Department), English was the medium of instruction. In the overall medical university, English was one of the mediums of instruction. People from all over the medical university came to the English workshops.

APPENDIX 8.1

To aid in planning the second workshop series, a small retrospective survey of participants' English language learning experiences was conducted at the conclusion of the first workshop. Instructions were printed in Chinese and questions were in English. The survey asked for: the participant's name and which sessions were attended (Part one); information reporting on a Likert Scale (1 equals strongly agree; 5 equals strongly disagree) for 46 questions (Part two); and open-ended responses (Part three). The questions (with mean result of 16 responses) are as follows:

1. Have you had specific "speaker training" (training as a public speaker) in Chinese? (2)
2. I have had adequate speaker training courses in Chinese. (4)
3. Previous to this workshop on English speaking and teaching in English, have you had specific "speaker training" (training as a public speaker) in English? (4)
4. I have had adequate speaker training course in English. (4)
5. I have studied English for _____ years.
6. My strongest skill in English is: Reading (12)
7. I have studied in an English-speaking environment.
   Specifically _____
   How many semesters _____ (1)
8. I have worked in an English-speaking environment.
   Specifically _____
   How many months _____ (1)
9. I have had adequate English training and orientation in these experiences. (2, 3)
10. I have had adequate, specific instruction in how to teach (pedagogy or methodology classes, whether in Chinese, English, or some other language). (3)

Speaking environments:

11. I feel comfortable lecturing in English. (2)
12. I feel comfortable in the Q & A (question and answer) time in English. (3)
13. I feel comfortable speaking English to perform classroom tasks (organizing groups, making class announcements, discussing course expectations with students). (3)

14. I feel comfortable speaking English to introduce myself to others at a conference. (3)
15. I feel comfortable speaking English in most professional situations. (2, 3)
16. I feel comfortable speaking English in most social situations. (3)

Speaking skills:

17. I have had adequate instruction in English pronunciation and intonation. (3)
18. I have made the switch from Chinese to English teaching successfully. (3)
19. I have confidence in my ability to create clear teaching materials in English. (2)
    a.   PowerPoint lectures (2)
    b.   Instructions for small group-based tasks (3)
    c.   Handouts or Web pages from which students can prepare or study (2)
    d.   Other (please specify) no answers
20. I am confident in my knowledge of appropriate medical lecture content. (2)
21. I am confident in my use of technical, medical English terms. (2)
22. I am confident in my use of English discourse organizers to signal the direction of my lectures. (3)
23. I am confident in my use of English to explain a process. (3)
24. I am confident in my use of English to define a term. (3)
25. I am confident in my use of English to expand or elaborate. (3)
26. I am confident in my use of English to clarify. (3)
27. I am confident in my use of English to answer students' questions. (3)
28. I am confident in my use of English to pose a question in a small group or seminar. (3)
29. I am confident in my use of English to pose a question in a lecture at an international conference. (3)
30. I am confident in my use of English to paraphrase or rephrase a point of concept in a lecture. (3)
31. I have anxiety about speaking English which tends to inhibit my performance. (3)

Lecture format versus workshop format:

32. I feel that a lecture format is adequate for developing my English skills. (2, 3)
33. I feel that lectures are efficient in terms of time spent and results derived. (2, 3)

34. I feel that lectures present information on WHAT to do in an English-speaking classroom, but not HOW to do it. (3)
35. I feel that workshops with highly trained skills-coaches will let us practice HOW to conduct English-language classes. (1,2)
36. I feel that workshops are more effective and therefore more efficient in terms of my time investment. (1)

Location/scheduling of workshops:

37. I feel that workshops should be offered in my work setting (hospital, office area, other). (2)
38. I feel that morning sessions are more convenient. (2)
39. I feel that afternoon sessions are more convenient. (3)
40. I feel that evening sessions are more convenient. (3)
41. I feel that Saturday sessions are more convenient. (5)

I would like help in these areas:

42. Information structure, discourse management (how to sequence information). (3)
43. Sentence-length intonation. (3)
44. Managing classroom tasks effectively (organizing groups, projects, feedback). (2)
45. Effectively conducting a discussion. (2)
46. Actively participating in a discussion. (1, 2)

Of the 16 participant responses, 5 (the mean) agreed ("tung yi") that they had "specific speaker training" in Chinese, but 7 (the mean) did not agree ("bu tung yi") that their training was "adequate." Most (12 of 16, 75%) did not agree that they had "adequate speaker training" in English. Only 4 of 16 (25%) respondents agreed or strongly agreed that they had "adequate" speaker training courses in English. As for their self-assessment of strongest skill in English, only 3 of 16 (18.75%) indicated speaking; none mentioned listening. Not surprisingly, 12 of 16 (75%) noted reading as their strongest skill. Three of 13 (23%) respondents had never studied or worked in an English-speaking environment. Of those with experience studying or working in English-speaking environments, only 5 of 16 (31%) agreed that they had adequate English training and only 3 of 16 (18.75%) reported agreement (2) or strong agreement (1) that they had had "adequate, specific instruction in how to teach ... whether in Chinese, English, or some other language." Mean values for level of comfort in using English to lecture, conduct Q & A time, perform classroom tasks, introducing self at conferences, and in social situations were consistently neutral (i.e., mid-range value of 3). Level of comfort for speaking English in "most professional situations" (Q. #15) was higher: 7 responded "neutral" (mid-range value of 3) and 7 "agreed" (value of 4). Other responses of significance for the current discussion include a preference for training workshops over lectures (Qs. #35 and #36) and a strong desire for help with "actively participating in a discussion" (Q. #46). Handwritten additional comments included two good summary statements of the pedagogical and language challenges facing the medical university: "teaching is interactive relationship between teacher and students. Teaching is a complicated process of learning as well. It's a culture change and language change" and "Teaching in English is a great challenge, but it is worthwhile doing so."

CHAPTER NINE

OVERCOMING LANGUAGE AND CULTURAL DIFFERENCES IN MEDICAL ENCOUNTERS: THE USE OF A LANGUAGE AND CULTURE TRAINING COURSE (LACT) IN EDUCATING IMGs IN AUSTRALIA

Marisa Cordella

ABSTRACT

The language and culture training course for international medical graduates (IMGs) draws upon a theoretical framework within discourse analysis and intercultural communication to understand how institutional/ professional discourse unfolds within multilingual and multicultural societies. Through this training course, IMGs play a threefold role, as observers, participants, and researchers. They observe how communication develops in different contexts and reflect upon it, actively participate in social activities and modulate their talk in response to recipients' contributions, and become researchers in the process of exploring the best communicative practices through the analysis and assessment of their own and others' communicative performances.

English Language and the Medical Profession: Instructing and Assessing
the Communication Skills of International Physicians
Innovation and Leadership in English Language Teaching, Volume 5, 175–210
Copyright © 2011 by Emerald Group Publishing Limited
All rights of reproduction in any form reserved
ISSN: 2041-272X/doi:10.1108/S2041-272X(2011)0000005015

INTRODUCTION

In recent years, human capital mobility, migration, and Internet communication have rendered many societies more ethnically diverse than before and brought a new outlook to multilingualism and multiculturalism. Ordinary verbal exchanges with people from different sociocultural and language backgrounds are becoming a daily experience for us all.

Communication between speakers of different language and cultural backgrounds presents challenges as misunderstandings and poor communication may occur, preventing the discourse from developing seamlessly. It is through language that cultural norms and values become visible in the discourse, permeating the verbal and nonverbal decisions speakers make. The negotiation of meaning among speakers then takes the center stage in any communicative event that seeks to be successful.

A medical consultation is a small-scale representation of a kind of cross-cultural exchange. Cultural differences between medical practitioners and their patients that emerge as expert knowledge, institutional procedures or protocols, health beliefs, religious beliefs, values, and norms subsequently create a gulf between those working within a medical institution and those who only possess lay medical knowledge (Beach, 2001; Candlin, 2002; Candlin & Candlin, 2002; Cordella, 2006, 2007, 2008, 2010; Linell, Adelswärd, Sachs, Bredman, & Lindstedt, 2002; Sarangi, Bennert, Howell, & Clarke, 2003; Sarangi & Clarke, 2002). The medical visit in many Western societies exhibits characteristics in the exchange between the doctor and the patient that show diverse ways of approaching the communicative event.

Currently, "there are few places in the world where the delivery of healthcare takes place in mono-cultural contexts" (Editorials, 2001, p. 186). Consequently, today's medical communication can turn into a complex event where both health beliefs and sociocultural expectations and assumptions intermingle and operate within the same exchange. In the last 20 years, Australia has become heavily dependent on International Medical Graduates (IMGs) to fill the national medical workforce shortage, which is partly due to the decline in the intake of students into medical courses (Birrell & Hawthorne, 2004, p. 85).

Today, 35% of rural medical practitioners and 20% of the total Australian national medical workforce is formed by IMGs (Flynn, 2006). An estimate of 13 years, according to Spike (2006), is required to become a medical practitioner; therefore, the demand will still be present in the foreseeable future. Previous studies have shown that the biggest challenges of working with IMGs is their different backgrounds in training, clinical skills, understanding of the health system, and communication skills

(McGrath, 2004; Roberts, Sarangi, & Moss, 2004; Whelan, 2006). Birrell and Hawthorne (2004) indicate that

> [p]ersons graduating from the diverse medical schools of Asia, the Middle East and Eastern Europe bring a variety of skills, knowledge and experience with them. There is however no guarantee that their training is relevant to the Australian setting ... including contemporary practice as regards to medical procedures, forms of therapy, awareness of the current repertoire of drugs and technical equipment. A good knowledge of English and the patient is also required for effective medical practice. (p. 96)

The study of communicative competence and performance of IMGs in Australia and the proposal of recommendations that could assist in their training is a much-needed requirement for the production of a better qualified medical workforce. The language and culture training course for IMGs (LACT-IMG) introduced in this chapter draws on a multidisciplinary theoretical perspective to establish the principles of intercultural communication in the medical encounter. The development of the LACT-IMG is based on research knowledge obtained through the analysis of an Australian and a Chilean medical corpus. The Australian data is composed of one OSCE recorded in 2007 and carried out by a group of IMGs enrolled in a bridging training course in Melbourne. The Chilean corpus is formed of natural recorded consultations that took place between 1997 and 2004 and were conducted in both an outpatient clinic and a cancer clinic in Santiago. Every conversation has been fully transcribed and analyzed following a discourse analysis (DA) approach (Cordella, 2004a; Cordella & Musgrave, 2009).

Traditionally, cross-cultural education has focused on identifying particular behaviors that provide an understanding of the attitudes, values, and beliefs of different ethnic groups. This approach has led to the establishment of stereotypes and an oversimplification of culture (Betancourt, 2003, p. 562), diminishing the complexities that exist within the same ethnic group. Medical educators have expressed their fear of "ghetto-izing" (Dogra & Wass, 2006, p. 686) and isolating a particular ethnic group.

One way to overcome these fears is to design a novel language and culture training course for IMGs which will make participants regularly explore and reflect upon their own cultural conventions and also examine and study the cultural practices of their new country of residence. The language and culture training course described here does not provide a "do-and-don't" list as there are too many training courses that already do that (Betancourt, 2003); instead, the course aims to teach, in ten hours spread over four weeks, *how* to improve competence in a multilingual and multicultural environment.

This chapter offers background for the development of a language and culture training course for IMGs. The first two sections provide the foundation to capture the complexities of intercultural communication and medical discourse. The following sections provide a set of exercises to be used with IMGs that aim to explore and understand how communication develops in different social settings. IMGs are asked to observe different social events, participate in some of them, and videorecord an OSCE performance. Through a multilevel assessment approach, IMGs explore, assess, discuss, and consolidate their language and cultural practices.

INTERCULTURAL COMMUNICATION

Intercultural communication is defined in this study as a communicative exchange between speakers from diverse language and cultural backgrounds. What makes intercultural communication different from other communicative events is that a set of additional potential conflicts may emerge in the discourse as a result of speakers not sharing the same sociocultural norms and values. Clyne (2005) indicates that

> Speakers tend to transfer cultural rules and norms from L1 [language 1] to their L2 [language 2]. Thus there are many situations where one needs to understand the cultural underpinnings of a message, or how a particular speech act is performed in the speaker's L1, in order to comprehend what he or she is trying to convey in English. An understanding of this enables one to gain something of an inside perspective, for language is the gateway to culture. (p. 59)

In previous studies conducted by Cordella (2002, 2003, 2004a, 2004b) in Chile in the area of medical discourse, a set of voices (*doctor voice, educator voice,* and *fellow human voice*) that health practitioners would engage in with their patients during the medical visit were identified. The categorization of each voice was done through a linguistic analysis that codified every turn in each consultation. Discourse analysis approaches (e.g., conversational analysis, interactional sociolinguistics) were utilized in this process. A description of the medical voice follows.

Medical Voices

Doctor Voice
The *doctor voice* is mainly reflective of a biomedical approach, looking for the factual evidence of the patient's ailment. Following Mishler (1984), this

voice represents health primarily as a biological phenomenon. In this voice, the medical practitioner seeks information about the medical condition through questions, assesses patients' test results, and manifests their alignment to the medical institution.

One of the main linguistic strategies in doctor–patient communication is *questioning*, in which the medical practitioner seeks information from the patient in order to deliver a diagnosis and/or assess the patient's well-being since the last visit. Questions are examples of adjacency pairs that call for an answer to be delivered in the next or later turns. The kind of answer given to a question is usually affected by how the question was asked in the first place, so there is a need to distinguish the type of questions used in the category of *doctor voice*. The *doctor voice* is formed of (1) questioning, (2) assessing and reviewing medical treatment, and (3) aligning to the medical institution. Examples of question seeking information are given in the chart below.

Question Seeking Information (QSI)		
QSI One	One question in search of information	Where does it hurt?
QSI Chain	A chain of questions in search of information	Where does it hurt? Does it hurt a lot? Can you rate how much it hurts?
QSI Multiple Choice	Questions in search of information delivered in a multiple-choice format	Does it hurt in the upper or lower region?
QSI Recycling/ Repetition	Recycling or repeating a previous question	So can you tell me again about how the pain started?
QIS + Summary, or Summary + QSI	The practitioner starts with a question and summarizes the key points already discussed in that consultation or previous visits. Practitioners can also initiate with a summary followed by a set of questions.	So are you constantly in pain? The pain started on last weekend, it is in the lower region and the area is swollen ...

Assessing and Reviewing Medical Treatment
The *doctor voice* also marks the assessment of test results or treatment recommended in previous visits and reviews the patient's compliance with and progress with that treatment.

Alignment to the Medical Institution
The physician's alignment to the medical institution is also portrayed in the *doctor voice*. The differential use of first person singular pronouns (*I*) and first person plural pronouns (*we*) can provide an insight into the degree of such alignment. There is a marked difference between saying, "I recommend you take X" and "we recommend you take X." The latter places the authority and responsibility on the institution or medical body the practitioner represents, whereas the former marks only the individual decision. It could be also said that the individual decision might have been prompted by institutional norms, but this cannot be unequivocally ascertained from the simple use of the first person singular.

Educator Voice
The *educator voice* works together with the *doctor voice* in its role in medical practice. In this voice, medical information is shared with patients to make them more knowledgeable about their health condition, thus providing the basis for preventative medicine and promoting adherence to medical treatment. The *educator voice* is formed of (1) communicating medical facts, (2) responding to patient discomfort, and (3) communicating medical treatment and management.

Communicating Medical Facts. Communicating medical facts includes communicating

(1) information regarding available test results;
(2) information regarding future tests; and
(3) information regarding the functioning of the human body.

Responding to Patient Discomfort. In responding to patient discomfort,

(1) doctors frame patient discomfort as a medical issue that requires a medical interpretation;
(2) doctors express confidence in the medical decisions taken in previous consultations, affirming either directly or indirectly that these were the right decisions; and
(3) doctors discuss the side effects associated with prescribed treatments.

Communicating Medical Treatment and Management.   The communication of medical treatment and its management take a dynamic format in many Western societies today through the negotiation that unfolds during the medical visit. The delivery of advice or a recommendation can be achieved in a variety of ways. For example, the recommendation can be marked by:

(1) *a marker of inevitability* (e.g., *have to*), which places an obligation on the patient to follow the doctor's instructions;
(2) *a marker of conditional inevitability* (e.g., *it would be good*), which stresses the desirability of following the doctor's instructions;
(3) the use or absence of an *impersonal form* when the agent is absent (e.g., *one sometimes prescribes this medicine, sometimes this medicine is prescribed*).

Previous studies have shown that a successful medical consultation also incorporates a humane touch (Mishler, 1984) to the institutionalized talk. The deconstruction of medical visits shows the presence of the *fellow human voice* (Cordella, 2004a, 2004b), which supports a mode of communication that is typically represented in many ordinary and friendly conversations.

Fellow Human Voice
The *fellow human voice* shows the human side of the health practitioner, who portrays a voice in which the interest falls on the individual who is going through some health problems rather than centering attention on the body part to be fixed. There are a number of linguistic strategies that can be used within this voice, including facilitating and assisting the telling of patient stories, creating empathy with the patient, showing special attentiveness to patient stories, and asking questions seemingly unrelated to patient health.

Facilitating the Telling of Patient Stories.   The development of patient talk is facilitated by the use of continuer markers (e.g., *uhm*) that give an indication to the patient that further elaboration is welcomed by the recipient (Jurafsky, Shriberg, Fox, & Curl, 1998).

Assisting the Telling of Patient Stories.   These strategies help patients to formulate their talk with the assistance of the recipient who contributes to the performance of a single proposition. For example, a recipient realizing that a speaker is struggling to find the right word may offer one to continue the discourse (Ferrara, 1992).

Creating Empathy with the Patient. Providing a sympathetic ear is paramount in the medical consultation (Frankel, 2000). The strategies practitioners use vary according to the gravity of the patient's medical condition. It has been shown that it is more effective to provide sound medical knowledge followed by empathetic utterances that support the patient's concerns and fears (Cordella & Musgrave, 2009) than simply uttering words that express empathy without providing the medical knowledge that support them. In fact "trained empathy" is highly inappropriate and shows poor communicative competence (Roberts, Wass, Jones, Sarangi, & Gillett, 2003).

Showing Special Attentiveness to Patient Stories. Linguistic strategies like mirroring (i.e., using the same words the patient has just used) and clarifying a previous utterance can indicate that the physician is closely following the patient's talk.

Asking Questions "Unrelated" to Patient Health. Every question asked in a medical visit plays a crucial role in assessing the patient's well-being. A question like "How was your weekend?" may reveal vital information to assess the patient's social network, use of leisure time, interests, and overall well-being. It is important to pay attention to the type of questions that would be appropriate to raise in a given sociocultural setting.

Institutional Knowledge/Knowledge of Governmental Medical Policies

The LACT-IMG calls for two extra categories to be included in the training. These are institutional knowledge and knowledge of government medical policies or procedures. Knowing about how the medical institution operates, what its norms and procedures are, and also what kind of government medical assistance is available to individuals is fundamental to provide the proper recommendations to patients.

Knowledge of Patient's Sociocultural Beliefs

It is also of vital importance to be aware of patient's sociocultural beliefs, especially in a multilingual and multicultural country, such as Australia. The physician should explore any cultural differences and ask for clarification if required. The patient also brings to the consultation a set of *voices* that engage with those used by the medical professional and which portray the patient's social identity within their community. The participatory roles of both doctor and patient and the possible outcomes of medical consultations are highlighted in Cordella's (2004a) *The dynamic consultation: A discourse analytical study of doctor–patient communication* (John Benjamins). I acknowledge that although the linguistic features that constitute a particular *voice* may be different among languages and cultures, it is how participants make use of these *voices* that is especially informative of the sociocultural group.

Conversational Rules and Intercultural Communication

Sacks, Schegloff, and Jefferson (1974), in their seminal work on the organization of talk, provide the basis to understand turn-taking in conversations. Sacks et al.'s (1974) study sparked significant interest in evaluating whether the turn-taking system proposed was valid for languages other than English. Clyne (1994), in a study conducted in intercultural workplaces in Melbourne, observed that:

> Content-based cultures such as Central and Southern Europeans (and to lesser extent South Asians) use an increase in tempo or simultaneous speech to indicate that the speaker wants to say all he or she needs to say. The harmony value is reflected in the turn-taking procedures of Vietnamese, ethnic Chinese and generally Southeast Asians who do not "fight" to maintain their turns and certainly do not increase the speed to do so. They also generally back down rather than engage in simultaneous speech. (p. 188)

In Chilean Spanish, the use of simultaneous speech is not only reserved for informal situations, but formal situations (e.g., medical visits) may also call for it. Examples of doctors and patients working together in the discourse by finishing each other's utterances were not uncommon in my previous work (Cordella, 2004a). Similarly, the use of silence, laughter, and backchanneling cues (Jefferson, Sacks, & Schegloff, 1977; Jurafsky et al., 1998) have to be understood within the sociocultural context in which they emerge, which is reflected in the discourse. By looking at them in isolation, we may risk misinterpreting them (Bowe & Martin, 2007).

Power Relations in Intercultural Communication

The power relation that is created in the event also indexes social, cultural, and contextual aspects of the discourse which are conveyed within the calendar time of the event (Cordella, 1999; van Dijk, 1996; Wodak, 1999). Medical communication of the past may not entirely assimilate the patient-oriented approach of today's visit. In Western societies, patients have many more rights than before, and contesting health practitioners' views is not as uncommon as in the past (Cordella & Musgrave, 2009).

Cultural Conceptualization

IMGs coming from a country where patients are viewed differently compared with the new country of residence, where society does not regard individual choice as a positive attribute, and/or where medical knowledge is hardly contested may be confronted with a "cultural conceptualization shock." According to Sharifian (2007):

> Cultural conceptualisations are *heterogeneously distributed* across the minds of a cultural group. That is, they are not equally imprinted in the mind of every individual member, but are rather shared in varying degrees between the members of a cultural group. (p. 34, emphasis in the original)

Cultural conceptualizations develop through *interaction* with members of a cultural group who regularly negotiate these conceptualizations in both the short term and in the longer term (e.g., across generations). In Sharifian's model, interaction with others is a key component. A cultural conceptualization is manifested at the level of cultural knowledge shared by the group. Any specific individual may have some of that knowledge, but not every set of cultural conceptualizations that everybody else has in the same cultural group will be equally shared by all (Sharifian, 2003, p. 90). This is an important consideration when training IMGs since their experiences in a new country will expose them to a variety of cultural conceptualizations (e.g., youth culture, masculinity/feminity, mateship, aging) that may not be noticed or understood at first. However, gaining knowledge about key cultural conceptualizations can only benefit their understanding of the society, turn their adjustment into a much easier process, and assist their communication practices within and outside the medical institution.

Cultural conceptualizations of health beliefs (Andary, Stolk, & Klimidis, 2003; Helman, 1994; Kleinman, 1980) are another factor to be taken into account, as a lack of understanding of health issues may well lead to communication breakdown.

Having established the basis for potential communicative conflicts leading to miscommunication and/or communication failure in intercultural exchanges, I now move on to a novel approach to train international medical graduates operating around the world. The LACT-IMG that I propose stems from a theoretical framework (presented above), empirical research in the area of doctor–patient communication, and a personal position that have all been developed over the past 15 years. The knowledge and expertise acquired throughout my research and teaching activities have inspired this communicative competence framework. Moreover, having migrated to Australia almost a quarter of a century ago in pursuit of my postgraduate studies in linguistics, I can now reflect on my own language and culture learning journey both as a linguist and as a migrant.

A briefer version of this training course has already been successfully trialed in Santiago, Chile, with a group of postgraduate medical students in a half-day workshop. In addition, students enrolled in a discourse analysis unit at Monash University in Australia have also effectively used the principles of this course to better understand, explore, reflect upon, and interpret intercultural communication.

THE LANGUAGE AND CULTURE TRAINING COURSE FOR IMGs (LACT-IMG)

Background

Much attention has been given to the differences that divide institutional talk—where the medical visit resides—and ordinary talk. However, little attention has been given to the commonalities that both discourses share. The first part of the training focuses on the recurrent features that are exhibited in institutional and ordinary conversations. The purpose is to sensitize and make IMGs aware of the basic rules of communication through the deconstruction of ordinary conversations. In this section of the training course, IMGs are observing different types of conversations and paying attention to the main structure of the talk, in addition to the participatory role that speakers engage in during the exchanges. A critical thinking approach is expected to provide an insight into the discourse within a sociocultural frame. IMG should also be encouraged to make comparisons with other familiar sociocultural groups to widen their perspectives on how the discourse operates the way it does in a given context.

Once this knowledge has been established, then the attention shifts to the IMGs' communicative performance (Modules Two through Four). In these activities, IMGs complete self-assessment, peer assessment, and ESL assessment tasks. Through debriefings, focus groups, and constructive feedback, IMGs can equip themselves to better function in the new language and cultural system. It is highly advisable that IMGs keep a diary and write down any new input they might come across, including keeping a list of new words and colloquial expressions that could be beneficial in the process of expanding their language and cultural competence.

There is an urgent need to design a training course for IMGs in a radically different way from those used in the past, when the emphasis has been on individuals' acquisition of a set of linguistic formulas which may not be fully understood without a sound knowledge of the culture (Roberts et al., 2003). It is through language that culture expresses itself, and therefore we cannot understand the language without also understanding the culture.

The exercise of just listing the key words of a language has been proven to be unbeneficial for IMGs, as many of them will use "trained" (Roberts et al., 2003) language chunks without fully engaging with the patient in the face-to-face exchange (Cordella & Musgrave, 2009). Following the Medical Board of Australia's requirement of language proficiency,

> [a]ll applicants must be able to demonstrate English language skills at IELTS™ academic level 7 or the equivalent, and achieve the required minimum score in each component of the IELTS academic module. (www.amc.org)

However, to maximize the chances for the patient's satisfaction and adherence to the medical treatment, IMGs' communicative performance will need to reflect both their English abilities and their sociocultural competence.

People generally do not become good communicators in a specialist area (e.g., medical profession) if they regularly fail to communicate effectively in other social settings. There is a degree of communicative ability transfer which needs to be accounted for. What is learned in one social setting can be transferred to another. Thus, the communicative skills of showing empathy to a friend who is going through a disconcerting path in his or her life can be transferred to the medical context when the medical practitioner needs to show support to his or her patient after an unwanted diagnosis has been delivered. Although these two scenarios are very different, both ask for empathy to be displayed, and some of the linguistic strategies may well be transferred (e.g., displaying supportive strategies).

Regardless of the IMGs' initial knowledge of the organization and construction of the discourse, it is recommended that all of them engage in the activities outlined below. Some IMGs may be better communicators and be more sensitive in recognizing how communication operates in different social settings. However, it is through the analysis of one's own and others' speech that participants will attain (better) knowledge about how to conduct themselves in future exchanges.

The theoretical background knowledge provided in the first part of this chapter should serve as the basis for the understanding of intercultural communication. Four modules are designed, and in each one of them a series of stages are organized to fully involve IMGs in their language and cultural acquisition. This 10-hour training course can be delivered in four weeks, focusing on one module per week. Appendix 9.1 provides an overview of the course structure.

Module One

Getting Started: You Already Know How to Communicate

The first module is composed of three stages. In each of them, a set of exercises and questions are designed for IMGs to gain an appreciation of how communication unfolds in different ordinary communicative encounters.

Stage 1: Class Activity.   The following are steps to this class activity:

(1) The ESL specialist presents the overall aims of the LACT-IMG training course outlining the key aspects of the training, the focus of which can be reviewed in the first section of this chapter. A concise explanation of the content of each module should follow.
(2) In the first session, IMGs are asked to fill in a survey that contains both demographic information and a self-assessment of their communicative skills (Appendix 9.2). A similar survey has already been trialed in Australia in a joint research project conducted at Monash University (Cordella & Spike, 2008; Mistica, Baldwin, Cordella, & Musgrave, 2008), between linguists, medical practitioners, and medical educators.[1]
(3) The ESL specialists provide information about those activities that need to be completed outside of class time and emphasize the importance of carrying them out before the next class.

Stage 2: Outside-Class Activity—How Are Ordinary Conversations Structured? (Ordinary Talk).   This activity aims at making IMGs reflect upon language in action in ordinary conversations by taking an ethnographic approach and making them observe how conversations between and among participants develop in two different social settings, a hospital cafeteria and a pharmacy. IMGs will be asked to take notes and to report back on their findings in the next class.

Exercise: Hospital Cafeteria (Ordinary Encounters)
Objective: To observe ordinary conversations by employing an ethnographic approach.
Background: A variety of conversations may be taking place at the same time and in the same place. Conversations may vary in their degree of formality and group composition.
The ESL specialists ask IMGs to pay attention to the following questions below:

• Observe the wide array of conversations that take place in the same social setting and at the same time. Enumerate them (e.g., conversation between professionals, family members).
• Observe how close/far they are standing or sitting to each other.
• Are they using any nonverbal communication (they probably are) as well? Can you describe how they use their body language?
• How could you categorize the conversation? Is it a conversation between equals/strangers/friends/intimates/colleagues/family members? Justify your response.

Exercise: Pharmacy or Equivalent Health Store (Service-Oriented Encounters)
Objective: To observe how the communication develops in a service-oriented encounter.
Background: Pharmacists in Australia and in other parts of the world play an important role in prescribing basic medicines that do not require a doctor's prescription. In addition, they provide health advice for simple medical ailments. IMGs may get some insight into seeking information, advice giving and delivering a prescription.
The ESL specialists ask IMGs to observe a conversation between a pharmacist and a client and pay attention to the following questions:

• Who initiates the communication? (e.g., Is it the client who addresses the pharmacist? Is it the pharmacist who approaches the client?
• What do they say to each other?
• How are people talking to each other? (e.g., Do they use formal/informal/ colloquial language?)

- Who is asking the questions? Who is responding? What types of questions are asked?
- Who is giving advice? How is the advice/recommendation given?
- How does the communication close? (e.g., What do they say to each other at the end of the conversation?)

ESL specialists are also advised to observe and participate in all the activities described above to bring along their informed views to the discussion.

Stage 3: Class Activity.   Objective: To reflect upon the conversations that took place at the hospital cafeteria and the pharmacy. The ESL specialists should focus on one social setting at a time, encourage IMG participation in the activity by comparing their answers and develop a degree of reflection upon language in action and the sociocultural expectations attached to a given context.

Once every exchange has been discussed (the questions listed above should help for this purpose), further questions are introduced to make IMGs acquire a broader knowledge about ordinary talk:

- What differences and similarities did you notice between the hospital cafeteria and the pharmacy? (e.g., To what extent were the conversations you observed in the pharmacy and hospital cafeteria similar/different? To what extent did the context of the conversation have a role here?)
- Can you identify the difference between service-oriented talk (pharmacy) and a friendly conversation observed in the hospital cafeteria?
- Which characteristics do these two conversations have in common?
- Did you observe instances at the hospital cafeteria or the pharmacy in which participants used laughter, interruptions, or change of volume in the talk? Why do you think this may have happened?
- To what extent would what you have observed be comparable with what would occur in your own sociocultural environment? What differences and similarities would you find in each of the above settings? Elaborate.

Possible Answers: Reflections.   The ESL specialists should prompt the IMGs to provide answers around the points described below.

(1) Many different conversations may be taking place at the same time in the same place. Conversations are made of verbal and nonverbal communication. In some language-culture communities the use of

nonverbal communication/body language is more prominent than others.

(2) People take turns in the conversation. One individual initiates the talk and another individual continues to the talk. Each of them contributes to the exchange depending on the role they occupy in the exchange and the purpose of the communication.

(3) The formality or informality of the conversation is manifested in the way people talk to each other and the social role each one of them occupies in the discourse (e.g., friendly conversation versus service-oriented conversation).

(4) The use of conversational features, including laughter, interruptions, and change of volume are contextually and socioculturally bound.

(5) Service-oriented encounters (see above) follow an orderly pattern (e.g., the use of questions and answers).

(6) Sociocultural rules and norms are manifested through the language (e.g., what to say, to whom to say it, and how to say it).

(7) Reading each other's discourse (inference) can be facilitated in those cases where participants negotiate meaning. Understanding each other requires a collaborative approach on both parties.

(8) Knowing how people communicate with each other gives us some knowledge about a given sociocultural group.

(9) Understanding how the discourse operates in one culture helps to appreciate other cultural groups' performances.

Module Two

Getting Inside the Medical Institution
The second module is composed of two stages that focus on institutional discourse, including a set of exercises and questions to consolidate knowledge.

Stage 1: Outside-Class Activity: How is Institutional Talk Organized?   Objective: To observe how professionals working in a health-care setting greet each other and pay attention to the patient's responses to his or her questions during a medical visit.

Background: Individuals greet each other depending on the relationship they have established or are negotiating with interlocutors. The role that each plays in the discourse, the time constraints, the context, and the setting also play a part in how the greeting is exchanged.

Greetings are relatively easy to observe and IMGs should be able to take notice of several greeting encounters in a day.

Greetings in Medical Peer Interactions.   The ESL specialists ask IMGs to pay attention to at least three examples of greetings in the workplace and to answer the following questions for each example they have observed.

- How is the greeting initiated?
- What do they say to each other?
- Does the greeting trigger the initiation of a brief exchange?
- Is the greeting used only as a politeness marker without the apparent intention of developing a conversation?

Medical Visit: Seeking Information.   Objective: To make IMGs aware of the effect that the type of question delivered has on the patient's disclosure of information.

Background: The way patients respond to questions depends greatly on the kind of questions they have been asked.

The ESL specialists ask IMGs to conduct a routine medical visit and to reflect on their language choices afterward by responding to questions below. IMG responses will be discussed in the next class:

- Identify the type of answers that the patient has given you (e.g., Has the patient answered with yes or no? Has the patient elaborated his or her response? Has the patient asked for clarification before answering?).
- Identify the types of questions that you may have used in the consultation. IMGs could write a list of questions that they recall to have used in the consultation.
- To what extent has focusing on questioning made you reflect on the effect that they have on the patient's contribution?

Stage 2: Class Activity.   Objective: For IMGs to reflect upon the above activities. The ESL specialists should focus on one exchange at a time, encouraging IMGs' participation in the activity by comparing answers and developing a degree of reflection upon language in action and sociocultural expectations.

Once questions for each section have been discussed, further questions are introduced to make IMGs acquire a broader and more comprehensive knowledge about institutional talk.

- What role do participants occupy in each exchange (e.g., doctor versus patient)?
- How does the participatory role of individuals modulate the talk in the exchange (e.g., doctors ask questions and patients respond)?
- How is asymmetry portrayed in the talk (e.g., those in higher status positions contribute differently to those with less power)?
- To what extent would what you have observed be comparable with what would occur in your own sociocultural environment. What differences and similarities would you find? Elaborate.

Possible Answers: Reflections. The ESL specialists should consolidate the following key points:

(1) Greetings differ significantly, depending on the relationship people have with each other.
(2) Some greetings lead to conversations while others are fleeting.
(3) There are factors that affect the development of a conversation after a greeting exchange (e.g., relationship between participants, lack of time). Also greetings have been shown to serve other communicative functions, for example, they can replace (in some cases) apologies by the mere fact of addressing the person and acknowledging their presence.
(4) Institutional talk, including medical discourse, is highly structured.
(5) There is asymmetry in the exchange, and this is shown in the way participants contribute to the discourse. Those in a higher position tend to control the course of the communication.
(6) The discourse is formed of sequences. For example, questions are followed by answers.
(7) Patients' answers are closely linked with the type of questions delivered (e.g., compare a simple question to a multiple choice question. How is the patient responding to them? To what extent do the doctor's questions affect the patient's responses?)
(8) Sociocultural rules and norms are manifested through the language that formulates and recreates them.
(9) There are a set of sociocultural expectations attached to every ordinary and institutional event.

Having outlined the principles that help drive a range of ordinary social exchanges and institutional/professional settings, in addition to the interface between language and sociocultural rules, norms, and expectations of a communicative event, we now move on to Module Three.

Module Three

The Skeleton Structure of the Medical Visit: Three Voices, One Consultation
The third module has the format of a workshop. The ESL specialists will be teaching how the medical consultation is usually structured and organized. A series of examples will be brought to the workshop to help the unfolding of the discussion.

Overall Objective: To expand on the knowledge acquired in Modules One and Two. In addition, in this module, IMGs will be taught to identify the key communicative components of the medical visit and will be equipped to acquire the necessary tools to assess medical exchanges.

Background: Medical discourse is broadly structured into three main discourses (i.e., *doctor voice, educator voice*, and *fellow human voice*) operating within the exchange and conveyed through doctor–patient interaction to different degrees (see above discussion).

This classification has already been applied in a training course for nurses in New South Wales, Australia (see www.icms.com.au/AMEP2006/abstract/49.htm) and in a half-day workshop designed for postgraduate students from the Faculty of Medicine in Chile. In that workshop, the same principles described in this manuscript were developed. However, participants did not have the opportunity to observe different exchanges as in Modules One and Two, and therefore their input was based only on how much they could recall from previous interactions.

This module is divided into three stages in which each of the medical voices is studied in detail. IMGs will have a chance to analyze each other's contributions to the event by concentrating only on one medical voice at the time.

Stage 1: Class Activity, Doctor Voice. Objective: To identify how the *doctor voice* is utilized in the medical exchange. To achieve this end, a role-play, performed by two volunteers, is presented to the rest of the group. The class at the time of the presentation will be taking note about the IMG's language choices (detailed information below).

Background: Seeking information constitutes one of the most recurrent strategies health professionals use in their visits. There is usually a close association between how the question is delivered and the response that it is given (see Module Two).

Role-Play	Five minutes
Participants	Two participants, one taking the role of the medical practitioner and the other taking the role of the patient
Scenario	The patient presents a severe stomachache. The physician seeks information to establish a diagnosis.

The rest of the group will take note of the physician's contribution to the talk by focusing on the questions below. It is fundamental that both parts of the questions are answered; thus, the IMG should notice if a particular strategy is used (e.g., Does the IMG ask open questions?) and how it is accomplished.

At the end of the role-play, a group discussion will follow, focusing on IMGs providing examples of the strategies exhibited in the discourse, identifying those strategies which assisted the patient in describing his or her condition, giving relevant information about the medical ailment and showing an alignment to the medical institution. For each area below, relevant questions are given to help focus the discussion on IMG communication.

Seeking Information from Patients about Their Health Condition

- Does the IMG ask open questions? How does he or she do it?
- Does the IMG fish for information? How does he or she do it?
- Does the IMG rephrase questions? How does he or she do it?
- Does the IMG summarize the main points and ask a relevant question? How does he or she do it?

Assessing and Reviewing the Medical Treatment. Does the IMG provide relevant information about the medical condition? How does he or she do it?

- Does the IMG provide an assessment of risk? How does he or she do it?

Alignment to the Medical Institution

- Does the IMG modulate institutional alignment?[2] How does he or she do it?

Group Discussion and Consolidation. Through a group discussion, the IMGs are asked to review, assess, and consolidate the *doctor voice*.
Stage 2: Class Activity, *Educator Voice*

Objective: To expand on the *educator voice* and identify how this voice is utilized in the medical exchange.

Background: To provide education to the patient is fundamental in medical discourse.

Role-Play	Instructions as above
Participants	As above
Scenario	The patient presents a severe stomachache because he or she has not been looking after his or her diet lately. The physician educates the patient in this regard.

The rest of the group will take note of the physician's contribution to the talk by focusing on the questions below. It is fundamental that both parts of the questions are answered; thus, the IMG should notice if a particular strategy is used (e.g., Does the IMG check patient understanding?) and how this is achieved (e.g., How does he or she do it?). At the end of the role-play, a group discussion will focus on IMGs providing examples of the strategies exhibited in the discourse. For each area below, relevant questions are given to help focus the discussion on the IMGs' communication.

Communicating Medical Facts

- Does the IMG provide accurate medical information (no jargon) about test results, future tests, functioning of the human body? How does he or she do it?
- Does the IMG give a clear detailed description of the medical condition? How does he or she do it?
- Does the IMG establish the patient's knowledge of the condition? How does he or she do it?
- Does the IMG check patient understanding? How does he or she do it?

Responding to Patient

- Does the IMG respond to the patient's questions? How does he or she do it?
- Does the IMG respond adequately to the patient's discomfort? How does he or she do it?

Communicating Medical Treatment and Management

- Does the IMG successfully communicate/negotiate medical treatment and management? How does he or she do it?

- Does the IMG develop a management plan (with the patient) short and long term? How does he or she do it?
- Does the IMG educate the patient about the medical condition? How does he or she do it?
- Does the IMG specifically explore preventative measures? How does he or she do it?

Group Discussion and Consolidation.   Through a group discussion the IMGs are asked to review, assess, and consolidate the *educator voice*.

Stage 3: Class Activity, Fellow Human Voice.   Objective: To expand on the *fellow human voice* and identify how it is utilized in the medical exchange.

Background: It has been shown that patients' satisfaction is closely associated with physicians displaying a voice that focuses on the individual rather than the patient.

Role-Play	Instructions as above
Participants	As above
Scenario	The patient presents a severe stomachache because he or she has not been looking after his or her diet lately due to intense obligations at work. The physician is asked to use the *fellow human voice.*

The rest of the group will take note of the physician's contribution by focusing on the questions below. As has been indicated above, IMGs should focus on both parts of the questions and write examples. At the end of the role-play a group discussion will follow focusing on IMGs providing examples of the strategies exhibited in the discourse. For each area below, relevant questions are given to help focus the discussion on IMG communication.

Facilitating the Telling of Patients' Stories

- Does the IMG provide support for the patient's development of their stories? How does he or she do it?

Creating Empathy with the Patient

- Does the IMG respond to the patient's emotional needs? How does he or she do it?

Showing Special Attentiveness to Patients' Stories

• Does the IMG use strategies that mark attentive listening skills? How does he or she do it?

Asking Questions Seemingly Unrelated to the Patient's Health

• Does the IMG use questions that are seemingly unrelated to the patient's health? How does he or she do it?

Group Discussion and Consolidation. Through a group discussion the IMGs are asked to review, assess, and consolidate the fellow human voice.

Institutional Knowledge and Medical Policies or Procedures
The LACT-IMG calls for two extra categories to be introduced into the training course to equip IMGs to be competent in medical practices which may differ from those they are used to. These are institutional knowledge and medical policies or procedures.

Knowing about how the medical institution operates, what its norms and procedures are, and also what kind of government medical assistance is available to individuals is crucial to provide the proper recommendations to patients within an institutional and sociocultural context.

Patient's Sociocultural Beliefs
Similarly, it is also of vital importance to be aware of the patient's sociocultural beliefs, especially in multilingual and multicultural countries where patients and health practitioners may come from very different health belief systems (e.g., Western versus non-Western medicine). The physician should explore any cultural differences and ask for clarification if required. In addition, IMGs should become familiar with state, provincial, or federal medical policies and practices (see above).

Module Four

Let's Get into Action: Now It's Your Turn!
The fourth module is composed of three stages, in which the participants will have a chance to put into practice what they have learned so far and to make a detailed analysis of their own and other colleagues' performances. A video camera is required to carry out this activity.

Stage 1: Class Activity. Objective: To put into practice the knowledge acquired in Module Three and consolidate the knowledge obtained in Modules One and Two by conducting an OSCE and debriefings.

Background: Cultural/racial diversity intensive workshops have contributed in making IMGs more aware of cultural differences (Dogra, 2001; Kai, Spencer, Wilkes, & Gill, 1999). Nevertheless, in some cases these programs (Betancourt, 2003) have furnished an oversimplified and stereotyped view of a particular social group by construing "do-and-don't" lists.

Communicative competence in medical settings has been mainly assessed through OSCE (Brazeau, Boyd, & Crosson, 2002; Dogra & Wass, 2006, Koop & Borbasi, 1994; Ross et al., 1988; Townsend, McLivenny, Miller, & Dunn, 2001), the results of which have informed teaching practices.

In this module, IMGs are asked to perform one OSCE which will be videorecorded to provide the material for assessment and instruction. The aim of this activity is to consolidate IMGs' critical-analytical approach to discourse, which will equip them to reflect upon diverse multilingual and multicultural exchanges and assist them with the development of their interactions with patients. The assessment chart which the IMGs are asked to fill in (Appendix 9.3) is composed of the key elements they have studied throughout this course. It is expected that the acquired knowledge will translate into a sound and informed assessment of their own and others' communicative skills and will make them reflect upon the effect that their contribution and the patients' participation may have in the development of the medical visit.

Stage 2: Class Activity (Videorecording). The class is divided in pairs. One IMG takes the role of a medical practitioner and the other, the role of a patient. If the role-play is conducted twice, then the participants will reverse their roles in the second round. The OSCE instructions are delivered to both participants (see Appendices 9.4 and 9.5). IMGs only have two minutes to read the instructions and eight minutes to perform the OSCE.[3]

Stage 3: Class Activity (Self-Assessment/Playback). Immediately after the recording has taken place, the IMG will self-assess his or her performance by playing back the OSCE.

Prompting IMG Self-Assessment: Playback. An ESL specialist can prompt the following questions to assist in the debriefing process:

(1) Were you satisfied with the overall conversation? Why?
(2) Which medical voices (i.e., *doctor, educator, and fellow human voice*) did you use in the exchange?

(3) Which voice did you mainly use in the encounter? Why do you think you made use of it? Which strategies did you use? Were they effective?
(4) Do you think the patient was satisfied with the consultation? Why?
(5) Did you notice any instance of communication failure or misunderstanding? If yes, what was the cause? What did you do to overcome the situation?
(6) Could you have done something differently?
(7) Overall, what mark out of 10 (being the highest) would you assign your performance?
(8) Which areas of the discourse should you pay more attention to in the future? Elaborate.

Prompting Simulated-Patient Assessment: Playback. The simulated patients are asked to assess both their own performance and the IMG contribution to the visit, using the following questions:

(1) Were you satisfied with the overall conversation? Why?
(2) Were you satisfied with how the medical voices were used? Was the strategy use and frequency adequate?
(3) Did you notice any instance of communication failure or misunderstanding? If yes, what was the cause? What did you do to resolve the situation?
(4) Could you and the physician have done something differently?
(5) Overall, what mark out of 10 (being the highest) would you give the IMG performance?

Peer Assessment/Playback. IMGs are asked to assess each others' performances by playing back the OSCE scenario and filling in the LACT-IMG assessment chart (Appendix 9.3).[4] This table highlights the main components of the three medical voices already introduced in Module Three and the communicative features that have emerged in subsequent studies (Cordella & Musgrave, 2009; Cordella & Spike, 2008). *Doctor* and *educator voices* are collapsed into one category to make the process of assessment easier and avoid the double counting of the same strategy, since some utterances may be classified under Doctor or Educator depending on its content.

IMGs are asked to assess each item independently from 1 (minimum) to 10 (maximum), indicate which linguistic strategy was used and write down a comment when appropriate.

The higher the score, the higher the occurrence of a given strategy in the consultation; nevertheless, the emergence of an item does not fully account for the effectiveness of its delivery. Therefore, the IMG will also need to indicate whether the language choice was adequate by reflecting upon the effectiveness of communication within the parameter of the sociocultural encounter and the type of consultation (e.g., first versus follow-up visits) conducted. To achieve this, IMGs are asked to use the LACT-IMG assessment chart and take notes while the OSCE scenario takes place, recall utterances or instances that may have caused problems in the consultation, and explore alternative languages choices which will be later addressed in the focus group. The assessment then will both quantify the presence or absence of any item and identify the category that is most likely to cause problems for the IMG. This information will prove beneficial for the ESL specialist and for the IMG, who will be working together to overcome those difficulties.

Stage 4: Class Activity (Focus Group). Once self-assessment, simulated-patient[5] assessment, peer assessment, and ESL assessment have been completed, the IMGs gather to exchange their impressions and review how the IMGs have assessed the OSCE scenario. It is recommended that a medical doctor/educator also be present in the focus group to highlight any medical matter that may be left unattended by nonmedical specialists.

During the focus group, any sociocultural aspects and health belief systems should be addressed and explored further. In the above OSCE the statement, *"I've lived my life doctor. I'm going to die anyway so what's the point?"* could serve as the basis to discuss the conceptualization of death and aging in different multilingual and multicultural communities.

Stage 5: Class Activity (Consolidation). At the end of the focus group, the ESL specialists should summarize the main points that have emerged in the modules studied in the LACT-IMG.

CONCLUDING REMARKS

The design of this LACT-IMG course draws upon a theoretical framework of discourse analysis, medical communication, and intercultural communication. Through observations and active participation in a range of ordinary and institutional/professional exchanges, it is expected that IMGs will become more sensitive and aware of the language choices available in ordinary conversations and medical discourses by observing, deconstructing, reflecting on, and exploring different linguistic strategies. This knowledge should equip them over time to become better communicators, which in turn will impact on their medical practices and patients' satisfaction.

NOTES

1. Research Team: Associate Professor Neil Spike, Dr. Marisa Cordella, Ms. Kara Gilbert, Professor Barry McGrath, Professor Gordon Whyte, Dr. Johannes Wenzel, Dr. Val Wass, and Dr. Simon Musgrave, from the Faculties of Arts and Medicine at Monash University; School of Medicine at Manchester University and the Centre for Postgraduate Medical Education, Southern Health.

2. Alignment to the medical institution refers here to the language choices people make in the verbal exchanges as a response to the institutional expectations and the medical guidelines. For example, as shown by Cordella (2004a), alignment to authority in Chileans Spanish is shown by the Spanish pronominal system that differentiates between formal and informal situations. Chilean physicians prefer addressing their patients using address forms that indicate formality such as "usted" (*you* formal) and by using patients' surnames. In contrast in Australia physicians tend to use patient's first name. In terms of medical guidelines, the institution is required to adhere to particular medical protocols depending on to the medical issues. Institutional expectations vary across languages and institutions. Therefore, inside knowledge was required to operate effectively.

3. This OSCE was one of the exercises that were used in a training bridging course conducted at Box Hill Hospital (Melbourne, Australia) and led by Associate Professor Neil Spike.

4. I acknowledge Dr. Simon Musgrave for his useful feedback on an earlier version of this chart.

5. Simulated-patient refers to the person who takes the role of the patient in a role-play or in an OSCE scenario.

ACKNOWLEDGMENTS

I am grateful for the valuable comments I received from the late Emeritus Professor Michael Clyne (1939–2010) from Monash University and Dr. Aldo Poiani from the School of Biological Sciences from Monash University on the earlier version of this manuscript.

APPENDIX 9.1

Schedule: The language and culture training course for IMG (LACT-IMG)

	Duration
Module One Getting started: You already know how to communicate. • Introduction	
Stage 1: Class activity Present overall aims of LACT-IMG and provide concise explanation about the content of each module.	1 hour
Stage 2: Outside-class activity (participants' own time) How are ordinary conversations structured? • Hospital cafeteria (ordinary encounters) • Pharmacy or equivalent health store (service-oriented encounters)	1 hour
Stage 3: Class activity • Possible answers: Reflecting	1 hour
Module Two: Getting inside the medical institution • Introduction	
Stage 1: Outside-class activity How is institutional talk organized? • Greetings in medical peer interactions • Medical visit: seeking information	1 hour
Stage 2: Class activity • Possible answers: Reflecting	1 hour
Module Three The skeleton structure of the medical visit: Three voices, one consultation • Introduction	
Stage 1: Class Activity: *Doctor Voice* • Class activity • Group discussion and consolidation	1 hour

Stage 2: Class activity: *Educator Voice* • Class activity • Group discussion and consolidation	1 hour
Stage 3: Class Activity: *Fellow Human Voice* • Class activity • Group discussion and consolidation	1 hour
Module Four: Let's get into action: Now it's your turn! • Introduction	
Stage 1: Class activity	15 minutes
Stage 2: Class activity • Videorecording	30 minutes
Stage 3: Class activity • Self-assessment/playback	1 hour
Stage 4: Class activity • Focus group	
Stage 5: Class activity • Consolidation	30 minutes

APPENDIX 9.2

Please mark with a cross your answers X.

1. Sex

   Female ☐   Male ☐

2. Age: In which category are you?

25–30 ☐	41–45 ☐	55–60 ☐
36–40 ☐	46–50 ☐	60–65 ☐
41–45 ☐	51–55 ☐	Other:

3. Language: Which language would you consider your strongest?

   _____

4. Enumerate all the languages you speak in order of fluency from most fluent to least fluent.

1. (most fluent)	4.
2.	5.
3.	6.

5. What is your cultural background?

   _____

6. Experience in practicing medicine: How long have you been practicing medicine before coming to this country?

   _____

7. Have you encountered any communication difficulties when interacting with locals in daily interactions (e.g., accent, jargon, humor, etc.)

   YES ☐   NO ☐

8. If your answer is YES
   8a. How did you notice that communication was not running smoothly?

   _____

   _____

   8b. What did you do to overcome the communicative difficulties?

   _____

   _____

9. Briefly describe two events where you've had some difficulties in communicating with a local speaker
   9a. _____

   _____

   9b. _____

   _____

10. Have you encountered any communication difficulties when interacting with local and nonlocal medical peers?

    YES ☐   NO ☐

11. If your answer is YES briefly describe two events when you've had some difficulties in communicating with them.
    11a. _____

    _____

    11b. _____

    _____

12. In order to become a competent communicator with medical peers and patients what do you think you need to pay attention to?

    _____

    _____

    _____

    _____

APPENDIX 9.3

LACT-IMG Assessment chart											
Communication of medical knowledge (*doctor* and *educator voice*).	1	2	3	4	5	6	7	8	9	10	Identify the strategy used. Write comments here.
Seeks information (allows patient to open up).											
Responds clearly to patient's questions.											
Checks understanding.											
Assesses and reviews tests results.											
Uses summaries.											
Educates patient on medical condition.											
Uses drawings or other visual technique to explain.											
Presents alternative treatments.											
Includes assessment of risk.											
Establishes patient's knowledge and reaction to condition.											
Assesses patient's adherence to treatment.											
Develops treatment plan.											

Develops management plan.											
Presents relevant information.											
Presents accurate information.											
Presents jargon-free information.											
Provides takeaway information.											
Arranges follow-up consultation.											
Fellow Human voice.											
Asks questions "unrelated" to patient's condition.											
Encourages questions from patient.											
Responds to patient's emotional needs.											
Checks patient's concerns.											
Uses active listening techniques.											
Reinforces key points.											
Sociocultural knowledge											
Demonstrates awareness of sociocultural differences (e.g., health beliefs).											

Asks patient's clarification of cultural practices.											
Negotiates meaning.											
Achieves the goals of the consultation despite cultural differences.											
Provides accurate institutional knowledge.											
Provides accurate information on government health-care initiatives.											
Total (Sum up the total number of points accrued.)											

APPENDIX 9.4

IMG instructions

Reading time: 2 minutes

Performance: 8 minutes

Station title: Management of patient diagnosed with bowel cancer

Sam Marks, aged 60, presents today for the results of his colonoscopy.

You saw him or her originally about two weeks ago when he presented with a history of a significant amount of PR bleeding for one week. You immediately recommended that he or she go for a colonoscopy. Ms. or Mr. Marks however, was initially reluctant to go, saying that he or she had had bleeding like this before and it turned out to be due to his or her hemorrhoids.

Today unfortunately, you have bad news for him or her because the colonoscopy showed a tumor, 2 cm in diameter, in the sigmoid colon and you now intend to refer him or her to a surgeon for further management.

The good news is that the biopsy indicates that the tumor is confined to the bowel mucosa.

APPENDIX 9.5

Simulated-patient instructions

Reading time: 2 minutes

Performance: 8 minutes

Station title: Management of patient diagnosed with bowel cancer

Your name is Sam Marks and you are aged 60. You are generally a healthy person and have infrequently had cause to go to the doctor. Your only problem is that you do get PR bleeding from time to time because of hemorrhoids that you have had for a long time and which play up whenever you eat too much takeaway food.

Two weeks ago in fact, you presented to your GP with a history of a significant amount of PR bleeding for one week. The doctor immediately recommended that you go for a colonoscopy. You were initially reluctant to go, saying that you had had bleeding like this before and that it turned out to be due to your hemorrhoids.

You have come to see your GP today for the results of the colonoscopy. The doctor tells you that a tumor, 2 cm in diameter, has been found in the sigmoid colon and that he will now refer you to a surgeon for further management. As soon as you hear this you say quite clearly to the doctor, "I've lived my life doctor. I'm going to die anyway so what's the point?"

CHAPTER TEN

ADDRESSING THE LANGUAGE AND COMMUNICATION NEEDS OF IMGs IN A U.K. CONTEXT: MATERIALS DEVELOPMENT FOR THE DOCTOR–PATIENT INTERVIEW

Marie McCullagh

ABSTRACT

This chapter outlines the language and communication challenges facing international medical graduates in the United Kingdom, and the potential for learning materials to help them meet these challenges. It provides an outline of the health system in which they need to operate, as well as the training and education framework within which they need to progress.

English Language and the Medical Profession: Instructing and Assessing
the Communication Skills of International Physicians
Innovation and Leadership in English Language Teaching, Volume 5, 211–228
Copyright © 2011 by Emerald Group Publishing Limited
All rights of reproduction in any form reserved
ISSN: 2041-272X/doi:10.1108/S2041-272X(2011)0000005016

INTRODUCTION: IMGs IN U.K. HEALTH SERVICES

Overview of the NHS

The National Health Service (NHS) is the means by which health care is provided to the population of the United Kingdom (see www.nhs.uk/ NHSEngland). It is a service which operates on the basis that health care is delivered without payment at the point of delivery. While the government has overall responsibility for the NHS, at the time of writing, acute and primary care services are delivered by semiautonomous trusts. There are a number of different types of trust, providing care in the fields of primary and acute care, mental health, and emergency service. The majority of doctors are employed in primary care as general practitioners, a role similar to that of family physicians in the United States. The trusts are the bodies which act as the legal employers of medical staff, and it is mainly within the acute and primary trusts that postgraduate medical trainees obtain their clinical experience. Because of regional governments within the United Kingdom, there are separate structures for the NHS in England, Scotland, Wales, and Northern Ireland.

The NHS relies heavily on international medical graduates (IMGs) for the delivery of the service. In 2009, approximately 36% of hospital doctors in the United Kingdom had obtained their primary medical qualification outside of the United Kingdom, 7% from institutions within the European Economic Area (EEA), and 29% from institutions elsewhere in the world (The NHS Information Centre, Medical and Dental, see www.ic.nhs.uk/ webfiles/publications/010_Workforce/nhsstaff9909/Medical/Medical_Den tal_Bulletin_1999-2009.pdf). In the case of general practitioners, GPs, the equivalent of the U.S. family and community practitioner, the proportion of IMGs is approximately 22% (The NHS Information Centre, General Practice, see Table 6 at www.ic.nhs.uk/webfiles/publications/010_Work-force/nhsstaff9909/GP/General%20Practice%20%20Bulletin%20Tables %201999%20-%202009.pdf).

Regulation of Medical Practice and Routes to Full Registration

In order to practice in the United Kingdom, all doctors, regardless of country of qualification or origin, have to register with the General Medical Council (GMC). Its function is "to protect, promote, and maintain the health and safety of the public by ensuring proper standards in the practice of medicine" (www.gmc-uk.org). U.K. medical school graduates are automatically eligible for initial registration on completion of their studies.

IMGs from within the EEA

Because of labor mobility legislation, those IMGs who come from within the EEA[1] are not required to undergo a standardized test for language or clinical competence. If they already have clinical experience, they are eligible for full registration by the GMC and their English language proficiency is checked on appointment by their prospective employer. Testing doctors from within the EEA is currently an issue under discussion following the death of a patient in the United Kingdom due to the negligence a Nigerian-born doctor. The doctor, trained in Germany, who was acting as a substitute for a regular GP, administered a lethal overdose of a painkiller ('Sufficient checks' on locum GP, 2010). While there have been discussions, no decisions have been made as yet on what form this testing of EEA doctors should take. Although the issue of testing of EEA doctors is an important one, the focus of this chapter is on how materials can help doctors to develop the communication skills they require.

Non-EEA IMGs

IMGs from outside the EEA are required to obtain a minimum score in an English test ((the International English Language Testing System™ (IELTS™), see www.ielts.org) and to pass a clinical and communication exam (the Professional and Linguistic Assessments Board (PLAB), 2010, see www.gmc-uk.org/doctors/plab.asp) before they can obtain initial registration. These exams, and their implications for IMGs, are discussed more fully below. Once they have obtained initial registration with the GMC, all IMGs can compete for training places in the Foundation Programme on the same basis as U.K. medical graduates (U.K. Foundation Programme Office, 2009). Starting in 2005, all newly qualified doctors are required to undertake the Foundation Programme, which delivers training within a range of clinical settings, in both acute and primary care. Having successfully completed the Foundation Programme, doctors can apply for advanced training in one of the specialist areas of medicine covered by the Royal Colleges (www.aomrc.org.uk/members.html).

IELTS

The International English Language Testing System (IELTS) is a four-part exam, administered by the British Council and partners. It focuses on reading, writing, listening, and speaking in an academic context. IMGs are required to achieve a score of 7 in each of the areas before they can take the PLAB. The general band level descriptor for IELTS 7 states that the candidate will have "operational command of the language, though occasional inaccuracies, inappropriacies and misunderstandings in some situations. Generally handles complex language well and understands detailed reasoning" (IELTS, 2010).

The IELTS score of 7 can be seen as broadly equivalent to TOEFL 600 (paper-based). However, the IELTS exam can only act as a yardstick to measure a speaker's general English language competence, so a score of 7 does not guarantee the same level of competence in a medical context.

Clinical Attachment

For many IMGs who have not completed an internship, a clinical attachment (an unpaid placement in a clinical setting under the supervision of a senior doctor lasting between two and six months) is a very attractive option. This is undertaken after acquiring the requisite IELTS score but before passing the PLAB. The clinical attachment provides a very good way of gaining experience regarding the legal, ethical, and cultural context of the practice of medicine in the United Kingdom. It can provide excellent experience of the U.K. clinical setting and of the scenarios which the PLAB is designed to test. Even when the experience involves limited exposure to clinical scenarios, the general exposure to the health-care setting can be useful in helping IMGs understand the cultural context. However, the changes in immigration legislation which have taken place since 2005 have made it more difficult for IMGs to obtain a clinical attachment. Even so, it remains an option for some, and for those who can undertake it, it provides an invaluable opportunity for learning.

The PLAB

The Professional and Linguistic Assessments Board (PLAB, www.gmc-uk.org/doctors/plab.asp) is a two-part exam which is broadly equivalent to the USMLE® Step 2 CK and CS exams in the United States. Part 1 is a written test of medical knowledge, which can be taken in a number of locations around the world. Part 2 is an Objective Structured Clinical Examination

(OSCE) and can only be taken in the United Kingdom. While communication skills are an important part of the exam, the focus is primarily on the candidate's ability to make an accurate diagnosis. Having passed the PLAB, IMGs can register with the GMC and apply for positions within the NHS.

In Part 2 of the PLAB, the candidate is required to undertake 14 clinical scenarios or "stations," where a simulated patient presents with various symptoms, from which the candidate is required to make a differential diagnosis. Symptoms can include diarrhea, palpitations, difficulty in swallowing, loss of consciousness, anxiety, weight loss, and pains in various parts of the body. Candidates are evaluated on their communications skills through observation of their interactions, usually with a simulated patient or the examiner. At some stations, however, communication is the main focus of the assessment, and the following areas may be tested: explaining diagnosis, investigation, and treatment; involving the patient in decision-making; communicating with relatives and health-care professionals; breaking bad news; seeking informed consent for procedures or consent for a postmortem; and giving instructions on discharge and advice on lifestyle, health promotion, or risk factors.

Entry to the Foundation Programme

Legislation passed in 2005 restricted the number of IMGs allowed into the United Kingdom, and while clinical attachments continue, the number in training has dropped. Also, in 2005, a major revision of postgraduate medical training established a common foundation program over two years ("F1" and "F2") for all newly qualified doctors, whether U.K. based or IMGs. It is a requirement for IMGs who have not had an internship in their own country to complete the Foundation Programme before they can progress to specialist training. The Foundation Programme has an online national application portal where graduate doctors can apply to a maximum of three training providers, with the aim of obtaining a training place with one of the providers. The training providers each have their own processes for evaluating applications. Currently, the proportion of EEA IMGs on the Foundation Programme is between 2% and 3%, and the proportion of non-EEA IMGs in training is around 8%.

Foundation Programme Assessment

All graduates who achieve a place on the Foundation Programme are required to undertake a range of work-based assessments during their training. Six instruments are used in this process. They include Team Assessment of Behavior (TAB), in which the ratings of medical and nonmedical colleagues are used to identify areas where potential behavioral issues may impact on professional practice. There is a considerable emphasis on trainees' ability to communicate with patients and to communicate effectively with colleagues. In terms of clinical skills, trainees are required to maintain a logbook of procedural skills, demonstrating their competence on 15 key procedures listed in the logbook.

Trainees are also expected to complete Mini Clinical Evaluation Exercises (mini-CEX) and at least six Case-Based Discussions, where clinical cases are discussed with a senior colleague. Trainees are also required to complete a "developing the clinical teacher assessment form," which outlines what contributions they have made in terms of teaching during the year and how their skills as teachers have improved. Taken together, these assessments place considerable demands on the communication skills of all Foundation trainees, especially for those IMGs who have not had communication skills training in their medical undergraduate program, unlike their U.K. counterparts.

Communication and Language Challenges for IMGs

As this section has outlined, there are a number of different possible entry points for IMGs, depending on their country of origin and the nature of their clinical experience before coming to the United Kingdom. For those who come from outside the EEA, there is the challenge of the IELTS exam and the need to pass the PLAB, whether with or without the experience of a clinical attachment. While those IMGs who come from within the EEA do not have to pass these two exams, there is still the challenge of the selection process for the Foundation Programme. Once this has been surmounted, there is the challenge of passing the formal assessments on the program, as well as fitting in as a team member within their workplace. These challenges show the broad range of contexts in which IMGs need to be able to use their language and communication skills effectively.

It is important to bear in mind that IMGs do not form a homogeneous group, and consequently, there is considerable variation in the amount of communication skills training which they will have received before coming to the United Kingdom. There are also likely to be considerable differences in the educational context in which their medical qualifications have been obtained, particularly in terms of the approach to patients, which can often contrast with the more patient-centered approach in the United Kingdom (Kergon, Illing, Morrow, Burford, & Bedi , 2009, p. 14).

In some cases, IMGs are more focused on the knowledge element of their training rather than the practical application of that knowledge (Kergon et al., 2009) which can present additional barriers to be overcome. The next section will describe how some of these challenges were addressed in a set of pedagogical materials which focused on communication in the doctor–patient interview. The final section will look at how these materials can be extended to meet the challenges of the broad range of contexts described above.

Materials Development

Beginning as my final project in a master's program in materials development, the initial aim of the pedagogical materials described below was to help IMG candidates meet the language and communication requirements of Part 2 of the PLAB examination. The emphasis of the exam was very much on clinical competence, and the language component was primarily focused on obtaining information from the patient in order to make a diagnosis. For the purposes of the master's project, this focus was felt to be too limiting, so that the objectives of the materials were broadened to help IMGs interact effectively with patients in a U.K. clinical setting.

The materials were produced in paper form in late 2004 as a thesis (McCullagh, 2004). In 2005, an opportunity arose to trial the materials at a local hospital with the first cohort of IMGs taking the new Foundation Programme. At that time, the provision of postgraduate training was undergoing extensive revision, which would place a greater emphasis on communication skills. The trial provided an opportunity to obtain feedback on some of the materials and to discuss some of the challenges that these IMGs had experienced. Following from this, my coauthor and I developed a proposal which was accepted by Cambridge University Press, and which led to the eventual publication of *Good Practice: Developing Communication Skills for the Medical Practitioner* in 2008 (McCullagh & Wright, 2008).

The initial needs analysis for the materials consisted of three parts: an analysis of the functional language required in the PLAB Part 2, an evaluation of published course books for medical English, and a review of the literature on doctor–patient communication. The starting point was to obtain a copy of the PLAB syllabus and look at the breakdown of tasks IMGs were required to carry out in the stations in the PLAB Part 2 exam. As stated earlier, the communicative element of the exam was very general in nature and was limited to talking to a patient, examining a patient, and demonstrating a procedure on an anatomical model. The use of standard medical texts (such as *Bates' Guide to Physical Examination and History Taking*, 9th edition) provided Bickley and Szilagyi (2005) an insight into the type of language which doctors would need to carry out a successful examination and obtain information for a diagnosis.

The evaluation of the existing medical English course books for IMGs was another important factor. All of the books examined included some focus on the doctor–patient interview, although some had more extensive coverage than others. From the evaluation, I observed that the main or exclusive focus of the existing books was on the development of medical lexis, functional language for the doctor–patient interview, and grammatical accuracy, especially in relation to the use of tenses and the development of vocabulary. From the review of literature on doctor–patient communication, the following areas emerged as important, but they were not specifically addressed by the course books. There was relatively little exposure to the type of language which would more commonly be used by patients, or to the variations in accents which are representative of the ethnically diverse nature of the U.K. population. The books made no reference to communication skills, either as a general topic or in the specific setting of the doctor–patient interview. In addition, there was very little focus on cultural issues, such as the discussion of sensitive topics with a patient. Finally, the range of activities did not directly reflect the range of tasks a doctor would need to carry out during a consultation.

Reviewing the medical communication literature was key to identifying a broader range of language and communication skills required for the doctor–patient interview. A core text, *Skills for Communicating with Patients*, by Silverman et al. (2005), provided considerable insight into the more detailed requirements of the doctor in the consultation, particularly the need for empathy and use of nonjudgmental language. In the course of exploring the broader aspects of the consultation, it became clear that the focus should not be solely on language, as there were other important elements which were involved in communicating meaning, such as nonverbal, paralanguage, active listening, and cultural elements. By focusing on these elements, IMGs would be able to understand communication in a more concrete way, and they could also use the elements to analyze communicative aspects of specific doctor–patient interactions. The elements could also be used by IMGs to evaluate their own performance and that of their peers.

Another key document in terms of doctor–patient communication was the Calgary-Cambridge observation guide (CCOG). A collaboration between U.K. and Canadian medical educators initially published in Kurtz and Silverman (1996), CCOG sets out the various stages which the doctor needs to follow in the interview to achieve a satisfactory outcome. CCOG is particularly useful for nonmedical ESP teachers, as it provides a very detailed breakdown of the different stages within each phase of the doctor–patient interview. For example, under the heading "negotiating treatment," the following subfunctions are listed: discussing options; providing information on treatment; obtaining the patient's view of need for action; perceived benefits, barriers, and motivation; eliciting the patient's reactions and opinions about plans and treatment; taking the patient's lifestyle, beliefs, cultural background into consideration; encouraging the patient to be involved in implementing plans; and asking about patient support systems. These provide a useful way of classifying the relevant language which doctors would need to carry out each function. Another document which was used to provide background to the context of doctor–patient communication was *Good Medical Practice: Duties of a Doctor* (see www.gmc-uk.org), the GMC guide to the requirements of good medical practice.

It is important to emphasize the iterative nature of the needs analysis process and the fact there was a steep learning curve for me as the researcher new to medical communication when understanding the complexities of the doctor–patient interview. Like many needs analyses, it was not a neat process into which all the elements fit at one time. It is also worth noting that the recognition of the role of communication skills in medicine has changed since the initial needs analysis was carried out. The increased sophistication of the PLAB in terms of its evaluation of the communication component of medical practice is one example of this. So too is the more fully developed set of assessments for the Foundation Programme, which reflect ongoing developments in communication skills training.

For the purpose of this chapter, I would like to focus on five key challenges in communicating with patients which the original materials addressed and to examine the continuing relevance of these challenges six years after their initial use. The first of these challenges is understanding colloquial language, or "patient speak." Second is developing an awareness of the language of politeness and respect. Third is nonverbal components of communication. Fourth is culture as a framework. The final challenge is the issue of reflection in learning.

"Patient Speak" (Colloquial Language)

The immediate challenge of "patient speak" is for doctors to understand colloquial or idiomatic terms used by patients to describe their symptoms and situations. The amount of colloquial language which is used is likely to vary according to the age and class of the speaker and the many regional variations which will need to be taken into account, depending on where the IMG is placed. At its most basic, "patient speak" is the use of idiomatic lexical items which are specific to the medical domain. Examples of this might be the use of the word *chesty* to describe a blocked chest. Another aspect, however, is the use of language which goes beyond the medical domain and is in everyday usage. An example is the use of phrasal verbs which occur in a very wide range of settings, for example, the expression *run down*, which means to be hit by a car but can also denote feeling generally unwell. In addition, there are examples of language which combine phrasal verbs with idiomatic language, for example, "my back is playing up" or "the pain has flared up again." As Polackova (2008) points out, these informal verb combinations can be found in authentic case studies, but they can be problematic for IMGs, who are unlikely to have had much exposure to them, even in their preparation for the IELTS.

A related category of "patient speak" is the use of euphemism to refer to issues or anatomical parts that the patient feels sensitive about discussing. For example, the term *down there* is often used by older patients to refer to their genitals. The IMG not only needs to understand what the patient is referring to but also needs to pick up on the sensitivity of the issue to the patient. The use of humor is another way in which a patient can indicate sensitivity about a topic, without openly displaying emotion. As Rughani and Davangere (2010) point out, this can often be a major challenge for IMGs. Humor can take the form of double entendres or sarcasm, and the doctor needs not only to understand what is being said and implied by the patient but also needs to be able to respond appropriately.

A further related factor is accent, which can be a major problem in preventing understanding, in terms of both the patient's pronunciation, and as Rughani and Davangere (2010) point out, the IMG's pronunciation also (see Labov & Hanau, this volume). While the IELTS and the PLAB should both identify major errors in pronunciation or screen out those with weak pronunciation, there is evidence that some IMGs in a GP setting cannot be understood by their patients at times. Sometimes, this is a question of moderating the speed of delivery, but it can also be a problem with pronunciation itself.

In responding to these challenges, *Good Practice* uses a range of idiomatic and euphemistic language in the audio and audiovisual recordings, as well as "patient speak" as a specific feature in each chapter. Learners are also exposed to a wide range of phrasal verbs. However, there is relatively little focus on the emotional content and meaning of the examples of "patient speak" in context. Likewise, while the role of humor within the medical interview is acknowledged, the materials do not explore how IMGs could deal with humor and how humor is viewed within a cultural context. With regard to accent, the materials expose learners to a variety of accents with an emphasis on understanding, but there is little specific focus on improving articulation. However, intonation and speed of delivery are addressed as part of the paralanguage element of communication. When a focus on articulation is required, a profiling of pronunciation features by country of origin could help to identify problem areas.

Politeness and Respect Forms

Adolphs, Brown, Carter, Crawford, and Sahota (2004) refer to the increased frequency of modal verbs used in health conversations to indicate politeness, and this is an area which represents a considerable challenge for IMGs in dealing with U.K. patients. An important example of where this may occur is when making requests; for example, "if you would like to remove your shirt, please" rather than "take off your shirt." The use of modals can also serve to reduce the awkwardness of a situation. Softeners, such as the use of the word *just*, for example, "If you could just take off your shirt," can also fulfill a similar role. However, for many overseas doctors, giving instructions requires the use of directive language, and they may not see that this type of language can make them appear to the patient as too direct and lacking in empathy, or in some cases as simply rude. Tone, speed of delivery, intonation, and pitch are also very important in conveying politeness, respect, and empathy. While these are very difficult to teach, it is important that IMGs appreciate how they play a role in developing and maintaining a relationship with a patient.

In addressing these challenges, the materials in *Good Practice* seek to highlight the importance of modal verbs, hedging, and indirect language and softeners in conveying respect and an awareness of the sensitivity of situations. The dialogues make extensive use of this type of language, and there are linked exercises to heighten awareness of their importance and appropriate use. For example, the phrase *come in* is repeated in a number of different tones so that doctors can begin to distinguish the meaning which patients could take from each. However, these types of activities are primarily intended to develop awareness, and the opportunities they provide to guide production are relatively limited. More exposure to authentic examples of this type would help IMGs appreciate more fully the effect that tone can have in this context and give them a greater opportunity for modeling their own production.

The Nonverbal Components of Communication

In carrying out the needs analysis in preparation for developing *Good Practice*, it became apparent that the nonverbal components of communication were of considerable significance in understanding patients, demonstrating active listening, and in establishing a relationship with them. The nonverbal components identified include eye contact, facial expressions, posture, proxemics, gestures, and touch. As Kurtz, Silverman, and Draper (2005) observe, nonverbal cues are "crucial to understanding patients' emotions and feelings," and they emphasize the need for doctors to be able to pick on these cues and to decode them. However, the decoding of these cues is not always straightforward, particularly for IMGs, who are operating in a different cultural context. In addition, as Bickley and Szilagyi (2005) point out, the channel is a two way one, and the IMGs themselves need to be aware of the messages that they are sending by their nonverbal cues.

In meeting this challenge, as outlined above, the materials include an explicit focus on nonverbal communication. In part, this is possible through the use of a video component in the materials. By using simulated patients and real doctors, *Good Practice* brings all of the different components of communication together. The use of semiscripted scenarios which can then be adapted by the participants to suit their own person means that authentic language can be used as well as appropriate nonverbal elements. In addition to helping IMGs appreciate the nonverbal cues of others, there are also a number of activities designed to help them develop awareness of their own nonverbal communication. These include role-playing in groups of three so that the observer can provide more objective feedback to the other two participants on their nonverbal communication. Further development of these exercises could involve the use of videotaping the role-play, and a systematic evaluation of the performances by all participants. The opportunity to watch their own performance can be a powerful tool in helping IMGs to reconcile their own perceptions of themselves as communicators and the feedback which they receive from others.

Culture as a Framework

Perhaps the most important component of the elements of communication which were identified is culture, providing the framework within which the other elements combine to create meaning. As Thompson (2003, p. 15) observes, "communication has to be understood in the context of the particular culture or intercultural network in which it occurs." This has a number of implications for the doctor–patient interview. Perhaps the most important is a broad understanding of the general norms of U.K. culture, which can be very different from those to which IMGs may be accustomed. This can be especially important for doctors when required to remain nonjudgmental in dealing with sensitive issues such as sexual health, drug addiction, or mental health issues. There is also the need to be aware of how factors such as ethnicity, age, and religious beliefs can affect these general norms in relation to specific patients.

For many IMGs, the difference between what is expected from doctors in their own culture and in the United Kingdom in terms of their approach to treating patients is a major challenge. The need to explore social issues, to consider the broader cultural context, and to involve the patient in the planning of their treatment can be alien concepts for many IMGs (Kergon et al., 2009). For this reason, it is important that IMGs have the communication and language skills to explore the broader cultural context of their patients, and to understand why there is a need to do this as well as to understand the medical benefits of negotiating treatment with patients. Dealing with situations which native doctors find challenging is also an area where an understanding of culture can help IMGs. These situations can include dealing with aggressive patients or breaking bad news in a diagnosis or on the death of a patient.

In addressing some of these areas, the *Good Practice* materials draw on sensitive issues such as breaking bad news, birth control, mental health issues, and addictions. Language and appropriate communication strategies are outlined, and opportunities are provided to role-play some of these scenarios. Some attention is given to examining the social context in which the discussion of sensitive issues can occur, such as in relation to underage birth control, to help IMGs identify cultural differences between the United Kingdom and their own culture.

Development of Reflective Practice

A final challenge which the materials address is the need for IMGs to develop their ability to reflect on their own learning and to give and receive feedback on their performance and that of their peers. The key objective of the book is to develop their ability to use communication and language skills effectively in the consultation; it is essential, therefore, that they have opportunities to check their understanding so they can measure their progress and obtain objective feedback on their performance. In addressing this challenge, the Calgary-Cambridge observation guide was used to provide one objective measure by which learners could begin to evaluate the success of a consultation. Used in conjunction with the audiovisual materials, the users of the materials could determine whether all the appropriate stages had been covered and in the correct order. As their knowledge of communication skills and language increased, they could evaluate the extent to which factors such as empathy and active listening were present in the consultation, and the extent to which they contributed to the outcome. Clear criteria were provided to enable IMGs to provide a relatively objective evaluation of each other's performance in role-play.

Implicit in addressing the self-learning challenge was the expectation that learners would already have some familiarity with the educational processes such as reflective practice, which are current in the United Kingdom. It was also assumed that their undergraduate education would have given them experience of giving feedback to and receiving it from their peers. While this is true of many IMGs, as Pilotto et al.(2007) point out, not all will have had this type of experience, and some explicit coverage of these skills may be required. In addition, they observe that negative feedback is particularly problematic in many non-Western cultures, in terms of loss of face. This is an important factor which needs to be born in mind when designing feedback activities.

FOUNDATIONAL PRINCIPLES OF THE MATERIALS DEVELOPMENT

In providing a principled approach to the materials development process, the work of two authors was particularly important. The first was Tomlinson (1998), whose work draws on principles of second language acquisition (SLA) to highlight features which should be included in learning materials. Five of these principles are particularly important for this learning context. These are that learning materials should (1) achieve impact, (2) be relevant and useful, (3) have authenticity, (4) promote confidence, and (5) provide opportunities for feedback on output. When considering what to include in the materials, these principles were used as a yardstick to guide the selection of texts and activities.

Our materials development process also relied on the work of Maley (2003), who examines materials in terms of their inputs, processes, and outcomes. Inputs refer to texts (written, visual, audiovisual) in their raw state, which are used to develop language. The processes are the activities devised around the inputs. In terms of outcomes from the inputs and processes, Maley identifies three types: pedagogical, educational, and psychosocial. The pedagogical outcomes are those which are relatively easy to measure in terms of the evidence of learning in clearly defined areas, such as the acquisition of specific lexis or grammatical structures. The educational outcomes are broader in scope, as in knowledge of the importance of cultural awareness in understanding communication. Psychosocial outcomes include increased self-esteem and confidence, and these can help learners with giving and receiving feedback.

All three types of outcomes are relevant to the development of materials for IMGs. At the pedagogical level, there are specific learning outcomes such as passing the PLAB. Meeting the assessment criteria for the Foundation Programme can also be seen as a pedagogical outcome. Supporting the ability of IMGs to talk about the role and importance of communication in medicine, with reference to authorities in the field, can be seen as an educational outcome. A similar outcome at a psychosocial level is the ability of the IMG to explain the importance of communication in medicine in relation to his or her own practice, to evaluate his or her own performance and demonstrating an awareness of how it could be improved. It is worth noting that over time, the communication skills component of the PLAB has been made more explicit and more important. The assessment criteria used by the Foundation Programme also make explicit reference to communication skills. These have helped IMGs to see the relevance of understanding the broader context of medical communication. While in the past, the more instrumental IMGs could focus almost completely on the clinical elements, there is now an explicit requirement for them to demonstrate at least a certain level of communicative competence in the medical setting. The challenge for materials, therefore, is to engage the learners to the extent that they can see the benefits of going beyond the requirements of simply passing the assessment.

Authentic Materials and Tasks

When developing the materials as outlined above, it was an essential consideration that they should have relevance, impact, and authenticity, in order to fully engage the learners. In addition, because the materials were intended to be used by language teachers who for the most part did not have a medical background, the relevance and authenticity needed to be supported by explanations which could be easily understood. For example, using the Calgary-Cambridge observation guide as part of the structure helped to provide learners with guidance for best practice in medical communication, but also provided teachers with a means of understanding where the exercises in language and communication skills fit in, and what they were building toward. Using authentic texts, such as patient information leaflets, as inputs to provide the basis for role-plays helped to enhance the realism of the exercise for both learner and teacher.

Other authentic inputs to the materials included reading texts taken from an ongoing column called "A patient who changed my practice" in the *British Medical Journal* (see www.bmj.com). The articles in the series provide a very personal account of doctor–patient encounters and the way in which they caused the doctors to reevaluate their relationship to patients. The articles selected for inclusion focused on successes and failures in communicating with patients, within the broader context of their role as a doctor, and are generally quite emotionally expressive. As inputs, they are intended to give IMGs insight into real communicative situations of considerable complexity, which they would not otherwise have the opportunities to experience. They also provide an opportunity for the IMGs to see reflective practice in action, as the doctors in the articles considered how their own practice had an effect on the patient, and whether their actions were justified. By using discussion activities to accompany the articles, an opportunity is provided for IMGs to discuss the articles with their colleagues for them to reflect on their own practice.

In terms of task authenticity, some activities may seem more directly relevant to the work of a doctor than others. For example, filling in patient information sheets could be seen by IMGs as immediately relevant to the activities they would be expected to perform in a clinical setting. Others, such as noticing the body language of a patient, may be less likely to be immediately seen as authentic. By putting these activities in the context of good professional practice, IMGs were enabled to understand their relevance. This also applied to the use of noticing exercises in "out and about" tasks, where learners were required to apply the theory they had learned to an everyday setting. This had the effect of reinforcing their learning of theory, and also of extending their knowledge to a broader context. For example, noting down examples of "softeners" or hedges that they encountered in everyday speech could help to develop their awareness of their new cultural context.

KEY LESSONS FROM THE MATERIALS, TRANSFERABILITY, AND FURTHER CHALLENGES

In looking at the lessons which can be drawn from the development of the materials for *Good Practice*, it is important to acknowledge that by focusing only on the doctor–patient interview, many of the areas presenting challenges, outlined above, have not been directly addressed. As the discussion has shown, mastery of communication and language skills is important in a much broader range of activities in which the IMGs will engage. However, by focusing only on the doctor–patient interview, an interaction with relatively clearly defined roles and time boundaries, IMGs have an opportunity to appreciate the importance of communication and language skills in a practical context, to see the positive impact that these can have on patients, and to begin to experience a sense of mastery as they develop their own skills. By focusing on the doctor–patient relationship, IMGs are given a foothold from which they can begin to explore the implications of communication and language skills for the other parts of their role within health-care settings. For example, the teamwork aspects of the role, outlined above, do not have the same boundaries of role and time which characterize the doctor–patient interaction, yet the communication and language skills which enable successful interaction in one can be transferred to the other.

By focusing on doctor–patient interaction, there is an opportunity for IMGs to begin to understand the complexities and nuance which are possible in a conversation, and the different elements of communication which are involved. Much of this knowledge is directly transferable to other communicative settings within health care, such as interacting within a team, on which IMGs are assessed as part of the Foundation Programme. A useful example of this relates to the use of politeness in the language of instruction. By gaining the knowledge of how modal verbs and other expressions are used as softeners in giving instructions to patients, the IMG should recognize that in a team context, something which sounds like a suggestion with an element of choice can be in fact a polite instruction by a superior to do something. However, because many IMGs have come from a very hierarchical system of medicine, in which extreme deference is shown to superiors and is shown to them by patients, the extent of the potential transferability of communication and language may need to be made explicit. As Kergon et al. (2009) observe, education supervisors reported that overseas doctors tended to be more subservient and reticent with the senior doctors while being more directive when communicating with patients.

Understanding the different ways in which respect is shown, particularly within a hierarchical relationship, is essential to good teamwork, which is such an integral part of IMG training. The difficulties which this poses for IMGs in terms of their cultural backgrounds have been outlined above. One way in which the cultural transition can be aided is by focusing on politeness and respect in the doctor–patient interview so that IMGs can identify the border between the legitimately assertive patient and the rude and aggressive one. By developing awareness within this context, the transfer of the relevant communication and language to working with colleagues is made much easier. Video clips which provide good examples of this type of interaction are essential for allowing the IMG to connect the theory and practice and to begin to integrate the knowledge into his or her own practice. Irony, humor, and sarcasm, mentioned by Rughani and Davangere (2010), are elements of language in which the issue of respect can be difficult to pin down. The use of good examples of this type of interaction within the doctor–patient interview can help IMGs recognize the boundaries in their interactions with colleagues.

From the discussion, it would appear that there is much which is transferable from the doctor–patient interaction to meet the wider communication and language needs of IMGs, as identified above. However, in order to fully achieve this transfer, it is important to ensure that IMGs have an explicit understanding of the process of learning in a U.K. context, in which significant emphasis is placed on giving and receiving feedback, on self-evaluation, and on the development of reflective practice. While these aspects were covered to some extent in *Good Practice*, more attention needs to be paid to the metalanguage which will enable IMGs to engage in discussion with their peers and their supervisors on the learning process in which they are engaged.

NOTE

1. Austria, Belgium, Bulgaria, Cyprus, Czech Republic, Denmark, Estonia, Finland. France, Germany, Greece, Iceland, Republic of Ireland, Italy, Latvia, Liechtenstein, Lithuania, Luxembourg, Malta, The Netherlands, Norway, Poland, Portugal, Romania, Slovakia, Slovenia, Spain, Sweden, and the United Kingdom. While Switzerland is not in the EEA, Swiss nationals have the same rights as EEA nationals.

CHAPTER ELEVEN

COURSES FOR HEALTH AND MEDICAL PROFESSIONALS

Carol Piñeiro

ABSTRACT

Designing courses for medical professionals requires knowledge of content as well as of environments in which these professionals will be working. Instructors should be prepared in both of these areas by studying, researching, and reading about topics their students are already familiar with in order to coach them in the language they will need to use to interact successfully in their respective environments. This chapter describes several courses that were developed with this purpose in mind.

INTRODUCTION

Designing English for specific purposes (ESP) courses for physicians can take many forms. In my role as an ESP instructor and course designer at an intensive English program at Boston University—the Center for English Language and Orientation Program (CELOP), I developed courses in English for international business and taught in the university's International Management Program in Japan. I also designed and delivered seminars and courses for nonnative teachers of English in other countries,

English Language and the Medical Profession: Instructing and Assessing
the Communication Skills of International Physicians
Innovation and Leadership in English Language Teaching, Volume 5, 229–259
Copyright © 2011 by Emerald Group Publishing Limited
All rights of reproduction in any form reserved
ISSN: 2041-272X/doi:10.1108/S2041-272X(2011)0000005017

sponsored through the Fulbright Program or other programs of the United States Information Agency or U.S. State Department.

In this chapter, I will describe four courses that I designed and taught for doctors and other health professionals who either came to the United States to pursue graduate degrees or who were currently working in a medical context, such as a clinic, hospital, or public health department. I taught these courses between 2004 and 2006, and they ranged from an intensive six-week course focusing on all skills with supplemental site visits to medical centers, to weekly classes focusing on oral and/or written skills taught in schools of public health.

For each course, I will provide a course description as well as discuss the following information: (1) the student population; (2) the process of curriculum development; (3) the course design and support materials for the instructor; (4) the syllabus and course schedule of activities; (5) the materials used, including textbooks, journals, articles, audio/video, and Web sites; (6) the assignments, such as readings, response papers, presentations, and research papers; (7) site visits, if scheduled, to Boston-area hospitals and medical centers; and (8) course assessments, including both faculty evaluation and students' performance.

The courses are discussed in the order in which they were developed and taught from 2004 to 2006, beginning with an intensive course designed for physicians and other medical professionals who, for the most part, came to the United States to enter master's in public health (MPH) programs at various universities. Similarly, the health-care workers in the other three courses were engaged either in study or research outside of a clinical setting. Therefore, the four courses emphasized, as Hamilton and Woodward-Kron (2010) did in their Clinical Communication Program, "the relationship between language, communication ... with the task of teaching language from within a specific content domain that has its own 'culture' such as the 'hospital culture'" (p. 1).

FOUR COURSES FOR DOCTORS AND OTHER HEALTH PROFESSIONALS

Course One: English for Health and Medical Professionals

Introduction
"English for Health and Medical Professionals" was a course I designed and taught for the first time in the summer of 2004 at CELOP. The Center

already offered ESP courses in business, begun in the 1980s, and in law, begun in the 1990s. These courses were started because of requests by students or sponsors and from a need that instructors as well as administrators noticed in the market. Besides the English for international business (EIB) sections that were part of the year-round English for academic purposes (EAP) program, we began offering courses in English for professional purposes (professional English) courses in the summer. These focused on business for pre-MBA candidates and law for practitioners and pre-LLM candidates. Prompted by direct requests from potential students and sponsors, faculty engaged in researching, proposing, designing, developing, and finally offering the courses. While there were only occasional requests for medical English, adding it to our professional offerings filled a niche and contributed a new dimension to our summer programs, while also boosting enrollment. Since I was interested in the topic and offered to develop the course, the Program Committee at CELOP approved offering a course for medical and health professionals (for further information on the range of professional English offerings, see www.bu.edu/celop/programs/summer/index.html).

The faculty for these courses were self-selecting, that is, they requested particular teaching assignments based on interest or knowledge. This knowledge was developed by periodic reading on topics in their fields of specialization in order to become familiar with them. Some even went so far as to take introductory courses in business or law so as to better prepare themselves for specialized teaching.

Having taught all levels and skills in my 30-year career as an ESL instructor, most recently in EAP and EIB, I was looking for a different area in which to expand my repertoire. Since I regularly informed myself about science and medicine, I felt capable of designing an ESP course in this area. I was also involved in IELTS™ testing and observed many nurses and health practitioners taking the exam in order to secure positions in American hospitals. Therefore, I approached the associate director in 2003 with the proposition, and after discussions with him and the director, I was asked to write a proposal for the university so that CELOP could obtain a course number and run a pilot in the summer of 2004.

Preparation
Belcher (2006) describes the ESP practitioner as "a combined needs assessor, specialized syllabus designer, authentic materials developer, and content-knowledgeable instructor, capable of coping with a revolving door of content areas relevant to learners' communities" (p. 139). These roles are

all challenging, so in preparation for this course, I began of my own accord, to study at Boston University's School of Medicine, taking undergraduate courses in medical terminology, biotechnology, technical writing for clinicians, and legal and ethical issues for clinicians, and even completing an externship in biomedical science at a local hospital. Those five courses earned me a Certificate in Biotechnology, the simplest qualification I could get in the shortest amount of time (for further information on this certificate, see www.bu.edu/met/programs/undergraduate/biotechnology).

The background I gained in medical science familiarized me with clinical and health-related topics, enabling me to give presentations and enter discussions with ease during the course. Since all full-time faculty and staff can take up to eight credits' worth of tuition-free courses per semester, CELOP did not have to pay for faculty preparation. I paid the registration fees associated with the courses, attended evening classes, did the assignments, and took the exams without any release time. The administration was pleased with these efforts, although they were by no means a requirement for teaching the course. Despite the considerable time commitment, I found it a substantive learning experience that increased my confidence level and added to my knowledge base and preparation for teaching medical professionals.

Course Summary
The 20-hour per week intensive course was scheduled for four weeks during the second summer term at the university, that is, from the middle of July to the middle of August in 2004. Based on feedback from the students, it was later divided into modules of two weeks each, so that those who could not attend the entire six weeks could enroll for either the first four or last four weeks, making it flexible for doctors with time constraints or for those required to attend August orientations for graduate students at other universities. In other words, the total number of hours was 80 (four weeks) during the first year, but they increased to a possible 120 (six weeks) in successive years. This meant that interested professionals had to apply for student visas like all the others at our language center. The classes were scheduled from 9:00 am to 1:00 pm, with a break in the middle.

Application Process
CELOP advertised by adding the course to its Web site, and the marketing manager designed print and Web-based flyers to send to scholarship agencies which administer Fulbright and Humphrey grants and to foreign universities with medical schools as well as to hospitals abroad. Students

who were attracted to the course were generally young professionals from Europe, South America, and Asia, who had a few years of working experience as physicians or health practitioners. Most of them had applied to graduate programs in the United States and were being sponsored by their government or another agency, although some were funding their own studies.

When students sent in their applications, we asked those interested in English for health and medical professionals to include a curriculum vitae (CV) and brief statement of purpose (SOP) for course development purposes. These were passed on to me by the admissions office so I would become familiar with students' backgrounds in order to prepare topics and site visits of interest. This method of screening allowed us to distinguish between undergraduates and graduates, and we accepted only those who had finished medical school in their country with possibly a few years of working experience. Those who were still in medical school (undergraduates in many countries) were steered into classes of academic English. As mentioned above, the students were mainly from Europe, South American, and Asia, and they had either seen the course listed on the CELOP Web site or were notified by their scholarship agency that it was appropriate for them.

With CVs and SOPs in hand, I could prepare a course that was instructive, timely, and suited to the purposes of the individuals in the class. Therefore, the course differed from year to year according to the needs and wants of the participants.

Participants
The first year brought only eight participants: three practicing physicians from Argentina, Japan, and Thailand; a recent medical school graduate from Belgium; a veterinarian from Chile; a nurse from Haiti; and two Ph.D. students, one in genetics from Taiwan and one in pharmacology from Paraguay. All but the Belgian planned to pursue graduate programs in the United States, and most had received scholarships to get a master's degree in public health or a doctorate in their particular field of study. Therefore, the information in the CVs and SOPs was invaluable insofar as it let me plan the curriculum that year with each student in mind. Because they were going to enter graduate programs, like the students I had previously taught in the professional business English courses, a focus on academic preparation was of primary importance.

Participants' English language proficiency varied in the course. Incoming Internet-based TOEFL® (iBT®) scores ranged from 80 to 100 (out of 120) taken before coming to the United States and Michigan Test scores between

75 and 95 (out of 100), taken after registering for the class in Boston. We did not set these levels, but we found that the screening process had been effective in that only upper intermediate to advanced students were included in the course. In general, the participants from Europe and Latin America had good English language skills; the doctor from Thailand and the nurse from Haiti needed coaching in accent reduction, while the doctor from Japan and the doctoral student from Taiwan had to hone listening and speaking skills. The European and Latin Americans were accustomed to using textbooks and reading journals entirely in English, while the Asians were not.

All participants had attended medical conferences where the medium of communication was English, and some had even given presentations and written articles for journals in English. Therefore, half of the class was somewhat skilled and at ease in the language, while the other half had to work more intensely on certain skills. That situation made the task of integrating activities and making sure all participants were engaged somewhat challenging, but the good nature and willingness of all the students throughout the course helped to accomplish these goals.

Needs Analysis and Curriculum Development

From my experience teaching other professional courses, as mentioned before, I assumed that as graduate students, physicians, or researchers, the participants would need fluent, comprehensible oral skills for socializing with peers, interacting with professors, making presentations, discussing cases, and giving lectures, much like the professionals in the fields of business and law at our center. Therefore, to develop these skills, I chose activities like dialog practice, role plays, impromptu speeches, group presentations, and short lectures, which strengthened listening and speaking skills. Additional comprehension exercises would include short online lectures and longer documentaries or DVDs on health-related topics, during which the participants would take notes and subsequently discuss. Therefore, the course was modeled on other courses we offered, with the main difference being that the focus was on medical and health topics and types of interaction.

In addition to oral skills, the participants needed grammatically accurate and contextually appropriate writing skills for sending e-mails, composing memos, drafting response papers, summarizing articles, describing diseases, and writing about research. Therefore, we would review and practice these types of communication, with students writing to me as if I were their supervisor, or writing to each other, peer to peer. In reading, they also needed to develop the skills of skimming and scanning short and long texts for information, differentiating between main ideas and details, choosing relevant information to identify a process or mechanism, and analyzing research.

Since the language skills of reading, writing, speaking, and listening intertwine in most contexts, I would attempt, as much as possible, to extend practice to all four skill areas in each exercise. However, for the sake of identifying the areas of focus, I have laid out the following chart.

Speaking/Listening Skills	Activities
Socializing with colleagues	Dialog practice
Interacting with patients	Role plays
Making/listening to presentations	Impromptu speeches/planned presentations
Discussing cases	Case discussion
Giving/understanding lectures	Short lectures/panel discussions
Reading/Writing Skills	Activities
Reading/writing e-mails	Writing/responding to e-mails
Reading/writing patient reports	Understanding/writing patient reports
Reading about visitation sites	Writing persuasive report about sites
Reading/writing journal articles	Reading/summarizing journal articles
Reading/writing about innovations	Reading/making graphic summaries

Materials
Because of the variety of backgrounds, interests, and goals of students, it was difficult that first year to find a textbook for the course. For the pilot program, I used *The Language of Medicine in English* by Tiersky and Tiersky (1992), which proved too easy for most of the students. For the second and third years of the course, I used other textbooks and materials to satisfy the differing needs of the members of the class. Table 11.1 contains a list of books and Web sites that have been used over the years, as faculty who teach it uncover even more sources to coincide with the interests and specialties of the students. Since Web sites contain information in audio,

Table 11.1. Materials for Course One (2004–Present)

Textbooks/reference books

Barnes-Svarney, P. (1995). *Science desk reference.* New York: Macmillan.
Burkit, H. G., Young B., & Heath, J. W. (1993). *Wheater's functional histology.* New York: Churchill Livingstone.
Cavusgill, S. (1995). *The road to healthy living.* Ann Arbor: University of Michigan Press.
Corbiel, J. C. (1986). *Visual dictionary.* New York: Facts on File Publications.
Gendinning, E. H., & Holmström, B. A. S. (2005). *English in medicine* (with CD). Cambridge: Cambridge University Press.
Gendinning, E. H., & Howard, R. (2007). *Professional English in use: Medicine.* Cambridge: Cambridge University Press.
Milnar, M. (2006). *English for health sciences* (with CD). Boston: Thomson ELT.
Penn, J. M., & Hanson, E. (2007) *Anatomy and physiology.* New York: Pearson/Longman.
Tiersky, M., & Tiersky, E. (1992). *The language of medicine in English.* New York: Pearson ESL.

Medical Journals

The Journal of the American Medical Association (JAMA)
The New England Journal of Medicine (NEJM)

Documentaries

Big bucks, big pharma: Marketing disease and pushing drugs. (2006). Media Education Foundation.
The medicated child. (2008). PBS, Frontline.
Selling sickness. (2004). Icarus: Ray Moynihan.

Films

Kenner, R. (2008). *Food, Inc.* Magnolia Home Entertainment.
Moore, M. (2007). *Sicko.* The Weinstein Company Home Entertainment.
Spurlock, M. (2004). *Supersize me.* Kathbur Pictures, Inc.

TV Shows

Grey's anatomy
House

Web sites

Avert (HIV/AIDS)—www.avert.org/aids.htm
Case Studies—www.casestudies.org
Center for Disease Control—www.cdc.gov
Department of Health and Human Services—www.hhs.gov
Health.gov—www.health.gov
Healthopedia.com—www.healthopedia.com
Kids Health—www.kidshealth.org
Medical Dictionary—www.medical.yourdictionary.com
National Institutes of Health—www.nih.gov
National Public Radio, Health—www.npr.org/sections/health
TED: Ideas Worth Spreading—www.ted.com/themes/browse
United Nations MDG—www.un.org/millenniumgoals
WebMD—www.webmd.com
World Health Organization—www.who.int/en

Medical Case Studies

Gross Anatomy—www.anatomy.med.umich.edu/courseinfo/clinical_index.html
Pathology—www.path.upmc.edu/cases.html
Science—www.ublib.buffalo.edu/libraries/projects/cases/ubcase.htm#medicine
Pulmonary—www.meddean.luc.edu/lumen/MedEd/medicine/pulmonar/cases
Academic Journals—www.academicjournals.org/MCS/index.htm

Sites visited

Boston Public Health Commission—www.bphc.org/Pages/Home.aspx
Boston University Medical School—www.bumc.bu.edu/busm
Boston University School of Public Health—www.sph.bu.edu
Children's Hospital—www.childrenshospital.org
Dana-Farber Cancer Institute—www.dana-farber.org
East Boston Neighborhood Health Center—www.ebnhc.org
Genzyme—www.genzymecenter.com
Harvard Initiative for Global Health—www.globalhealth.harvard.edu
Harvard Medical School—www.hms.harvard.edu/hms/home.asp

Harvard School of Public Health—www.hsph.harvard.edu
Joslin Diabetes Center—www.joslin.org
Mass. College of Pharmacy—www.mcphs.edu
Mass. General Hospital—www.massgeneral.org
Novartis—www.novartis.com
Partners in Health—www.pih.org
Tufts University—www.hnrc.tufts.edu

video, and print format, they are invaluable tools for strengthening skills in listening, reading, and research.

Assignments
Typically, a survey was given out the first day of the course, and students rated their abilities in the different skills and their preparedness for the types of activities they would be required to perform in their future study or work. They were also asked to list three topics and one site visit relevant to their interests. This assessment of needs was then used to plan the areas of focus during the course as well as the site visits. The resources listed in Box 11.1 were also consulted to see how the class could serve the needs of the particular group of students that year.

During class, participants did a variety of assignments both in groups and individually. The speaking exercises were conducted in pairs or in small groups; these included dialogs, role plays, and impromptu speeches. Other speaking activities were conducted with the whole group; these included presentations, case discussions, and lectures. Listening exercises could be conducted individually in the multimedia lab or with the group via podcasts in class. These included current events or news items about health topics; if students listened to the same one, they compared notes and answered questions. If they listened to different ones, they reported on them to the group.

Other assignments were focused on reading and writing skills. At the start of the course, I gave students in pairs articles from different newspapers or magazines to read and summarize and report on to the class. Later, they looked on the Internet for articles to read, summarize, and report on. After each tour or site visit, they had to write a memo to a certain person such as a colleague, a supervisor, or the minister of health in their country reporting what they had seen with the purpose of enlightening, suggesting, or persuading the reader, if appropriate, to introduce an intervention or implement a similar program in their country. For their final project, students had to choose a research topic and write a five-page paper, make a set of PowerPoint slides, and give a presentation to the group the final week of the course. The titles of their projects show the range of specializations of the first year's participants:

- Bovine mastitis and herd health
- Conducting clinical trials in developing countries: Risk or relief?
- Imaging techniques for the detection of myocardial hibernation
- Saving lives after cardiac arrest with defibrillators
- The impact of free trade in services on healthcare reform in Thailand
- The search for evidence of effective health promotion
- The use of Caco-2 cell monolayer as intestinal model for drug absorption assessment
- The world of RNAi: Mechanisms and applications

Invited Speakers
I searched for speakers who would come, free of charge, to give the class an informal talk on their specialty, which included topics like HIV/AIDS, maternal healthcare, drug development, epidemiology, and so on. In subsequent iterations of the course, other instructors augmented the list and were able to attract well-informed speakers to the class or find medical lectures in the city for the participants to attend.

Site Visits
Being in Boston meant that there were numerous world-class hospitals and medical centers that students could visit, and at the beginning of each course, I showed the participants a list of these and asked them to choose three of them, along with topics they would like to learn about during the visit. From hospitals to community health centers, each visit was arranged with the students' interests in mind. Before the visit, they would look on the Internet at the hospital or healthcare facility and make up a list of questions to ask. The format of the trip was usually a tour of the site and then a mini-lecture by one of the doctors or specialists—at which point the participants could ask their questions. As mentioned above, the students' follow-up assignment was to write a memo to someone in their country reporting what they saw and suggesting that it be implemented (see Box 11.1 for a list of sites visited for Course One).

Course Regularization
As mentioned above, the first summer course had only eight students for four weeks, but in subsequent years, the number gradually increased, and

the course was lengthened. It has been offered every summer since 2004 for six weeks, from the beginning of July to mid-August, in two-week modules, as previously explained. When the Institute for International Education (IIE) learned that Boston University offered English for health and medical professionals, they began sending students from other countries to CELOP to prepare them for graduate studies at American universities. A few years ago, the enrollment peaked at 30 students, which was enough for two sections; last year, however, only about a dozen students were enrolled, enough for only one section. While we are not certain of the reason for this, it could be due to shrinking funds at the agencies that sponsor these students.

Another change, prompted by the evaluations that students filled out at the end of the first year, was to lengthen the summer program from four to six weeks, although we had to adjust the length the way we did in the past with other professional courses. That is to say, some students can study for only four weeks, due to work commitments or other circumstances. Therefore, we developed three, two-week "stand-alone" modules, allowing students to enroll for the first four weeks, the last four weeks, or all six weeks. This solved the problem of students who were able to attend for only a month and pleased the sponsors, who were reluctant to pay for two weeks of a course that students were unable to attend.

Assessment and Evaluation

Student Assessment. At the end of the program, students received an evaluation from their instructor of their linguistic strengths and weaknesses using a standard CELOP program form. This evaluation assessed their speaking, listening, reading, and writing skills, as well as their readiness for the graduate programs that most were going to enter. They were also given a grade for their final paper and presentation, which was completed in a satisfactory manner in most cases. If the students took the paper-based TOEFL offered at CELOP in the final weeks of the summer program, that score was also listed on the form.

Course Evaluation. During the last week, students were given an opportunity to assess the program, rating classroom activities, materials, field trips, and office staff, as well as commenting on the course, instructor, and classroom experience, and suggesting changes. The summary of the first course evaluation can be seen in Appendix 11.1; the lowest rating (3.5 out of 5) was given to the course text, indicating that it was not appropriate for the course. Those who had studied medicine in their countries found it too easy, while others found that it contained terminology that would not be of use to them in the future.

Two other ratings that were relatively low (3.8) were given to time spent in the multimedia lab on listening comprehension exercises and the afternoon spent at Longwood Medical Area on a field trip. The students may not have valued the individual nature of the lab work, instead preferring the interactive parts of class. As far as the field trip was concerned, the comments concerned visiting too many places in one day; we went to four sites at the Longwood Medical Area the last week of class.

Higher ratings were given for News Articles/Discussions (4.5), Videos/ Listening Comprehension (4.6), Final Presentations (4.8), and Research/ Writing (5). Overall, the course rating was 4.7, which meant that students were satisfied with the offerings of the first year, although there were areas to reconsider and improve upon for the future.

Changes Made as a Result of Evaluation Feedback
To address the issue of choosing an inappropriate textbook, the next year we did not use a textbook; rather, I showed the students several university textbooks in different areas and allowed them to choose chapters that they wanted to read and present to the class. The first week, I did the presentation to model the skills needed and the techniques that could be used. The second week, I allowed the students to sign up to do the presentations and gave them feedback on their performance. By the third week, the students were critiquing each other, and by the fourth week, they were being graded on their performance. This way of handling the textbook issue proved more effective than choosing a text that all of the students would have to buy and use. Because of their different fields and interests, it would have been difficult to find a book appropriate for all. Rather, the course put the onus of reading and assimilating material on the students, as they had to choose the topics and teach their peers about them.

The other two areas, the multimedia lab and field trips, were improved in these ways. Instead of asking the students to listen to only lectures, I searched for videos, so that visual input would provide support for the audio input, and at the same time, be more interesting. I also revised the field trip schedule and took the class to different areas of Boston once a week, visiting only one site at a time.

I continued the activities that received high ratings—news articles/ discussions, videos/listening comprehension, final presentations, and research/writing—knowing that they served to prepare the students for graduate work in the future.

Subsequent instructors have modified other aspects of the course, while maintaining the basic format of teaching classes using materials on health and medical topics, such as textbooks and online multimedia, with the goal of strengthening academic and social skills.

Besides the assessment of the course, I also collected testimonials from some of the students in the 2004–2006 programs to put up on the CELOP Web site. These can be seen in Appendix 11.2. The testimonials indicate that, in general, the students were satisfied with the course because it provided solid preparation for the graduate programs that most were about to enter at American universities. In particular, it improved their writing and public speaking skills, introduced them to the healthcare system in the United States through site visits, enabled them to participate in group discussions, and further developed their reading and listening skills.

After three years, I derived much personal and professional satisfaction from redesigning and improving the course. The personal satisfaction stemmed from the variety of students with diverse backgrounds and areas of expertise that I encountered over the three years. I gained knowledge about medical practices and systems in developing countries, pharmaceutical advances and genetic techniques, and many other areas of research. The professional satisfaction arose from my own reading and learning about medical topics in order to provide rich resources that included news reports, journal articles, audio/video materials, and lectures. I also gained knowledge about the medical centers in the Boston area and came into contact with generous professionals willing to share their expertise with international students. I will begin to teach the course again this year and look forward to learning about new developments from the other instructors.

Course Two: Writing for Graduate Students in Public Health

Writing for Graduate Students in Public Health was a course proposed to CELOP by the School of Public Health (SPH) at Boston University for its international graduate students in the fall of 2004. Because I had just taught the summer EHMP course, I was the logical candidate to teach at SPH as well. Therefore, I traveled across town to the Medical Campus, where I taught for three years. The following sections will describe the course, students, curriculum, assignments, and assessments during that time period.

Course Description

The writing class was a concurrent support course held weekly for two hours throughout the fall semester on Friday mornings with subsequent half-hour tutorials with each student. The primary goals were to give international students a foundation in academic writing and assist them with writing assignments from the courses they were concurrently taking in the Master's in Public Health (MPH) program. The emphasis in the two-hour class was on presenting and having students practice different rhetorical styles, like the narrative for objective reporting, analysis for data interpretation, persuasion for requesting funds or services, and representation of graphic data for research purposes.

The weekly half-hour tutorials served the purpose of addressing individual students' needs, and I would tutor four students for another two hours after each class on a revolving basis. If they did not have a piece of writing to show me at their scheduled session, they could save up that time and e-mail sections of papers to me before the due date. I would review and comment on these papers, occasionally editing parts if there were mistakes that obscured meaning. The students valued this feedback before they turned the papers in to their professors, most of whom understood the students' language limitations and graded them on content more than style.

Student Population

A few of the students were physicians, like those in the summer EHMP course, sent by the governments of developing countries or scholarship agencies to major in some aspect of public health. They were expected to seek an opportunity for professional training (OPT) after completing their coursework to gain experience in the United States before returning to their country to improve the aspects of public health they had studied. The concentrations were in HIV/AIDS care and prevention, maternal and child healthcare, or epidemiology. Studying public health seemed to put them in a different category than clinicians, who in developing countries did not earn much and worked long hours. With an MPH, they might work for the ministry of health, an international agency, or an NGO to have a better chance to further their career, as I was told by some of them anecdotally.

Syllabus and Curriculum Development

Because this course arose out of a request to CELOP from SPH at Boston University, the textbook and class structure had already been decided beforehand. My role as instructor was to evaluate the writing of international students who had been referred to the course after completing an impromptu writing sample and then to choose chapters from the book I was given that would best address their needs. I was also asked to read the students' written assignments during the semester and either make comments or directly help them correct mistakes in paragraph-level organization and sentence-level syntax and lexis. During the first semester, my role became clearer as I performed these tasks and tried different approaches to shift the responsibility for self-correction onto the students.

Materials

The textbook, *Academic Writing for Graduate Students*, by Swales and Feak (2004) was required for the course, and it contained lessons with model paragraphs and exercises along with guidelines for writing. Unable to cover all the lessons, I chose those that were pertinent to the assignments on the syllabi that the students provided me with.

I also helped the students to analyze the course syllabi given by their professors so that they could understand the reading, writing, and research assignments they had been given for the semester. This exploration was helpful for students, as was explaining the rubrics that were handed out for grading papers. This was a basic orientation activity that gave them a clearer understanding of the requirements for the course and the expectations of the professors.

After the individual tutorials, I also recommended to students that they review certain areas of grammar, word formation, complex sentence structure, paraphrasing, and citation conventions on the Purdue Online Writing Lab (OWL), which they could do independently. This saved time that would have otherwise been devoted to sentence—or paragraph—level corrections and allowed me to focus on more global issues of organization, analysis, and interpretation in their papers. Other useful Web sites on particular topics were made available to the students for their reference during the semester (see Table 11.2 for materials used in Course Two).

Assignments

Formal instruction included guidelines for assignments given by SPH professors on their syllabi, such as abstracts, book reports, policy memos, site visit reports, papers, and even articles for publication in professional journals. Informal instruction included engaging in peer critique in a workshop format; that is, students would bring in segments of papers, like introductions or conclusions, with enough copies for their classmates. Sitting in a circle, students other than the writer would read aloud and make corrections or revisions to what was written, offering constructive criticism.

Table 11.2. Materials for Course Two

Textbooks

Swales, J., & Feak, C. (2004). *Academic writing for graduate students: Essential tasks and skills.* Ann Arbor: University of Michigan Press.

Web sites

American Medical Association—www.ama-assn.org
Purdue Online Writing Lab—www.owl.english.purdue.edu
World Health Organization—www.who.int/en

In this fashion, writers received positive comments as well as suggestions for greater accuracy or clarity in their writing—and were thus encouraged to improve.

Course Regularization
This noncredit course has been offered every fall since 2004 for a new group of international students each year. The students are identified as those who were accepted into the master's program with lower TOEFL scores, or those who, during the August orientation for international graduate students, displayed deficient writing skills. In other words, any student who might have difficulty with MPH assignments is required to attend the course. If the instructor can demonstrate in the first few weeks that a student is actually a skillful writer, he or she can be excused from taking the course. However, when the students learn that they will receive tutorials that provide individualized help with papers, they usually opt to stay. A full-time faculty member from CELOP is given release time to go to the Medical Campus each week to teach the course, which is funded through the dean's office at the School of Public Health. In other words, SPH pays CELOP, and the course is counted as part of the teaching load of the instructor.

Assessment and Evaluation
The course is evaluated by students through evaluations distributed at the end of the semester at SPH. When I was an instructor, course evaluations were kept at the School of Public Health rather than being sent to CELOP. It seems fair to say, however, that the students have evaluated the course

favorably since SPH has continued to offer the course and to ask CELOP to supply the instructor. I have also been told that the SPH faculty are aware of and appreciative of the course, as it allows them to spend office hours discussing the substance of a paper or research project with a student instead of correcting errors and trying to construct meaning from a student's words. Although a semester is hardly enough time to improve one's writing, it does allow students to learn the fundamentals of academic discourse. Feedback from students includes expressions of appreciation and sharing of grades that they have received on papers that the instructor has reviewed. An acknowledgment also comes from the dean of SPH via the associate director of CELOP to the instructor at the end of the term. The fact that Writing for Graduate Students in Public Health continues to be offered is another indication that it is meeting students' needs.

Course Three: Medical and Scientific Writing

Description
Medical and Scientific Writing was another course I taught during the summer of 2004 at a request to CELOP from the Dana-Farber Cancer Institute (DF) in Boston. The course was taught at the Institute for eight weeks with two-hour classes on Tuesday and Thursday afternoons for a total of 32 hours. DF had set aside funds and hired me through CELOP to pilot the course. Their goals were to improve the level of English production skills, that is, speaking and writing, of international researchers and postdoctoral grantees at DF. Although the emphasis was on the improvement of writing skills, I was also asked to address the oral communication skills of the participants as well, since they played a vital role in contributing to the teamwork required by research.

   Formerly, they had paid an ESL freelance instructor to conduct small group tutoring on different days of the week, but they decided to pilot a course to determine if a university instructor could improve the skills of a larger group more effectively. After discussing the parameters of the course with the continuing education coordinator in the human resources department, I agreed to pilot the course in addition to teaching a full academic load of 15 hours per week. At the time, I was teaching Course One at CELOP, as described above.

Student Population
A dozen students were recommended for the course, and after giving short speaking (oral interview about their work at DF) and writing (summary of

responsibilities in the lab) assessments on the first day, I determined that it was a mixed-level class, ranging from intermediate to low-advanced. Among them were a few doctors conducting research, some Ph.D. students, and a few postdoctoral students. The languages of the participants were Chinese, Korean, Spanish, Italian, and Russian; I realized that I would have to deal with the differences in language ability in diplomatic ways while attempting to advance the writing and speaking skills of all students.

Syllabus and Curriculum Development
The continuing education coordinator gave me two books to use for the course, *On Being a Scientist* (Committee on Science, Engineering, and Public Policy, National Academy of Sciences, National Academy of Engineering, and Institute of Medicine, 1995) and *Graduate Research* (Smith, 1998), but neither was appropriate for classroom use; rather, they were reference books that might serve as guides for research writing. One of the professors at DF had recommended them to the coordinator, so she passed them to me. What some of the students needed, however, was oral and written sentence-level grammar practice. Having recently developed the curriculum for the course at CELOP for health and medical professionals, I was able to incorporate some of its content into the syllabus and thus address the needs of the group at DF. I used the same grammar lessons from the CELOP course, which was running concurrently, and provided exercises on items like word forms, verb tenses, passive voice, adverb clauses, and unreal conditionals, to name a few.

I also started with simple writing exercises like e-mails and proceeded to more complex ones like summary writing and research reports. For e-mail topics, I used lab equipment catalogs from suppliers like Fisher Scientific magazines (e.g., *Lab Reporter*), which would be familiar to the students, and gave functional writing assignments like placing and sending an order, making and apologizing for a complaint, reporting on and acknowledging either progress or lack of it in an experiment, and so on. The students were assigned a different partner for each exercise; for example, one would send an e-mail, while the other would respond, both copying me so I could print out and correct their writing and return it at the next class. Subsequently, they would make the corrections to their e-mails and resend them to me. These interactive exercises not only taught them useful language like the format and expressions of e-mails but also contained communication gaps to which they had to respond authentically. More advanced functional writing included describing an experiment, reporting results, and explaining charts or graphs, among other tasks.

Materials

As mentioned before, two texts were bought for the students by the human resources department, but I was unable to use them during the course since they were reference guides for native speakers. What the students needed were handbooks with exercises to improve the writing of nonnative speakers, so I simply made handouts on my own. Had I been asked to teach the course again, I would have chosen a more practical text that contained models of functional writing along with short grammar lessons, phrasal verb usage, and practical exercises the students could complete and check outside of class.

Because these texts could be used only indirectly in class, the onus was on me to find, among my ESL materials, appropriate exercises that would assist the students in improving their writing so as to conduct, document, and publish their research. This proved problematic for the students at the intermediate level, some of whom had studied medicine in other countries but who had come to the United States to obtain graduate degrees and do research instead of engage in clinical practice. (Reasons given me by students were that the United States Medical Licensing Examination® (USMLE®) was very difficult to pass, and that lab work was a less stressful than clinical work.) Because most of the course participants functioned in lab settings and did not have direct contact with patients, it was less urgent to improve oral language, although they did have to discuss research with colleagues, to comment on the papers that were being written, and to assist at presentations at conferences.

Therefore, in order to improve oral as well as written skills, I gathered news articles on medical and scientific topics written for lay people from magazines such as *Newsweek*, *Time*, and *U.S. News and World Report* and made up exercises to use in class. These activities included reading and responding to questions as well as work on pronunciation, word forms, grammar, and complex sentence structures.

I also brought videos made for the general public on medical or scientific topics that I showed in half-hour segments to improve listening comprehension and vocabulary usage. I would make a worksheet with previewing, viewing, and postviewing activities, which culminated in discussions (see Table 11.3 for materials used in Course Three).

Assignments

After determining their particular fields and research interests, I looked online for short articles that the course participants could read and discuss in class and summarize for homework. I copied sentences from their

---

Table 11.3. Materials for Course Three

Books

Committee on Science, Engineering, and Public Policy, National Academy of Sciences, National Academy of Engineering, and Institute of Medicine. (1995). *On being a scientist: Responsible conduct in research.* Washington, DC: National Academy Press.
Smith, R. V. (1998). *Graduate research: A guide for students in the sciences.* Seattle: University of Washington Press.

Films

Cracking the code of life. (2001). PBS, NOVA.
Fetal alcohol syndrome and other drug use during pregnancy. (1994). Films for Humanities.
Harvest of fear: Exploring the growing fight over genetically modified food. (2001). PBS, NOVA.

Magazines

Fisher Scientific Catalog—www.fishersci.com
Lab Reporter Magazine—www.fishersci.com
Newsweek—www.newsweek.com/tag/health.html
Time—www.healthland.time.com
U.S. News—www.health.usnews.com

---

summaries and distributed them in class, so that the students could do error correction in pairs as a way of working on grammar indirectly. Afterward, I put the sentences on an overhead projector for a final check with the whole class. I also asked the students to do short presentations on everyday as well as medical or scientific topics to practice oral grammar. For both the writing and speaking assignments, I made up a short checklist on which I noted errors in syntax, lexis, and pronunciation, handing these checklists back after the presentations (see Appendix 11.3).

Assessment of Course
The continuing education representative from the human resources department reported that the course received good evaluations from the students, but because of their wide range of abilities and the limited number of hours, the

lower-level students did not make notable progress in the eight-week duration of the course. In my assessment, the class should have been divided into intermediate and advanced students so that each group could have worked on making improvements at their level. It is unclear how DF addressed this situation—whether they reverted to the previous model of small-group sessions given by freelance ESL teachers to assist with research writing or hired an independent instructor to continue the course, which may have been more cost-effective than hiring a faculty member from a nearby university.

Certainly, a need existed among international researchers for such a course, and teaching one in-house afforded me a perspective that I could not have gained at a university. What might be more helpful in the future is to group the students into English levels, that is, intermediate or high-intermediate, so they can work on similar structures and make more progress. Granted, this is easier said than done, given the time constraints of people working in research groups with rotating schedules and given the limited funds that may be available for language training. But if I were to teach similar course in the future, I would make certain suggestions so as to assure students that the time was well spent and that progress was possible.

Course Four: Writing for Researchers in Public Health

Writing for Researchers in Public Health was a series of individualized weekly writing consultations for doctors, Ph.D. students, and postdoctoral researchers in the Department of Nutrition at the Harvard School of Public Health (HSPH). I served as writing consultant at HSPH for two years, between 2004 and 2006, when a colleague who had been doing the tutorials obtained a teaching position in Korea. When she returned, the consultancy reverted back to her.

Course Summary
The Department of Nutrition thought it very important that its international researchers speak and write English well enough to give presentations at conferences and submit articles to professional journals. Therefore, funds had been set aside to give any student who wanted or needed tutorials the opportunity to have them. When I taught there, the sessions were scheduled on Friday afternoons, and each student would have a 30-minute session to practice discussion or presentation skills in order to improve grammar, vocabulary, or pronunciation. They could also bring in their research reports or journal articles for review and editing.

Student Population
A few of the students were doctors who were getting a Ph.D. in nutrition, although they were in the minority. Most were Ph.D. students or postdoctoral students interested in the connection between nutrition, health, and the etiology of disease. Several were working under professors who were examining longitudinal studies such as the Framingham Heart Study, the Health Professionals Follow-Up Study, and the Nurses' Health Study, which are referenced at the end of this chapter.

The students would begin by explaining their research topic to me, and I would ask questions to clarify what I did not understand. We would discuss the progress of their work from week to week, and they would bring the articles they were working on with their research group for review and feedback. The papers, which formed part of their ongoing study, were reviewed section by section each week. Occasionally, they would bring a set of PowerPoint slides for me to go over that explained their research in order to prepare for a departmental meeting or a presentation at a national or international conference.

Syllabus and Curriculum Development
Since these were private tutorials, what the students were working on dictated what we did in class. There was no real need to develop a curriculum or write a syllabus, although I tracked what each student did during each session and turned in the record to the department at the end of each month for bookkeeping purposes. I also filled out an evaluation form assessing the students' speaking and writing skills for the Department of Nutrition at the end of the fall and spring semesters.

Materials
As the purpose of the classes was to assist each student in improving his or her English language skills, there were no prescribed materials. Rather, I was able to choose grammar, writing, or pronunciation exercises from my library to address each individual's needs. For my own acquisition of knowledge in the field, I read a book written by the chair of the Department of Nutrition, Dr. Walter Willett, entitled *Eat, drink and be healthy* (Willet, 2001). I also looked at the Web sites of the Framingham Heart Study, the Nurses' Health Study, and the Health Professionals Follow-Up Study referred to above for information on the material that the students were investigating in their quest for links between diet and health (see Table 11.4 for materials used in Course Four).

> **Table 11.4.** Materials for Course Four
>
> Willett, W. C. (2001). *Eat, drink and be healthy: The Harvard medical school guide to healthy eating.* New York: Simon & Schuster Source.

Assignments
The students were not assigned work outside of the tutorials, as their primary purpose was to advance oral and written skills so that they could document their research cogently and professionally.

Assessment of Course
The value of the course was the individualized nature of the classes, that is, the oral skills instruction and the assistance with revision of written work. The students themselves acknowledged the value of this instruction and assistance at the end of each semester when they filled out evaluation forms and turned them in to the Department of Nutrition. Although I did not see the results, the coordinator assured me that they were positive. The professors, principal investigators (PIs), and graduate student advisors also recognized the value of the tutorials in helping nonnative speakers collaborate with native speakers in research groups and share the responsibility of writing and presenting the work of the group equally. It was satisfying to go through the process of observing a paper being completed section by section and to witness the satisfaction of the researcher as he or she announced that the PI had deemed that it was ready to submit to a journal. It was also gratifying to be cited in the acknowledgments as a person who had contributed to the editing of the paper. If I were to be hired for a similar consulting position, I would gladly accept it.

CONCLUSION

The courses that I have described in this chapter allowed me to enter an intriguing world of knowledge and research, one that has continued to pique my interest and enrich my academic development. Although demanding because of the steep learning curve, designing and executing courses for health and medical practitioners is an exercise that has rich rewards. After a several-year hiatus from teaching medical English because of the faculty rotation policy at our language center, I am due to commence this type of ESP course again. I look forward to working with physicians and other health professionals as they come to the United States to seek opportunities in educational and research contexts. Like many ESL professionals, by "addressing newly identified learner needs and [my] own needs in pedagogical contexts," I find myself "able to face the prospect of reappraising the role of English language teaching in a rapidly globalizing world with a ready array of professional resources" (Belcher, 2006, p. 151).

APPENDIX 11.1 CELOP PROFESSIONAL PROGRAM EVALUATION

"English for Health and Medical Professionals" (EN009) was a four-week intensive English program designed to help you develop the language skills necessary to be successful in an American graduate health or medical program. We hope that you found the curriculum interesting, useful, and challenging, and we would appreciate your advice on improving it.

This form has two sections. The first section asks you to rate the usefulness of the various activities and materials used to meet the objectives of this program. Please rate each item on a scale of 1 to 5: 1 = not useful, 5 = extremely useful, 6 = not applicable, or did not participate. The second section asks you to comment on different aspects of the program.

Section 1: Rate the program

A. Classroom Activities	Not useful		Extremely useful	Average
Dialogue Practice	1	2 3 4	5	4.2
Grammar Lessons	1	2 3 4	5	4.2
News Articles/Discussions	1	2 3 4	5	4.5
Research and Writing	1	2 3 4	5	5.0
Final Presentations	1	2 3 4	5	4.8

Comments:

B. Materials	Not useful		Extremely useful	Average
The Language of Medicine	1	2 3 4	5	3.5
Multimedia Lab Practice	1	2 3 4	5	3.8
Videos/Listening Comp.	1	2 3 4	5	4.6

Comments:

C. Field Trips	Not useful		Extremely useful	Average
Longwood Medical Area	1	2 3 4	5	3.8

Comments:

D. Office Staff	Not useful		Extremely useful	Average
Assistance and advice	1	2 3 4	5	4.5

Comments:

E. Overall Rating	Not useful		Extremely useful	Average
EHMP EN009	1	2 3 4	5	4.7

Section 2: Comment on the program

1. Please explain the reason for your overall rating.
   - A lot of chances to speak, write, listen to English.
   - Excellent course, good materials, even better classmates, and wonderful teacher.
   - Generally, it was very useful, but too short. If there were more time, it would get a better rating score.
   - I think this course was very well done. Maybe it would be better if the classes began at 9:00 am and finished at 4:00 pm every day.
   - Short course, but very good in preparing skills in university life in research or graduate courses for medical professionals.
   - This program gave me some materials to review vocabulary and English expressions related to this field. However, this program should be a bit longer.
2. What comments would you make about your instructor and your classroom experience?
   - A lot of experience and she knew directly about most of our countries.
   - Maybe the teacher can give more practice correcting the mistakes we made in writing and speaking.
   - Remarkable guide and teacher.
   - Small class motivated us to participate in class activities.
   - Wonderful teacher with lots of experience and pedagogical skills.
3. If you could change anything about the program, what would you change?
   - I have no idea about changing program; there are no problems.
   - I think it's OK, but maybe four weeks is an extremely short course; six weeks would be better.
   - I would like to work more hours in class (9:00 am to 4:00 pm all days)
   - Longer, and I would change the textbook *Language of Medicine* for another with more complex readings.
   - Maybe we can divide the program into several topics, and we can practice each topic evenly.
   - The course duration should be six to eight weeks.
4. How did you find out about this program? Would you recommend it to colleagues?
   - From CELOP front desk. Yes, I learned a lot.
   - I found this program because one of my friends recommended CELOP and one of the officers recommended EN009.
   - I got information from the CELOP Web page. Of course I will recommend this course to my colleagues or friends.

- I was told by my sponsor (maybe Harvard recommended it). Yes, I'll recommend it to colleagues.
- Through LASPAU and Fulbright, these programs are part of the experience.
- Yes, absolutely!

APPENDIX 11.2

Comments for Boston University Web site about "English for Health and Medical Professionals":

I think that international students need grammar review and writing assistance before entering an American graduate program; this course provided that for us.

Physician, Dominican Republic
MPH Program, Boston University School of Public Health

I learned a lot about the healthcare system in the United States, and I was able to improve my research writing and public speaking ability.

Physician, Saudi Arabia
University of Jeddah

Even though I just finished Medical School and do not plan to study in the United States at present, I found the course helpful in activating my latent English language skills. We each gave a PowerPoint presentation on our area of interest, which was a useful experience.

Physician, Belgium
University of Ghent

I would definitely recommend this course to colleagues who are coming to study in the United States. They will improve their language skills and be better prepared for graduate study.

Physician, Thailand
MPH Program, Harvard School of Public Health

This course not only introduced us to various healthcare facilities in Boston, but also gave us the skills we need to be successful in our graduate health programs.

Physician, Haiti
MPH Program, University of South Florida

This course was a good preparation for doing graduate work at an American university. Besides studying academic English, we read articles and watched videos on medical topics and then discussed important issues in class.

Pharmacist, Chile
Ph.D. Program, University of Maryland

As medical writer, I was familiar with most of the topics presented, but I became better at discussing and writing about them during the course.

Medical Writer, Japan
MPH Program, Boston University School of Public Health

The instructor's advice on how to write research papers was useful, and her editing helped us correct our mistakes. We were able to improve our scientific writing skills in this course.

Geneticist, Taiwan
MS Program, Tufts University

The program was very useful for international students. We had a chance to practice reading, writing, speaking, and listening in the areas of health and medicine. The small class size allowed us to participate actively in discussions.

Physician, Japan
MPH Program, Harvard School of Public Health

This course is a very good preparation for MPH graduate students even if you don't have a medical background.

Japan International Cooperation Agency, Japan
MPH Program, Boston University School of Public Health

Excellent course, interesting material, knowledgeable instructor. Although it was short, I felt better prepared to begin an academic program after attending it.

Veterinarian, Chile
Ph.D. Program, Cornell University

The instructor had a lot of experience, and she was familiar with the public health situation in our countries. Even though it was short, the four-week course was still a valuable learning experience.

Physician, Chile
MPH Program, Harvard School of Public Health

I strongly recommend this course to graduate students; you can learn how to discuss current topics, write reports, and make presentations. The field trips to healthcare organizations are also very interesting.

Physician, Japan
MPH Program, Harvard School of Public Health

I recommend this course to anyone coming to the United States to study in the health or medical fields. It will help you understand academic expectations in graduate school.

Pharmacist, Vietnam
MS Program, Massachusetts College of Pharmacy

APPENDIX 11.3

Medical and Scientific Writing
Writing and Speaking Evaluation
Writing
Arguments, Ideas, Evidence: *how well your writing sets forth arguments, discusses ideas, and gives the evidence from articles.*

(poor)   1   2   3   4   5   (excellent)

Communicative Quality: *how well you communicate the above in your writing.*

(poor)   1   2   3   4   5   (excellent)

Vocabulary and Sentence Structure: *how varied, correct, and advanced the vocabulary and grammar you use are.*

(poor)   1   2   3   4   5   (excellent)

Speaking
Fluency and Coherence: *how fast you speak without pauses, repetition or rephrasing and how well connected your ideas are.*

(poor)   1   2   3   4   5   (excellent)

Lexical Resource: *how varied and precise the words you use to express your ideas are.*

(poor)   1   2   3   4   5   (excellent)

Grammatical Range and Accuracy: *how correct and advanced the grammar you use is.*

(poor)   1   2   3   4   5   (excellent)

Pronunciation: *how well you approximate the American sound system and intonation/stress patterns.*

(poor)   1   2   3   4   5   (excellent)

Name: _____ Date: _____

Scores: Speaking ____ Writing ____ Vocabulary ____
Composite Score: ____

CHAPTER TWELVE

PRONUNCIATION AS LIFE AND DEATH: IMPROVING THE COMMUNICATION SKILLS OF NON-NATIVE ENGLISH SPEAKING PATHOLOGISTS

Joanna Labov and Cheryl Hanau

ABSTRACT

Many hospitals in the United States are under pressure to demonstrate an improvement in the English proficiency of international medical doctors. This chapter describes an English for professional medical communication course that was designed for international pathology residents but could be used effectively in any medical specialty. The effectiveness of the course, which focused on pronunciation, was measured by an authentic, on-the-job communication measure—a dictation of pathology specimens for transcription by medical secretaries. This type of course will be increasingly in demand to meet the needs of the numerous teaching hospitals that have international resident doctors on staff.

English Language and the Medical Profession: Instructing and Assessing
the Communication Skills of International Physicians
Innovation and Leadership in English Language Teaching, Volume 5, 261–285
Copyright © 2011 by Emerald Group Publishing Limited
All rights of reproduction in any form reserved
ISSN: 2041-272X/doi:10.1108/S2041-272X(2011)0000005018

INTRODUCTION

This chapter reports on the effectiveness of an innovative course designed to improve the English pronunciation of international medical graduates (IMGs) who are non-native English speaking pathologists. The doctors were required to attend the pronunciation course by their pathology department because their pronunciation was often incomprehensible to the medical secretaries who transcribed their dictations. Pathologists dictate reports that describe specimens removed by surgeons during surgery from patients' bodies as healthy or tumorous and, therefore, their accurate pronunciation is critical. In medical practice, a single mistake in transcription is unacceptable because it could mean the difference between life and death for a patient, for example, *anterior* understood as *inferior*. In addition, the transcriptions of the doctors' dictations of specimens are legal documents which are admissible in court and can be used in malpractice lawsuits.

An important aspect of pathologists' responsibilities is to describe all specimens in terms of their size, length, weight, color, and texture. This procedure is called a *gross examination* because the doctors examine the specimens visually and without the use of a microscope. The doctors dictate to a tape recorder their descriptions of the specimens while examining and measuring them. Their medical secretaries transcribe the dictations from the tapes, often listening to them multiple times. If the medical secretaries are unsure of the accuracy of their transcriptions, they submit them to the doctors to correct any errors they may have made in transcription. For this procedure to be effective, the doctors need to be able to recognize their mistakes in the transcriptions. The dictations can be considered to be "verbal photographs" because the transcriptions will be used later by other doctors to make medically important decisions after the specimens have been discarded. Therefore, it is critical for the health of the patient that the dictations are accurate and comprehensible. However, the dictations of pathologists for whom English is not the first language may be difficult to comprehend by their medical secretaries.

An internal review by the pathology department of an urban university's College of Medicine determined that a number of its nonnative English-speaking doctors were not always understood by the other doctors and the medical secretaries. Seven doctors in this category were required to attend the course "English for Professional Medical Communication" in order to improve their English communication skills, including their ability to dictate clearly to medical secretaries. The Accreditation Council for Graduate Medical Education (ACGME) required the university pathology department to evaluate its residents' interpersonal and communication competencies (see ACGME General Competencies) in order to maintain its accreditation as a teaching institution. The interpersonal and communication skills required by the ACGME for all residents include the ability to present information to consultants, referring physicians, and colleagues (Robertson, 2006). One of the specific interpersonal and communication competences pathology residents need is the ability to dictate in a comprehensible manner.

The intensive 10-week course was designed to improve the doctors' English pronunciation with a particular focus on their ability to dictate clearly their specimen reports. Transcriptions of these doctors' dictations were used as one of the course texts in order to improve the doctors' abilities to communicate while dictating and to increase their motivation to improve their pronunciation. This English for specific purpose (ESP) course was one of many ESP courses offered by a university-based intensive English language program for nonnative English-speaking doctors in Philadelphia (Hoekje, 2007).

A review of the research that has been conducted on the challenges that nonnative English-speaking medical doctors face in communicating on the job in hospitals in the United States is provided below. Following the review, a description of the ESP course, its course design, and the teaching method used will be given. The research questions, the methodology, and the results of a research study of the effectiveness of the course will then be presented.

Communicating Medical Information

Background

In 1999, the ACGME made the decision to require teaching hospitals to document their attempts to improve their native and nonnative English-speaking doctors' communication skills (Larkin, McKay, & Angelos, 2005). This decision was based on the current concern in the medical field for reducing doctors' language errors and the adverse effects of those errors on patients' health (Brennan et al., 2004; Delbanco & Bell, 2007; Kohn, Corrigan, & Donaldson, 1999; Leape et al., 1991; Martinez & Lo, 2008; Massachusetts Coalition for the Prevention of Medical Errors, 2006; Phillips & Bredder, 2002; Phillips, Christenfield, & Glynn, 1998). The ACGME's decision was also a result of the current concern in the medical field about the performance of the large number of IMGs who are training in hospitals in the United States (Bates & Andrew, 2001). In 2005, a quarter of all doctors (25.3% of 902,053) in the United States were IMGs coming from 127 countries such as India (9,468), Philippines (1,814), Mexico (807), China (96), and Columbia (46) (American Medical Association, 2007). In 2006, there were a total of 6,361 IMG pathologists in the United States comprising 33% of the pathologists in the United States (19,171) and 2.7% of the IMGs in the United States (236,669) (American Medical Association, 2008).

Teaching hospitals in the United States are required to demonstrate an improvement in their nonnative English-speaking doctors' interpersonal and communication skills (Robertson, 2006). According to Wilner (2007), IMGs face this challenge of learning effective communication skills in order to master the competencies required by the ACGME: (1) Patient Care, (2) Medical Knowledge, (3) Interpersonal and Communication Skills, (4) Professionalism, (5) Practice-Based Learning and Improvement, and (6) System-Based Practice (see ACGME General Competencies). Wilner (2007) states that the misinterpretation of intent or critical information resulting from IMGs' ineffective communication skills can result in "life threatening and potentially litigious ramifications" (Wilner, 2007, p. 14). He notes the important role of the accurate interpretation of intonation in the doctor–patient relationship and the accuracy of IMGs' pronunciation in communicating effectively when conveying medical information. Wilner (2007) provides examples of words which if misunderstood by IMGs could be critical to the health of their patients (*15 mg* vs. *50 mg*, *bleeding* vs. *breathing*) (p. 14). Other types of communication problems faced by doctors are (1) an inability to converse colloquially due to a lack of an informal style of speaking, (2) a lack of medical knowledge of technical words, and (3) perceptions of male/female gender roles which differ from the accepted North American gender role (Bates & Andrew, 2001).

Moreover, it has been found that IMGs' communication problems with patients and hospital personnel affect their clinical performance as a result of cultural differences, expectations, and procedural knowledge (Fiscella, Bothola, Roman-Diaz, Lue, & Frankel, 1997; Kales et al., 2006; Searight & Gafford, 2006; Whelan, 2006); discourse styles and communication styles (Bates & Andrew, 2001; Hoekje, 2007); and adherence to asymmetrical power relations (Erickson & Rittenberg, 1987). The English skills of IMGs have been shown to affect patient satisfaction and are considered as a weakness by IMGs' faculty and colleagues (Eggly et al., 1999). The results of these studies are relevant for IMGs who specialize in primary care, such as family medicine, pediatrics, and general internal medicine, and who need to interact with patients daily.

In contrast, since pathologists spend much of their time examining specimens, it might seem that their communication problems are less important than for other types of physicians. Nevertheless, it is critical that pathologists have competent interpersonal and communication skills when interpreting laboratory results and conveying this information to other doctors as well as other hospital personnel. For this reason, the focus of this chapter is on reporting the results of a research study that was conducted on the English pronunciation of a group of IMGs.

The IMG Pathologists' Communication Needs

The high-stakes tasks required of pathologists include the following: (1) interpreting laboratory data, (2) dictating specimen reports, and (3) speaking via intercom with doctors during surgery. According to the ACGME Program Requirements for Graduate Medical Education in Anatomic Pathology and Clinical Pathology (effective July 1, 2007), the competencies required of resident pathologists are: (1) Patient Care, (2) Medical Knowledge, (3) Interpersonal and Communication Skills, (4) Professionalism, (5) Practice-Based Learning and Improvement, and (6) System-Based Practice (see ACGME General Competencies). Of the ten interpersonal and communication skills required, there are two skills that relate directly to the dictation of specimen reports: (1) communicating effectively with physicians, other health professionals, and health related agencies, and (2) maintaining comprehensive, timely, and legible medical records, if applicable (ACGME, 2007a, p. 15).

Smith et al. (2006) propose curriculum content and evaluation guidelines for resident competencies in clinical pathology to include the following two communication skills: (1) the ability to provide a clear and informative report, and (2) the ability to provide direct communication to the referring physician or appropriate clinical personnel when interpretation of a laboratory test result reveals an urgent, critical, or unexpected finding, and to document this communication in an appropriate fashion. The mastery of both of these skills is essential for pathologists since the health of their patients is based on the doctors' use of clear and comprehensible speech.

THE ENGLISH FOR PROFESSIONAL MEDICAL COMMUNICATION COURSE

Introduction

In spring 2001, the director of the English Language Center in the same university system was contacted by a professor of pathology and laboratory medicine at the University College of Medicine, the second author. Based on the internal review, there was a perceived need for increased communication training for several nonnative English-speaking resident pathologists. During spring 2001, ESP specialists of the English Language Center met with representatives of the pathology department to observe critical tasks that the doctors are required to perform. The ESP specialists' goal was to use this information as a basis to design a course centered on the doctors' communication needs. Their pronunciation was seen as a critical skill since it is crucial for the patients' health that medical secretaries comprehend the doctors' specimen reports. Prior to the beginning of the class, the instructor met with the pathology department director and doctors at the hospital to explain the course.

The goal of this course was to improve the comprehensibility of the doctors' dictations of their specimen reports by achieving greater clarity and accuracy of their speech. Thus, the instructor's goal was not for the doctors to produce native-like English accents that would enable them to sound like native English speakers when they dictated their reports. Instead, the instructor's goal was to improve the doctors' comprehensibility as measured by the medical secretaries' comprehension of the dictations.

According to the second author, the return rate of the transcriptions of the University College of Medicine medical secretaries was about 5% of the total transcriptions. The hospital does not offer any formal training to the doctors on how to conduct dictations. However, the residents receive feedback as to when they should slow down or speak clearly. The medical secretaries replay any unclear segments of the dictations for reclarification by the doctor.

Course Design

The ESP course consisted of seven group class sessions and three individual sessions designed to provide individualized attention to the doctors' presentations of their dictations. The organization of the course required the doctors to present to the class a dictation three times.

Class 1: Introductions, diagnostics, goal-setting, tutoring schedules
Class 2: Individual tutorials
Class 3: Dictation presentation 1
Class 4: Overview of common issues in communication (segmentals)
Class 5: Individual tutorials (midterm conference)
Class 6: Dictation presentation 2
Class 7: More issues in communication (suprasegmentals)
Class 8: Individual tutorials
Class 9: Dictation presentation 3
Class 10: Conferences, certificates, wrap-up

The duration of each English class session was 90 minutes, which resulted in a total of 15 hours of class time. The course was held at the main facility of the university English Language Center and not at the hospital site. The first author was the instructor of the course.

Students

The doctors enrolled in the course were seven highly motivated and fluent nonnative English-speaking pathology residents whose speech was fossilized, or in more recent terminology, stabilized. The doctors' speech was determined to be fluent based on diagnostic oral interviews conducted on the first day of the course. The term *fossilization* refers to fixed features of first language phonology and grammar in the second language that are resistant to development (Selinker, 1972). The more recent term *stabilization* used by Long (2005) refers to fossilization as nonmovement, which can imply the possibility of future change in language forms.

The doctors had begun learning English 10 to 20 years before taking the course and had fixed phonological and grammatical patterns in their second language. An example of a fixed phonological pattern is a Chinese-speaking doctor's deletion of the /n/ in the final position of the second syllable of the word *abundant* as heard in a dictation.

Two Chinese doctors and one Peruvian doctor were enrolled in the course in the winter term of 2001. Three Chinese doctors and a Peruvian doctor were enrolled in the course in the spring term of 2002. The group comprised three female and four male doctors whose ages ranged from 30 to 40 years. The Chinese doctors were raised in Beijing, Shanghai, and Shandong, and the Peruvian doctors were raised in Lima. These pathology residents had already graduated from medical schools in their respective countries and were enrolled at the time of the study in their first and second years in a five-year pathology residency program. After completing the program, the doctors would be eligible to take the board examinations required to become certified pathologists in the United States.

Teaching Method

The method used to teach the course was task-based, communicative, and student-centered. Visual, tactile, and experiential methods were used to teach the doctors how to articulate English phonemes and to differentiate between them in terms of production and perception. A communicative approach was used as shown by the doctors' in-class presentations of their dictations throughout the semester, in which the focus was on the communication of meaning.

The transcriptions of the doctors' dictations of their specimen reports were an integral component of the course because they played an important role in the course requirements, format, and the teaching methodology of the course. (See Appendix 12.1 for an example of the transcription of a Chinese-speaking doctor's dictation.) The transcriptions were used as course materials, and the words taught in the course were in the transcriptions. The decision to use the transcriptions as course materials was based on the doctors' communication needs for their professional practice.

The content of the class included the following topics, which were also used to improve the doctors' pronunciation during instruction: the height and duration of vowels, vowel contrasts, place and manner of articulation, voicing, and consonant contrasts. The suprasegmental features of intonation, stress, pausing, prosody, and rate of speech were also presented to the doctors to increase comprehensibility.

The pronunciation textbook selected was Orion (1999) because the author's use of graphics was particularly appropriate for medical personnel. This text displays sagittal views of the oral and naval cavities for pairs of consonants and vowels. The graphics display vowel contrasts, consonant contrasts, and a list of instructions for the articulation for each phoneme. This visual approach to teaching pronunciation proved to be useful for the doctors, given their knowledge of the articulatory organs, and helped them to learn the places of articulation for consonants quickly. Tactile activities were also used in the course.[1]

Other techniques and materials used in the course were tissues to teach syllable-initial aspiration, mirrors to view the oral cavity, and rubber bands to demonstrate vowel duration preceding voiced and voiceless consonants (see, e.g., Acton, 1997; Gilbert, 1993). The Chinese-speaking doctors were familiar with the International Phonetic Alphabet (IPA), which was used during the course as a tool to teach them to pronounce English vowels and consonants accurately. The Peruvians were taught the IPA symbols that they needed to know to participate in the class activities.

The doctors were asked by the instructor to bring to the first day of class a transcription of a dictation and an audio recording of themselves reading it. They were required to record themselves reading the same transcription at three times throughout the semester (Weeks 1, 6, and 9). The purpose of the recordings was to create a record for assessment of their ability to dictate that was as realistic as possible to the tasks which are required of their job. The recorded dictations were used to determine which words the doctors had problems pronouncing and to assess their progress in improving their pronunciation during the semester. The instructor (first author) listened to the original dictation to determine the main pronunciation problems and plan the teaching program. She created a list of the words which had been pronounced incorrectly by all or most of the doctors. This list of words was used as course material for the doctors to practice in class individually and as a group. The accurate pronunciation of technical and nontechnical medical words found in the dictations which the doctors pronounced inaccurately was also taught explicitly in class.

The activities used in the course included making three recordings, two in-class oral readings of the doctors' written dictations and instruction on the words which they had pronounced inaccurately. Three tutorial sessions for individual doctors were held throughout the semester so that each doctor received individual attention regarding the pronunciation of his or her dictations. Intensive work was conducted during the tutorial sessions on the production of specific vowels and/or consonants. The same topics used in the individual sessions were then used in the following group session with the whole class. For example, the native Chinese-speaking doctors practiced in class /l/ and /r/ words from their dictations such as *plunging* and *red* as well as nasals in word-final position such as *firm*, which proved to be difficult for them and many other Chinese speakers to pronounce (Swan & Smith, 2001). The native Spanish-speaking doctors practiced in class palatals and affricates in word-initial position, such as *yellow* and *gelatin* which proved to be difficult for them and many other Spanish speakers to pronounce accurately (Swan & Smith, 2001).

An important component of the course was to heighten the doctors' awareness that although they speak, read, and write English fluently, their pronunciation was often unintelligible to their listeners. These busy doctors were committed to spending an hour and a half in class once a week which they would normally have spent in other ways relevant to their practice. Therefore, it was important that the doctors understood that the improvement of their pronunciation was critical for their professional practice. This understanding increased the doctors' motivation to improve their pronunciation because of their desire to become competent medical professionals and their interest in practicing medicine in the United States. The doctors applied themselves to learn the course content and completed all assignments diligently. They had positive evaluations of the course, enjoyed it, and believed that their pronunciation had improved as a result of the course.

EVALUATING THE EFFECTIVENESS OF INSTRUCTION: THE RESEARCH STUDY

At the time of the course, there was interest on the part of the university English Language Center and the College of Medicine's pathology department to document improvement in the comprehensibility of the doctors' pronunciation on a phonemic level. Because of the need for research studies that investigate the comprehensibility of nonnative English-speaking pathologists' dictations and the types of comprehensibility problems that may affect the accuracy of their transcriptions, a research study was designed to assess this issue. The research study also addressed the need for research to determine whether doctors who have clear evidence of stabilized phonology can improve their English pronunciation through intensive study. This present study addresses the above needs.

One of the goals of the study was to determine the extent to which non-native English speaking pathologists have problems communicating in English. A second goal was to determine the specific types of communication problems that doctors have when dictating specimen reports to the medical secretaries. A third goal was to assess the effectiveness of a 10-week course designed to improve the doctors' ability to dictate clearly in English.

Research Questions

The research questions posed in this study were the following:

(1) How frequently do IMGs have communication problems in dictating reports on specimens to medical secretaries?
(2) What are the types of communication problems that IMGs have in dictating reports on specimens to medical secretaries?
(3) Was the course "English for Professional Medical Communication" effective in improving IMGs' ability to dictate clearly reports on specimens?

The Methodology of the Study

Subjects

After the course was completed, the research study was initiated in order to determine the effectiveness of the course. The tapes of four Chinese and one Peruvian doctor were selected as research data from the seven doctors who had participated in the course. The other tapes were not chosen because one doctor had recorded a speech he had given at a conference instead of selecting a dictation and another doctor's dictation tape had poor clarity due to technical problems.

Data Collection

The doctors recorded themselves reading dictations of their own specimen reports three times during the semester (Weeks 1, 6, and 9). The same dictations were read and recorded by the doctors in each of the three weeks. The five dictations and the doctor's first languages are shown in Table 12.1.

Medical Secretaries. Four experienced medical secretaries who work in pathology departments in Philadelphia hospitals were paid to transcribe the dictations. Their length of experience transcribing dictations ranged from 6 to 23 years. All of the medical secretaries were native English speakers, had a minimum of a high school education, and no formal medical education. The medical secretaries did not work at the university's College of Medicine and thus did not know the doctors who participated in this study.

Transcriptions. Each of the five doctors dictated specimen reports in Weeks 1, 6, and 9. Transcriptions of the doctors' dictations of their reports in Weeks 1 and 9 were examined in order to document the doctors'

Table 12.1. Five Pathologists' First Languages and Specimens Examined.

Doctor's First Languages	Specimens
1. Chinese	Breast
2. Spanish	Colon
3. Chinese	Colon
4. Chinese	Heart
5. Chinese	Placenta

improvement from the beginning to the end of the course. The reports taped by the doctors totaled ten reports. The tapes were randomized and given to the medical secretaries without the doctors' names being identified so that they would not be influenced by the speaker's identity while transcribing the dictations. A first set of five tapes was given to each secretary containing reports from either Week 1 or 9 in random order. After completing this set of tapes, the secretary returned the five tapes to the pathology program director. Then, a second set of five tapes which also contained reports from Week 1 or 9 in random order was given to each secretary. Thus, each secretary transcribed all of the 10 reports but in different randomized order. This process resulted in 40 transcriptions.

The medical secretaries were given the following instructions for transcribing the dictations: Leave a blank when you did not understand a word; circle the words with a blue pen that you have difficulty understanding; and circle the words with a red pen that you have difficulty understanding but understood with the help of the context surrounding the word.

Data Analysis

The doctors' production of words which were judged unintelligible and which were misunderstood by the medical secretaries were categorized and totaled according to the type of error produced (Table 12.2). The term *unintelligible* was operationalized to mean that the medical secretaries left a blank in the transcription because they did not understand the word and could not guess what it meant. The term *misunderstood* was operationalized to mean that the medical secretaries transcribed incorrectly the word that they thought they understood but were later shown to be incorrect by the doctors. Two other types of words were also categorized and totaled: (1) words that the medical secretaries had difficulty understanding but were understood after they listened to them; and (2) words that the medical secretaries had difficulty understanding but were understood after the lexical contexts were relistened to multiple times (i.e., the preceding and/or following words).

The words in each category were subdivided into technical and nontechnical words by the instructor of the course. Words characterized as technical words are words that are normally used exclusively in a medical context—for example, *cotyledons, hemicolectomy, infarction, intraventricular,* and *histological.* The following are examples of nontechnical words: *designated, flat, tan, parenthesis, possible, size,* and *yellow.*

Table 12.2.   Types of Judgments of Doctors' Dictations.

Medical Secretaries' Judgments	Example
1. Unintelligible	(left blank)
2. Misunderstood	*patch* as *plaque*
3. Difficult to comprehend but comprehensible	*appendix*
4. Difficult to comprehend but understood by context	*unremarkable*

Research Findings

Findings for Research Question 1

Tables 12.3 and 12.4 provide data that show whether and to what extent the doctors' dictations were comprehended by medical secretaries. Table 12.3 presents the comprehensibility of the five doctors' dictations in Week 1 as determined by the medical secretaries. The text of the dictations totaled 907 words. Since the dictations were listened to by the medical secretaries four times each, the result was 3,628 judgments.

Table 12.3 demonstrates that a total of 72 (2%) of the words produced by the doctors were unintelligible to the medical secretaries. There were a total of 52 (1.4%) occurrences in which the medical secretaries misunderstood the doctors' words. At first glance, a total of 3.4% of the words that were incomprehensible to the medical secretaries may seem to be a small percentage. However, the incomprehension of 124 words is critical in the medical profession because one mistake in comprehension in this high-stakes environment could affect a patient's health dramatically.

Incomprehensible and Difficult to Comprehend Words.   Table 12.4 provides an analysis of 65 words produced by the doctors which were incomprehensible to the four medical secretaries. The combined four medical secretaries' judgments of the 65 words totaled 150 judgments because they include each of the medical secretaries' judgments of the words and some of the words occurred multiple times. These judgments are a subset of the combined medical secretaries' judgments (3,628) of the doctors' dictations (907 words) shown in Table 12.3. Recall that the term *difficult to comprehend* is used for words which the medical secretaries understood after listening to them several times, or by relistening to the words preceding and/or following them.

Table 12.3. Medical Secretaries' Comprehensibility of Five Doctors' Dictations in Week 1 of the Course ($N = 3,628$).

Comprehensibility of Words	Judgments of Words N (%)
Comprehensible	3,504 (96.6)
Incomprehensible	
Unintelligible	72 (2.0)
Misunderstood	52 (1.4)
Total	3,628 (100)

Table 12.4. Judgments of Doctors' Productions ($N = 65$ words; $N = 150$ judgments).

Comprehensibility of Words	Judgments of Words N (%)
Incomprehensible words	
Unintelligible	72 (58)
Misunderstood	52 (42)
Total	124 (100)
Difficult to comprehend words	
Understood by relistening to the word	14 (54)
Understood by the context of the word	12 (46)
Total	26 (100)
Total judgments of doctors' productions	150

Table 12.4 shows that more than half of the incomprehensible words (58%) were unintelligible to the medical secretaries, which indicates that the doctors' pronunciation was so unclear that the medical secretaries could not guess their meaning. However, it is less probable that the unintelligible words would result in a medical error than the words which were misunderstood by the medical secretaries. Unlike the misunderstood words, the words which were unintelligible to the medical secretaries would be explained to the medical secretaries by the doctors because it would become clear to the medical secretaries that they had not understood the words and would need clarification from the doctors. In the normal process of transcription review, the doctors read the secretaries' transcripts to check for accuracy. However, the words which were misunderstood by the medical

secretaries would need to be caught by the doctors themselves upon reviewing the transcript in order to be clarified. This would require that the doctors realize that certain words were incorrect in the dictation.

A total of 54% of the words that were difficult for the medical secretaries to understand were only understood by their listening to them multiple times. Nearly half of the words were only understood also by listening to the context, the words before or after the questionable word. These findings show the extent to which the doctors' dictations were difficult for the medical secretaries to comprehend.

Summary of the Findings for Research Question 1. Communication is a severe problem for the doctors as shown by the findings displayed in Tables 12.3 and 12.4. The large number of unintelligible, misunderstood, and difficult to comprehend words produced by the doctors could result in numerous medical errors.

Research Question 2

Research Question 2 focused on the type of communication problems that doctors have when dictating specimen reports to medical secretaries. Table 12.5 provides the medical secretaries' comprehensibility of the doctors' productions of technical and nontechnical words. Table 12.6 presents a phonological analysis of the medical secretaries' comprehension of the Chinese-speaking and Spanish-speaking doctors' dictations.

Technical and Nontechnical Words. Table 12.6 presents an analysis of the combined medical secretaries' judgments of the doctors' production of technical words and nontechnical words that were incomprehensible to the medical secretaries. These words consist of the same words which were judged by the medical secretaries, shown in Table 12.4.

Table 12.5. The Comprehensibility of Technical Words Produced by Doctors as Judged by Medical Secretaries.

Type of Words	Unintelligible Words *n* (%)	Misunderstood Words *n* (%)	Total *N* (%)
Technical words	18 (25)	10 (19)	28 (22)
Nontechnical words	54 (75)	42 (81)	96 (77)
Total	72 (100)	52 (100)	124 (100)

Table 12.6. An Analysis of Selected Incomprehensible Words Produced by Chinese-Speaking and Spanish-Speaking Doctors.

Types of Problems	Chinese-Speaking Doctors		Spanish-Speaking Doctor	
	Unintelligible Words[a]	Words Misunderstood	Unintelligible Words[a]	Words Misunderstood
/æ/, /ɛ/, /I/	edge	flat as bright		thin as seen, ascending as descending
/l/-/r/		length as mass flat as bright red as gray		
Consonant clusters	plunging			
Palatals		patch as plaque		thin as seen, ascending as descending, yellow as gelatin
Syllable-final nasals /n/, /m/		firm as full, chambers as changes		
Combinations including /n/, /m/, /l/ and /v/ in the syllable codas of multisyllabic words; stress patterns	uninvolved invaded designated parenthesis ascending abundant unremarkable circumference valve	anterior as inferior	unremarkable	

[a]Upon review of the transcription these words were identified.

Table 12.5 shows that the comprehensibility of the doctors' dictations is greater when they dictate technical words than nontechnical words. Out of the total judgments, only 22% of the doctors' incomprehensible words were technical words whereas 77% were nontechnical words. This is an important finding because many medical specialists may assume that doctors have problems accurately pronouncing mainly technical words.

Of note, only 4% of the words in the texts of the five dictations (907) were categorized as technical words. A number of these 35 words occurred multiple times but were only counted once. Thus, 87% of the combined medical secretaries' judgments (3,628) of the doctors' five dictations were of nontechnical words whereas only 13% were of technical words. These findings indicate the disproportionate number of nontechnical to technical words that occurred in the dictations.

For the purpose of illustration, Table 12.6 provides a phonological analysis of selected incomprehensible words produced by the Chinese-speaking and Spanish-speaking doctors. The selected examples are provided for illustrative purposes and are not exhaustive.

Table 12.6 shows that a combination of phonological factors contributed to the Chinese and Spanish-speaking doctors' problems in dictating clearly such as vowels /æ/, /ɛ/, /I/; the consonants /l/ and /r/, consonant clusters, and syllable-final nasals. Of note is the finding that the doctors have problems producing accurate word-internal combinations, including /n, /m/, and /v/ in the final syllables of multisyllabic words such as the word *uninvolved*. The word *uninvolved* used in the sentence "The uninvolved colonic mucosa is gray, tan, and unremarkable," is challenging for the doctors to pronounce accurately because it has two syllable-final nasals, /v/, and /l/, and three syllables with stress on the first and third syllables (see Appendix 12.1). One can see that the incomprehensible words in Table 12.6 are nontechnical words that are often used on a daily basis.

Nature of Misunderstandings. The following two examples illustrate the seriousness of the nature of the doctors' problems in pronouncing English accurately and thus producing comprehensible dictations. The medical secretaries misunderstood two words spoken by two Chinese doctors that are critical in the medical field: *infarction* and *firm*. The potential for medical error is serious in the following examples.

Example 1: A Placenta Specimen
Infarction (dead tissue)—transcribed as *infection*.
Example: "Examination of the parenchyma [tissues surrounding the fetus] reveals an area of *infection* measuring 4.8 × 3.2 × 14 cm."
It is critical that doctors distinguish clearly between the words *infarction* and *infection* because their meanings differ greatly. *Infarction* means dead tissue and *infection* refers to the infiltration of tissue by microorganisms. Placental pathology reports are often requested in cases where an infant or child has deficits that are alleged to have occurred during delivery. A lesion in the placenta indicates that a problem was present before delivery, which means that no error was conducted by hospital staff during delivery. If the abnormal tissue was infected during delivery, it would indicate that an error had been made by medical personnel. The accurate transcription of the

specimen description could be used by hospitals to defend themselves against malpractice suits.

Example 2: A Breast Specimen

Firm—transcribed as *full*.

Example: "A $5 \times 4 \times 4$ cm *full* mass [lump] is located in the center involving four quadrants."

Doctors need to pronounce the word *firm* accurately because they use the term to convey their suspicions that a lump in a breast specimen may be malignant. The substitution of the word *full* in this context causes this important information to be lost. The inaccurate pronunciation of the word *firm* could result in a medical error if the transcription of the word were not caught by the secretary as an error. If this were to happen, it is possible that a woman who has breast cancer might not receive treatment.

Summary of the Findings for Research Question 2. The problems that doctors face in dictating clearly in English are not confined to their pronunciation of technical vocabulary because a large number of nontechnical words were incomprehensible to the medical secretaries. Important phonological problems found in this study were: (1) inaccurate stress in complex words especially when coupled with the mispronunciation of consonants (e.g., *circumference*); (2) inaccurate pronunciation of vowels such as /æ/ and /ɛ/(e.g., *flat* and *edge*); and (3) inaccurate combinations of /n/, /m/, and /l/ in the syllable codas of multisyllabic words (e.g., *uninvolved*).

Findings for Research Question 3

The third research question focused on whether the ESP course was effective in improving the doctors' abilities to dictate clearly their specimen reports. Tables 12.7 and 12.8 provide data that document that the ESP course was effective in this regard.

Table 12.7 presents improvement in the comprehensibility of the doctors' pronunciation of 11 words that had been taught explicitly to the doctors and 23 words that had not been taught explicitly. The combined medical secretaries' judgments of the 34 words total 57 judgments in Week 1 and 24 judgments in Week 9. The medical secretaries' judgments of the 57 words are a subset of their judgments of unintelligible and misunderstood words in Table 12.4. Of particular interest to the instructor-researcher was the improvement in the pronunciation of words that were explicitly taught and practiced in the course. "Explicitly taught" refers to those words that were taught and practiced in the course. Of the 57 words that were judged incomprehensible in Week 1, nine were later explicitly taught in the course.

Table 12.7. Improvement in the Comprehensibility of Words Taught Explicitly to Doctors as Judged by Medical Secretaries.

Words Produced	Incomprehensible Words	
	Week 1	Week 9
Taught explicitly	23	5
Not taught explicitly	34	19
Total	57	24

Table 12.8. Improvement in the Comprehensibility of Words Produced by the Doctors in Weeks 1 and 9 ($N = 3,628$).

Comprehensibility of Words	Judgments of Words	
	Week 1	Week 9
Comprehensible	3,504	3,537
Incomprehensible	124	91
Total words	3,628	3,628

Table 12.7 shows a decrease of 33 words in the number of incomprehensible words produced by the doctors to the medical secretaries in Week 9. This finding demonstrates improvement in their ability to dictate clearly to the medical secretaries. The doctors' productions of incomprehensible words that had been taught explicitly in the ESP course decreased by 78% from Weeks 1 to 9 (23 to 5 words). The decrease in the number of incomprehensible words produced by the doctors that were taught explicitly was significant at the $p < .01$ level.

There was also improvement in the comprehensibility of words which were not explicitly taught to the doctors. The doctors' productions of incomprehensible words in Week 9 which were not explicitly taught decreased by 44% from Week 1 (34 to 19 words). It is possible that the doctors improved their pronunciation of the words that were not explicitly taught to them because they applied the concepts and skills they learned in the course to the pronunciation of these words.

Table 12.8 presents the comprehensibility of the doctors' dictations as determined by the combined four medical secretaries' judgments (3,628) of the total words read by the five doctors (907 words) in Weeks 1 and 9.

Table 12.8 shows an increase in the doctors' production of comprehensible words in Week 9 from Week 1 as determined by the medical secretaries (3,504 to 3,537 words). As shown in Table 12.7, the doctors' production of incomprehensible words decreased by 33 words. Thus, the doctors' production of incomprehensible words decreased from 124 words in Week 1 to 91 words in Week 9. The decrease in the number of incomprehensible words produced by the doctors in Week 9 was significant at the $p < .0001$ level.

Summary of the Findings for Research Question 3. The findings demonstrate a significant decrease in the doctors' productions of incomprehensible words, including the words taught explicitly to the doctors as well as those words not taught explicitly to them. The significant increase in the comprehensibility of the doctors' abilities to dictate clearly demonstrates the effectiveness of the ESP pronunciation course.

DISCUSSION

The improvement in the doctors' pronunciation demonstrates the effectiveness of the ESP course in increasing their ability to clearly dictate reports on specimens. The course design, curriculum, teaching approach, and materials used were designed to improve the doctors' English pronunciation as much as possible in a short amount of time. Thus, the ideal teaching situation was created for doctors who were motivated and took the course seriously. It is surprising that this course was as successful as it was shown to be given the challenges that adult second language learners face in improving their pronunciation (Macdonald, Yule, & Powers, 1994; Stenson, Downing, Smith, & Smith, 1992; Vardanian, 1964). However, it is encouraging to know that given an ideal teaching situation, students of this type can improve their pronunciation so that they can be understood by others who need to do so on a daily basis.

The methodology used in the ESP course was repetition of the same dictation before, during, and after instruction with a focus on the key terms used in the doctors' field. These dedicated doctors were highly motivated people who were used to excelling in their field. Their motivation was high to excel in the ESP course because of a possible fear of having poor evaluations and failure. One can imagine that it would be harder to see such results when the vocabulary is varied in spontaneous speech or the student is less internally and/or externally motivated.

Of significance is the finding that the doctors transferred their improvement of the words taught in the ESP course to words that were not taught explicitly in the course (see Table 12.7). The success of this method has potential for improving the pronunciation of a large number of words for learners who do not have time to spend many hours in class. They could potentially learn to improve their pronunciation of a selected list of words in class and then continue to practice them at home. This could be a very effective methodological outcome of the results of this study which could be useful for IMGs and other users of English who need to improve their pronunciation but have busy schedules that prevent them from spending a great deal of time in class.

The dictation by doctors of their specimen reports is a high-stakes situation because even one error made could prove fatal to the patients' health during surgery or over an extended period of time if the wrong diagnosis is reported. It can be argued that the transcription errors that can cause a medical error result from misunderstandings and not unintelligible words. Misunderstandings are caused by the medical secretaries' tendency to find meaningful but incorrect interpretations of the words they transcribe. The cases in which the medical secretaries think they have succeeded but in fact have not because they have misunderstood the doctors' intent are the most important and interesting cases.

The following example is such a case. The word *patch* correctly used was found in the following sentence in Dr. T's dictation of a specimen from a patient's heart: "The epicardium which is smooth but covered with the anterior right ventricle appears to be composed of artificial patch-like material." However, in Week 1, Dr. T's pronunciation of the word *patch* was understood by all four medical secretaries as *plaque*. This misunderstanding was the result of the insertion of /l/ by Dr. T and possibly the multiple meanings of the word *plaque* in English. At the beginning of the semester all four medical secretaries transcribed the phrase "patch-like material" as "plaque-like material" whereas at the end of the semester each of them transcribed it accurately. In Week 1, Dr. T's pronunciation of the word *patch* as [plæk] shows that she overproduced /l/ and velarized the palatal /tʃ/ to /k/. In Week 9, Dr. T's production of [pætʃ] reflects her accurate pronunciation of the palatal /tʃ/ and nonuse of /l/. An independent listening by the first author of Dr. T's pronunciation of the word *patch* in her dictation in Weeks 1 and 9 confirmed the above analysis.

The medical secretaries may have found it plausible that the heart's epicardium would have artificial plaque-like material on it because the word *plaque* refers to a deposit of material in a bodily tissue or organ. The medical secretary's job as transcriber is to create a text that is meaningful to the reader rather than to transcribe sounds into isolated words without regard to context. In other words, the transcription creates a schema (Anderson, 2004) for interpreting the words. The more plausible a word appears to the medical secretaries, the more likely it is that it will escape detection and result in a medical error. Words that are transcribed incorrectly because they appear to be plausible, such as *plaque*, may not be detected even by reviewers or doctors themselves as incorrect and thus may result in a medical error.

The medical secretaries' transcription of difficult words is a mark of the doctors' success whereas the secretaries' failure to transcribe words that are unintelligible can be considered a mark of the doctors' lack of success. It is clear that the doctors need to focus on improving their pronunciation of the words which were unintelligible to the medical secretaries and difficult to comprehend. However, the most important types of words which are needed for pronunciation training are those which were misunderstood because they may be the most likely to cause medical errors.

The general public expects that pathologists and other doctors will not fail in their work. Thus, it is essential to teach pronunciation to doctors in a high-stakes situation where the outcome of success is critical. This approach to teaching pronunciation contrasts with the general approach that exists in teaching pronunciation to second language learners because pronunciation teachers generally do not consider the teaching of pronunciation to be literally a life and death issue. They also do not expect to find a significant decrease in the incomprehensibility of students' pronunciation in a 10-week period of time. However, this possibility depends on the specialized range of vocabulary and the motivation of the learner. Specialists in the field of teaching pronunciation will be heartened to learn about the successful results of this intensive, communication-oriented, professional needs-based course designed for success.

Pedagogical Implications

The use of authentic, professional task-based materials is effective in the teaching of pronunciation to second language learners. Dictations, transcriptions, and vocabulary lists can be used to teach motivated students who desire to improve their pronunciation. Doctors can be advised to spell words that have been shown to be difficult to comprehend while dictating (e.g., words beginning in /l/ and /r/, /θ/ or /ð/). The techniques used in the pronunciation course can be applied to nonnative English-speaking professionals in specialties other than pathology. This type of course will be increasingly in demand in order to fulfill the needs of numerous teaching hospitals which have many international residents on staff. It was designed for international pathology residents but can be effective for any specialized area of medicine as well as for teaching pronunciation in nonmedical contexts.

Suggestions for Future Research

It would be useful to replicate this study using a greater number of native Chinese-speaking and Spanish-speaking doctors as well as doctors from other language backgrounds. It would be valuable to teach these doctors the words found to be challenging for the doctors in the current study—*designated, uninvolved, plunging*—in order to investigate their progress in improving pronunciation of the words. It would also be valuable to use as subjects doctors in medical areas other than pathology to determine what types of pronunciation problems they have when communicating with patients and hospital personnel.

CONCLUSION

Accurate pronunciation by medical doctors is a life and death issue. The high improvement rate of the doctors' pronunciation skills in this study demonstrates the effectiveness of the pronunciation course, "English for Professional Medical Communication." Highly motivated doctors whose speech has stabilized can improve the comprehensibility of their English pronunciation in a short period of time by attending an ESP course tailored to their needs and interests. The use of dictations as task-based instruction proved to be an effective method of improving the doctors' communication skills. Pre- and post-evaluation of the doctors' oral dictations by medical secretaries revealed an improvement in the comprehensibility of the pronunciation of the doctors' dictations. The improvement of stabilized, adult second language speakers' pronunciation can occur given the correct pedagogical situation.

NOTE

1. For example, a tactile activity was used to teach the accurate pronunciation of apical /l/ and /r/, enabling the doctors to feel the tip of their tongues when pronouncing words that have /l/ in syllable-initial position. The doctors were asked

to place a chopstick in their mouths horizontally while they said four sentences that contain words that have /l/ and /r/ in contrasting position (see Appendix 12.2). By doing so, the doctors could feel the contrast between the words that require the articulation of the tip of the tongue for /l/ and /r/ and those which do not.

ACKNOWLEDGMENTS

I would like to thank the following people for their support, encouragement, and suggestions for my manuscript: Teresa Labov, William Labov, Barbara Hoekje, and Chia-ying Pan.

APPENDIX 12.1

Text Previously Dictated, Transcribed, and Corrected Used to Test a Chinese Doctor's Dictation Ability in Weeks 1 and 9

(1) Three polyps in the colonic mucosa are identified and named P1, P2
(2) and P3. P1 measures $0.6 \times 0.5 \times 0.4$ cm and is 3.5 cm from the
(3) tumor and 12 cm from the ileum margin. P2 measures $0.25 \times 0.2 \times$
(4) 0.2 cm and is 3.5 cm from the tumor, 7 cm from the ileum
(5) margin. P3 is flat and measures $0.6 \times 0.5 \times 0.1$ cm and is 23 cm
(6) from the tumor, 16.5 cm from the distal margin. The uninvolved
(7) colonic mucosa is gray, tan and unremarkable.

APPENDIX 12.2

Four Sentences With /l/ and /r/ Alterations in Contrasting Position

(1) I correct wrong sentences.
(2) I collect long sentences.
(3) I collect wrong sentences.
(4) I correct long sentences.

Written by Manami Suzuki (from PennTesolEast presentation; cited with permission).

ACGME GENERAL COMPETENCIES

General Competencies
Minimum Program Requirements Language
Approved by the ACGME, September 28, 1999
Educational Program
www.acgme.org/outcome/comp/compMin.asp

The residency program must require its residents to obtain competencies in the 6 areas below to the level expected of a new practitioner. Toward this end, programs must define the specific knowledge, skills, and attitudes required and provide educational experiences as needed in order for their residents to demonstrate:

a. Patient Care that is compassionate, appropriate, and effective for the treatment of health problems and the promotion of health
b. Medical Knowledge about established and evolving biomedical, clinical, and cognate (e.g., epidemiological and social-behavioral) sciences and the application of this knowledge to patient care
c. Practice-Based Learning and Improvement that involves investigation and evaluation of their own patient care, appraisal and assimilation of scientific evidence, and improvements in patient care
d. Interpersonal and Communication Skills that result in effective information exchange and teaming with patients, their families, and other health professionals
e. Professionalism, as manifested through a commitment to carrying out professional responsibilities, adherence to ethical principles, and sensitivity to a diverse patient population
f. Systems-Based Practice, as manifested by actions that demonstrate an awareness of and responsiveness to the larger context and system of health care and the ability to effectively call on system resources to provide care that is of optimal value

WEB SITES

Academy of Medical Royal Colleges	www.aomrc.org.uk
Accreditation Council for Graduate Medical Education	www.acgme.org
Adult Migrant English Program Research Centre	www.icms.com.au/AMEP2006/abstract/49.htm
American Board of Internal Medicine	www.abim.org
American Medical Association, International Medical Graduates	www.ama-assn.org/ama/pub/about-ama/our-people/member-groups-sections/international-medical-graduates/imgs-in-united-states.shtml
Australian Medical Council, International Medical Graduates	www.amc.org.au
Boston University, Center for English Language and Orientation Programs	www.bu.edu/celop
British Medical Journal	www.bmj.com
Council of Europe	www.coe.int/lportal/web/coe-portal
Educational Commission for Foreign Medical Graduates	www.ecfmg.org
English Medium Education in China	www.chinaenglishmedium.com
General Medical Council	www.gmc-uk.org

International English Language Testing System™ (IELTS™)	www.ielts.org/default.aspx
International Medical Travel Journal	www.imtj.com
Kaohsiung Medical University	http://www.english2.kmu.edu.tw
Kaohsiung Medical University, Faculty of Medicine for Post-Baccalaureate	www.kmu.edu.tw/~spbm/eng-web/ programs/overview.html
Kaplan Medical	www.kaptest.com/Medical_Licensing/ Step-2-CS/index.html
Ministry of Education, Republic of China (Taiwan)	http://www.english.moe.gov.tw
National Health Service, Health and Social Care Information Centre	www.ic.nhs.uk
Taiwan Medical Tourism Development Association	www.tmtda.org/en
United States Medical Licensing Examination® (USMLE®)	www.usmle.org
USMLEWorld, LLC	www.usmleworld.com
Virtual Mentor, American Medical Association Journal of Ethics	www.virtualmentor.org

REFERENCES

A patient who changed my practice. *British Medical Journal*, Ongoing column.

Accreditation Council for Graduate Medical Education. (2007a). *ACGME program requirements for graduate medical education in anatomic pathology and clinical pathology.* Retrieved from www.acgme.org/acWebsite/downloads/RRC_progReq/300pathology_07012007.pdf. Accessed on July 28, 2008.

Accreditation Council for Graduate Medical Education. (2007b). *ACGME standards.* Retrieved from www.acgme.org/outcome/Comp/compFull.asp. Accessed on December 7, 2007.

Accreditation Council for Graduate Medical Education. (2009). *Outcome project: Enhancing residency education through outcomes assessment.* Retrieved from www.acgme.org/outcome. Accessed on June 23, 2009.

Acton, W. (1997). Seven suggestions of highly successful pronunciation teaching. *The Language Teacher Online.* Retrieved from langue.hyper.chubu.ac.jp/jalt/pub/tlt/97/feb/seven.html. Accessed on July 28, 2008.

Adolphs, S., Brown, B., Carter, R., Crawford, P., & Sahota, O. (2004). Applying corpus linguistics in a health care context. *Journal of Applied Linguistics, 1*(1), 9–28.

Ainsworth-Vaughn, N. (2001). The discourse of medical encounters. In: D. Schiffrin, D. Tannen & H. Hamilton (Eds.), *Handbook of discourse analysis* (pp. 453–469). Malden, MA: Blackwell.

Alguire, P., Whelan, G., & Rajput, V. (2009). *The international medical graduate's guide to U.S. medicine and residency training.* Philadelphia, PA: American College of Physicians.

American Medical Association. (2007). *International medical graduates in the U.S. workforce: A discussion paper.* Retrieved from www.ama-assn.org/ama1/pub/upload/mm/18/img-workforce-paper.pdf. Accessed on September 5, 2008.

American Medical Association. (2008). *Physician characteristics and distribution in the U.S.* Chicago, IL: American Medical Association.

American Medical Association. (2009). *Member groups and sections: International medical graduates.* Retrieved from www.ama-assn.org/ama/pub/about-ama/our-people/member-groups-sections/international-medical-graduates.shtml. Accessed on June 23, 2009.

Andary, L., Stolk, Y., & Klimidis, S. (2003). *Assessing mental health across cultures.* Bowen Hills: Australian Academic Press.

Anderson, R. C. (2004). Role of the reader's schema in comprehension, learning and memory. In: R. R. Ruddell & N. J. Unrau (Eds.), *Theoretical models and processes of reading* (pp. 594–606). Newark, DE: International Reading Association.

Arthur, G. K., Brooks, R., & Long, M. L. (1979). A language-cultural course for foreign psychiatric residents. *American Journal of Psychiatry, 136*, 1064–1067.

Astor, A., Akhtar, T., & Matallana, M. A. (2005). Physician migration: Views from professionals in Colombia, Nigeria, India, Pakistan, and the Philippines. *Social Science and Medicine, 61*, 2492–2500.

Atkinson, P. (1995). *Medical talk and medical work: The liturgy of the clinic.* London: Sage.

Auerbach, E., & Wallerstein, N. (1984). *English for the workplace. ESL for action: Problem posing at work.* Reading, UK: Addison-Wesley.

Bailey, K. (1983). Foreign teaching assistants at U.S. universities: Problems in interaction and communication. *TESOL Quarterly, 17*, 308–310.

Bailey, K., Pialorsi, F., & Zukowski/Faust, J. (Eds). (1984). *Foreign teaching assistants in U.S. universities.* Washington, DC: NAFSA.

Bates, J., & Andrew, R. (2001). Untangling the roots of some IMGs' poor performance. *Academic Medicine, 76*, 43–46.

Beach, W. (2001). Lay diagnosis. Special issue of *Text, 21*(1/2), 221–250.

Beach, W., & LeBaron, C. (2002). Body disclosures: Attending to personal problems and reported sexual abuse during a medical encounter. *Journal of Communication* (September), 617–639.

Beckman, H., & Frankel, R. (1984). The effect of physician behaviour on the collection of data. *Annals of Internal Medicine, 101*, 692–696.

Belcher, D. (2006). English for specific purposes: Teaching to perceived needs and imagined futures in the worlds of work, study and everyday life. *TESOL Quarterly, 40*(1), 133–156.

Belcher, D. (2009). Problem-solving for nursing purposes. In: D. Belcher (Ed.), *English for specific purposes in theory and practice* (pp. 205–228). Ann Arbor, MI: University of Michigan Press.

Bellet, P., & Maloney, M. (1991). The importance of empathy as an interviewing skill in medicine. *Journal of the American Medical Association, 266*(13), 1831–1832.

Belz, J. (2002). The myth of the deficient communicator. *Language Teaching Research, 6*(1), 59–82.

Betancourt, J. R. (2003). Cross-cultural medical education: Conceptual approaches and frameworks for evaluation. *Academic Medicine, 78*(6), 560–569.

Bevis, T., & Lucas, C. (2007). *International students in American colleges and universities: A history.* New York, NY: Palgrave Macmillan.

Bickley, L. (1999). Critical thinking: From data to plan. In: B. Bates, L. Bickley & R. Hoekelman (Eds.), *Bates' guide to physical examination and history taking.* (7th ed., pp. 705–750). Philadelphia, PA: Lippincott.

Bickley, L. S., & Szilagyi, P. G. (2005). *Bates' guide to physical examination and history taking* (9th ed.). Philadelphia, PA: Lippincott.

Birrell, B., & Hawthorne, L. (2004). Medicare Plus and overseas-trained doctors. *People and Place, 12*(2), 83–99.

Bishop, S. (Ed.). (2008). Medical education in the USA. *Education USA Connections* 2. Retrieved from www.educationusaconnections.iienetwork.org/file_depot/010000000/2000030000/26726/folder/63728/Medical+Education+in+the+USA.FINAL3.pdf. Accessed on June 23, 2009.

Blake-Ward, M. (2008, April). Instructing the long-term resident. Colloquium on Assessing and Instructing International Physicians' Communication Skills. Paper presented at the 42nd Annual TESOL Convention and Exhibition, New York City, NY.

Bosher, S., & Smalkoski, K. (2002). From needs analysis to curriculum development: Designing a course in health-care communication for immigrant students in the USA. *English for Specific Purposes, 21*, 59–79.

Boulet, J., Bede, C., & McKinely, D. (2007). An overview of the world's medical schools. *Medical Teacher, 29*(1), 20–26.

Boulet, J., McKinley, D., Whelan, G., van Zanten, M., & Hambleton, R. (2002). Clinical skills deficiencies among first-year residents: Utility of the ECFMG clinical skills assessment. *Academic Medicine, 77*, S33–S35.

Boulet, J., Smee, S., Dillon, G., & Gimpel, J. (2009). The use of standardized patient assessments for certification and licensure decisions. *Simulation in Healthcare, 4*, 35–42.

Boulet, J., van Zanten, M., McKinley, D., & Gary, N. (2001). Evaluating the spoken English proficiency of graduates of foreign medical schools. *Medical Education, 35*, 767–773.

Bowe, H., & Martin, K. (2007). *Communication across cultures: Mutual understanding in a global world.* Cambridge: Cambridge University Press.

Braasch, D. (2009). From antihyperalgesic to zona pellucida: Teaching the pronunciation of scientific vocabulary. Paper presented at the 43rd Annual TESOL Convention and Exhibition, Denver, CO.

Brazeau, C., Boyd, L., & Crosson, J. (2002). Changing an existing OSCE to a teaching tool: The making of a teaching OSCE. *Academic Medicine, 77*(9), 932.

Brennan, T. A., Leape, L. L., Laird, N. M., Hebert, L., Localio, A. R., Lawthers, A. G., Newhouse, J. P., Weiler, P. C., & Hiatt, H. H. (2004). Incidence of adverse events and negligence in hospitalized patients: Results of the Harvard Medical Practice Study I. *Quality and Safety in Health Care, 13*(2), 145–151.

Brotherton, S. E., & Etzel, S. I. (2009). Graduate medical education, 2008–2009. *Journal of the American Medical Association, 302*, 1357–1372.

Brown, A. (2003). Interview variation and the co-construction of speaking proficiency. *Language Testing, 20*, 1–25.

Brown, K., Fishman, P., & Jones, N. (1990). *Legal and policy issues in the language proficiency assessment of international teaching assistants.* University of Houston Law Center, Institute for Higher Education Law and Governance, Houstan, Texas.

Bruce, N. (1992). Enhancing the status of communication in health science education and professional practice. Paper presented at the 34th Annual TESOL Convention and Exhibition, Vancouver, Canada.

Burns, A., & Roberts, C. (2010). Migration and adult language learning: Global flows and local transpositions. *TESOL Quarterly, 44*(3), 409–419.

Cameron, R. (1998). A language-focused needs analysis for ESL-speaking nursing students in class and clinic. *Foreign Language Annals, 31*, 203–218.

Canale, M., & Swain, M. (1980). Theoretical bases of communicative approaches to second language teaching and testing. *Applied Linguistics, 1*(1), 1–47.

Candlin, C. (1987). Explaining moments of conflict in discourse. In: R. Steele & T. Threadgold (Eds.), *Language topics: Essays in honour of Michael Halliday* (pp. 413–429). Amsterdam: John Benjamins.

Candlin, C. (Ed.) (2002). *Research and practice in professional discourse.* Hong Kong: City University of Hong Kong Press.

Candlin, C., Bruton, C., Leather, J., & Woods, E. (1981). Designing modular materials for communicative language learning, an example: Doctor-patient communication skills. In: L. Selinker, E. Tarone & V. Hanzeli (Eds.), *English for academic and technical purposes: Studies in honor of Louis Trimble* (pp. 105–133). Rowley, MA: Newbury House.

Candlin, C., & Candlin, S. (2002). Discourse, expertise, and management of risk in healthcare settings. *Research on Language and Social Interaction, 35*(2), 115–137.

Candlin, C., Maley, Y., Crichton, J., & Koster, P. (1994). *The language of lawyer-client conferencing.* New South Wales: The Law Foundation.

Candlin, S. (1995). *Towards excellence in nursing. An analysis of the discourse of nurses and patients in the context of health assessments.* Lancaster, UK: University of Lancaster.

Carter, R. (2004). *Language and creativity. The art of common talk.* London: Routledge.

Char, W. F. (1971). The foreign resident: An ambivalently valued object. *Psychiatry, 34*, 234–238.

Chen, C., Lai, C., Lu, P., Tsai, J., Chiang, H., Huan, I., & Yu, H. (2009). Performance anxiety at English PBL groups among Taiwanese medical students: A preliminary study. *The Kaohsiung Journal of Medical Sciences, 24*(3), S54–S58.

Chia, H.-U., Johnson, R., Chia, H.-L., & Olive, F. (1999). English for college students in Taiwan: A study of perceptions of English needs in a medical context. *English for Specific Purposes, 18*(2), 107–119.

Chur-Hansen, A., Elliott, T. E., Klein, N. C., & Howell, C. A. (2007). Assessment of English-language proficiency for general practitioner registrars. *Journal of Continuing Education in Health Professions, 27*, 36–41.

Chur-Hansen, A., & Vernon-Roberts, J. (1999). Using standardized patients to evaluate undergraduate medical students' proficiency in speaking English. *Academic Medicine, 74*, 829–834.

Chur-Hansen, A., Vernon-Roberts, J., & Clark, S. (1997). Language background, English language proficiency and medical communication skills of medical students. *Medical Education, 31*, 259–263.

Clyne, M. (1994). *Inter-cultural communication at work: Cultural values in discourse.* Cambridge: Cambridge University Press.

Clyne, M. (2005). *Australia's language potential.* Sydney: University of New South Wales Press.

Cohen-Cole, S. (1991). *The medical interview: The three-function approach.* St. Louis, MO: Mosby.

Committee on Science, Engineering, and Public Policy, National Academy of Sciences, National Academy of Engineering, and Institute of Medicine. (1995). *On being a scientist: Responsible conduct in research.* Washington, DC: National Academy Press.

Connor, U. (1999). How like you our fish? Accommodation in international business communication. In: M. Hewings & C. Nickerson (Eds.), *Business English: Research into practice* (pp. 71–99). Harlow, UK: Longman.

Connor, U., Goering, B., Matthias, M., & MacNeill, R. (2009). Information use and treatment adherence among patients with diabetes. In: M. Ruiz-Garrido, J. Palmer-Silveira & I. Fortanet-Gomez (Eds.), *English for professional and academic purposes.* Amsterdam: Rodopi.

Connor, U., Goering, E., Hamilton, H., & MacNeill, R. (2007, June). Exploring health literacies in relation to prescription medication. Paper presented at the Communication, Medicine, & Ethics conference (COMET), University of Lugano, Switzerland.

Connor, U., & Rozycki, W. (2007, October). Health literacy and disease knowledge. Preliminary findings from interviews with diabetes patients. Paper presented at the International Conference on Communication in Healthcare (ICCH), Charleston, SC.

Connor, U., Rozycki, W., & Ruiz-Garrido, M. (2006, June). Intercultural study of health literacy and medicine labels. Paper presented at the Fourth Interdisciplinary Conference on Communication, Medicine & Ethics (COMET), Cardiff University, Wales.

Connor, U., Ruíz-Garrido, M., Fortanet, I., & Palmer, J. (2006). Análisis contrastivo de la comunicabilidad del prospecto de los medicamentos en España y en Estados Unidos [Contrastive analysis on the communicability of medication information from Spain and the United States]. In: B. Gallardo Paúls, C. Hernández Sacristán & V. Moreno Campos (Eds.), *Lingüística Clínica y Neuropsicología Cognitiva. Actas del Primer Congreso Nacional de Lingüística Clínica. Vol. 3. Lingüística Interaccional en Ambitos de Salud* (pp. 140–152). Valencia: Universitat Jaume I.

Connor, U., Ruiz-Garrido, M., Rozycki, W., Goering, E., Kinney, E., & Koehler, J. (2008). Intercultural study of patient-directed medicine labeling: Text differences between the United States and Spain. *Communication and Medicine, 5*(2), 27–42.

Cordella, M. (1999). Medical discourse in a Hispanic environment: Power and simpatía under investigation. *Australian Review of Applied Linguistics, 22*(2), 35–50.

Cordella, M. (2002). La interacción médico-paciente en escrutinio: Un estudio de sociolingüística interaccional. *Onomazein: Revista de Lingüística, Filología y Traducción del Instituto de Letras de la Pontificia Universidad Católica de Chile, 7*, 117–144.

Cordella, M. (2003). En el corazón del debate: El análisis del discurso en la representación de las voces médicas. *Oralia: Análisis del Discurso Ora, 6*, 147–168.

Cordella, M. (2004a). *The dynamic consultation: A discourse analytical study of doctor-patient communication.* Amsterdam: John Benjamins.

Cordella, M. (2004b). You know doctor, I need to tell you something: A discourse analytical study of patient's voices in the medical consultation. *Australian Review of Applied Linguistics, 27*(2), 92–109.

Cordella, M. (2006). 'No, no I haven't been taking it doctor': Compliance, face threatening acts and politeness in medical consultations. In: M. Placencia & C. García (Eds.), *Linguistic politeness in the Spanish-speaking world* (pp. 191–212). Mahwah, NJ: Lawrence Erlbaum Associates.

Cordella, M. (2007). Unveiling stories to the oncologist: a matter of sharing and healing. *Panacea@: Medicine and Translation, 9*(26), 230–238.

Cordella, M. (2008). Two experts and one patient: Managing medical practices and religious beliefs. *Monash University Linguistics Papers, 6*, 19–28.

Cordella, M. (2010). Negotiating religious beliefs in a medical setting. *Journal of Religion and Health,* Retrieved from www.springerlink.com/content/n31j128073224t30. Accessed on July 14, 2011.

Cordella, M., & Musgrave, S. (2009). Oral communication skills of international medical graduates: Assessing empathy in discourse. *Communication and Medicine, 6*, 129–142.

Cordella, M., & Spike, N. (2008). Working toward a better communication between international medical graduates and their patients in Victoria. *Health Issues, 96*, 28–29.

Crespi, I. (1977). Attitude measurement, theory, and prediction. *Public Opinion Quarterly, 41*(3), 285–294.

De La Croix, A., & Skelton, J. (2009). The reality of role-play: Interruptions and amount of talk in simulated consultations. *Medical Education, 43*(7), 695–703.

Delbanco, T., & Bell, S. K. (2007). Guilty, afraid and alone: Struggling with medical error. *The New England Journal of Medicine, 357*, 1682–1683.

Desai, S. (2003). *101 biggest mistakes 3rd year medical students make and how to avoid them.* Houston, TX: MD2B.

Dogra, N. (2001). The development and evaluation of a programme to teach cultural diversity to medical undergraduate students. *Medical Education, 35*, 232–241.

Dogra, N., & Wass, V. (2006). Can we assess students' awareness of cultural diversity? A qualitative study of stakeholders' views. *Medical Education, 40*, 682–690.

Drew, P., & Heritage, J. (Eds). (1992). *Talk at work: Interaction in institutional settings.* Cambridge: Cambridge University Press.

Dudley-Evans, T., & St John, M. J. (1998). *Developments in English for specific purposes.* Cambridge: Cambridge University Press.

Duff, P., Wong, P., & Early, M. (2002). Learning language for work and life: The linguistic socialization of immigrant Canadians seeking careers in healthcare. *The Modern Language Journal, 86*, 397–422.

Duncan, J., & Parker, A. (2007). *Open forum 3*. Oxford: Oxford University Press.

Editorials. (2001). *Medical Education, 35*, 186–187.

Educational Commission for Foreign Medical Graduates. (2009a). *The one dozen things you might not have known, realized, or understood about American medicine*. Retrieved from www.ecfmg.org/acculturation/dozen.html. Accessed on June 27, 2009.

Educational Commission for Foreign Medical Graduates. (2009b). *Above all—Professionalism analysis*. Retrieved from www.ecfmg.org/acculturation/12/analysis.html. Accessed on June 27, 2009.

Educational Commission for Foreign Medical Graduates. (2009c). *IMG advisors network (IAN)*. Retrieved from www.ecfmg.org/acculturation/ian.html. Accessed on June 28, 2009.

Eggly, S., Musial, J., & Smulowitz, J. (1999). The relationship between English language proficiency and success as a medical resident. *English for Specific Purposes, 18*(2), 201–208.

Engeström, Y. (2005). Between professional and organizational: The changing discourses of medicine. *Journal of Applied Linguistics, 2*, 351–356.

Erickson, F., & Rittenberg, W. (1987). Topic control and person control: A thorny problem for foreign physicians in interaction with American patients. *Discourse Processes, 10*, 401–405.

Fadiman, A. (1997). *The spirit catches you and you fall down: A Hmong child, her American doctors, and the collision of two cultures*. New York, NY: Noonday.

Federation of State Medical Boards, Inc., & National Board of Medical Examiners. (2011). *USMLE bulletin of information*. Retrieved from http://usmle.org/General_Information/bulletin/2011/2011%20BOI.pdf. Accessed on June 13, 2011.

Ferrara, K. (1992). The interactive achievement of a sentence: Joint productions in therapeutic discourse. *Discourse Processes, 15*, 207–228.

Fiscella, K., Bothola, R., Roman-Diaz, M., Lue, B. H., & Frankel, R. (1997). "Being a foreigner, I may be punished if I make a mistake": Assessing transcultural experiences in caring for patients. *Family Practice, 14*, 112–116.

Fisher, S., & Groce, S. (1990). Accounting practices in medical interviews. *Language in Society, 19*, 225–250.

Flynn, J. (2006, August 17). Media release. Australian Medical Council.

Frankel, R. (2000). The (socio)linguistic turn in physician-patient communication research. In: J. Alatis, H. Hamilton & A.-H. Tan (Eds.), *Linguistics, language, and the professions education, journalism, law, medicine, and technology* (pp. 81–103). Georgetown: Georgetown University Round Table on Languages and Linguistics (GURT).

Frankel, R. (2009). Empathy research: A complex challenge. *Patient Education and Counseling, 75*, 1–2.

Friedman, M., Sutnick, A. I., Stillman, P. L., Norcini, J. J., Anderson, S. M., & Williams, R. G. (1991). The use of standardized patients to evaluate the spoken-English proficiency of foreign medical graduates. *Academic Medicine, 66*, S61–S63.

Friedman, M., Sutnick, A. I., Stillman, P. L., Regan, M. B., & Norcini, J. J. (1993). The relationship of spoken-English proficiencies of foreign medical school graduates to their clinical competence. *Academic Medicine, 68*, S1–S3.

Friedman, T. L. (2005). *The world is flat*. New York, NY: Farrar, Straus & Giroux.

Gaston, P. L. (2010). *The challenge of Bologna*. Sterling, VA: Stylus.

Gee, J. (1990). *Social linguistics and literacies: Ideology in discourses*. Philadelphia, PA: Farmer.

Gee, J. (1999). *An introduction to discourse analysis*. London: Routledge.

Gibbs, W. W. (1995). Lost science in the third world. *Scientific American, 273*(2), 76–83.

Gilbert, J. (1993). *Clear speech. Pronunciation and listening comprehension in American English.* New York, NY: Cambridge University Press.

Glendinning, E., & Holmstrom, B. (2005). *English in medicine* (3rd ed.). Cambridge: Cambridge University Press.

Glendinning, E., & Howard, R. (2007). *Professional English in use.* Cambridge: Cambridge University Press.

Goffman, E. (1959). *The presentation of self in everyday life.* New York, NY: Doubleday.

Good, B. (1994). *Medicine, rationality, and experience: An anthropological perspective.* Cambridge: Cambridge University Press.

Good, B., & Good, M.-J. (2000). "Fiction" and "historicity" in doctors' stories: Social and narrative dimensions of learning medicine. In: C. Mattingly & L. Garro (Eds.), *Narrative and the cultural construction of illness and healing* (pp. 50–69). Berkeley, CA: University of California Press.

Goodwin, C. T., & Nacht, M. (1983). *Absence of decision: Foreign students in American colleges and universities.* New York, NY: Institute for International Education.

Graddol, D. (2000). *The future of English.* Retrieved from www.britishcouncil.org/learning-elt-future.pdf. Accessed on April 28, 2010.

Graddol, D. (2006). *English next.* Retrieved from www.britishcouncil.org/learning-elt-future.pdf. Accessed on April 28, 2010.

Grant, L. (2009). *Well said* (3rd ed.). Boston, MA: Heinle Cengage Learning.

Gropper, R. (1996). *Culture and the clinical encounter: An intercultural sensitizer for the health professions.* Yarmouth, ME: Intercultural Press.

Gumperz, J. (1982a). Fact and inference in courtroom testimony. In: J. Gumperz (Ed.), *Language and social identity* (pp. 163–195). Cambridge: Cambridge University Press.

Gumperz, J. (1982b). *Discourse strategies.* Cambridge: Cambridge University Press.

Gumperz, J. (1999). On interactional sociolinguistic method. In: S. Sarangi & C. Roberts (Eds.), *Talk, work, and institutional order* (pp. 453–471). Berlin: Mouton de Gruyter.

Haas, W. J. (1988). Botany in republican China: The leading role of taxonomy. In: J. Z. Bowers, J. W. Hess & N. Sivin (Eds.), *Science and medicine in twentieth-century China: Research and education.* Ann Arbor, MI: Center for Chinese Studies, University of Michigan.

Halliday, M. (1985). *An introduction to functional grammar.* London: Edward Arnold.

Hallock, J. A., Stephen, S. S., & Norcini, J. J. (2003). The international medical graduate pipeline. *Health Affairs, 22,* 94–96.

Halpern, J. (1993). Empathy: Using resonance emotions in the service of curiosity. In: H. Spiro, M. McCrea Curnen, E. Peschel & D. St James (Eds.), *Empathy and the practice of medicine* (pp. 160–173). New Haven, CT: Yale University Press.

Hamilton, J., & Woodward-Kron, R. (2010). Developing cultural awareness and intercultural communication through multimedia: A case study from medicine and the health sciences. *System, 38*(4), 560–568.

Harden, R. M. (2006). International medical education and future directions: A global perspective. *Academic Medicine, 81*(12), S22–S29.

Harik, P., Clauser, B. E., Grabovsky, I., Margolis, M. J., Dillon, G. F., & Boulet, J. R. (2006). Relationships among subcomponents of the USMLE Step 2 Clinical Skills Examination, the Step 1, and the Step 2 Clinical Knowledge Examinations. *Academic Medicine, 81,* S21–S24.

Hawkins, R. E., Swanson, D. B., Dillon, G. F., Clauser, B. E., King, A. M., Scoles, P. V., Whelan, G. P., Burdick, W. P., Boulet, J. R., & Homan, A. G. (2005). The introduction of clinical skills assessment into the United States Medical Licensing Examination (USMLE): A description of USMLE Step 2 Clinical Skills (CS). *Journal of Medical Licensure and Discipline, 91*(3), 22–25.

Heath, C. (2002). Demonstrative suffering: The gestural (re)embodiment of symptoms. *Journal of Communication, 52*(3), 597–616.

Helman, C. G. (1994). *Culture, health and illness: An introduction for health professionals* (3rd ed.). Oxford: Butterworth-Heinemann.

Hoekje, B. (2007). Medical discourse and ESP courses for international medical graduates. *English for Specific Purposes, 26,* 327–343.

Hoekje, B. (2008, April). Discussion. Colloquium on Assessing and Instructing International Physicians' Communication Skills. Paper presented at the 42nd Annual TESOL Convention and Exhibition, New York City, NY.

Hoekje, B., & Williams, J. (1992). Communicative competence and the dilemma of international teaching assistant education. *TESOL Quarterly, 26,* 243–270.

Hornby, A., & Wehmeier, S. (2004). *Oxford advanced learner's English-Chinese dictionary* (6th ed.). Oxford: Oxford University Press.

Horvath, K., Coluccio, G., Foy, H., & Pellegrini, C. (2004). A program for successful integration of international medical graduates (IMGs) into U.S. surgical residency training. *Current Surgery, 61,* 492–498.

Hu, H. C. (1944). The Chinese concept of "face". *American Anthropologist, 46*(1), 45–64.

Hutchinson, T., & Waters, A. (1987). *English for specific purposes: A learning-centered approach.* Cambridge: Cambridge University Press.

Hwang, T.-L. (2006). The current medical education system in Taiwan. *Asia Pacific Biotech News APBN, 10,* 812–814.

Hydén, L.-C., & Mishler, E. (1999). Language and medicine. *Annual Review of Applied Linguistics, 19,* 174–192.

Hymes, D. (1972). On communicative competence. In: J. B. Pride & J. Holmes (Eds.), *Sociolinguistics* (pp. 269–293). Harmondsworth, UK: Penguin Books.

Hymes, D. (1974). *Foundations of sociolinguistics.* Philadelphia, PA: University of Pennsylvania Press.

Ibrahim, Y. (2001). Doctor and patient questions as a measure of doctor-centredness in UAE hospitals. *English for Specific Purposes, 20,* 331–344.

Institute for International Education. (1960). *Open doors.* New York, NY: Institute for International Education.

Jefferson, G., Sacks, H., & Schegloff, E. (1977). *Preliminary notes on the sequential organization of laughter.* Cambridge: Cambridge University Press.

Jurafsky, D., Shriberg, E., Fox, B., & Curl, T. (1998). Lexical, prosodic, and syntactic cues for dialog acts. *Proceedings of ACL/COLING-98 Workshop on Discourse Relations and Discourse Markers.* Retrieved from www.stanford.edu/~jurafsky/ACL98discourse.pdf. Accessed on July 5, 2011.

Kai, J., Spencer, J., Wilkes, M., & Gill, P. (1999). Learning to value ethnic diversity: What, why and how? *Medical Education, 33,* 616–623.

Kales, H. C., DiNardo, A. R., Blow, F. C., McCarthy, J. F., Ignacio, R. V., & Riba, M. B. (2006). International medical graduates and the diagnosis and treatment of late-life depression. *Academic Medicine, 81*(2), 171–175.

Kashani, A. S., Soheili, S., & Hatmi, Z. N. (2006). Teaching English to students of medicine: A student-centered approach. *Asian ESP Journal, 2*, 85–98.

Kendon, A. (1986). Some reasons for studying gesture. *Semiotica, 62*(1/2), 3–28.

Kendon, A. (1990). *Conducting interaction: Patterns of behaviour in focussed encounters.* Cambridge: Cambridge University Press.

Kergon, C., Illing, J., Morrow, G., Burford, B., & Bedi, A. (2009). *The experiences of U.K., E.U. and non-E.U. medical graduates making the transition to the U.K. workplace.* Swindon, UK: ESRC.

Kleinman, A. (1980). *Patients and healers in the context of culture: An exploration of the borderland between anthropology, medicine and psychiatry.* Berkeley, CA: University of California Press.

Kleinman, A. (1995). *Writing at the margin: Discourse between anthropology and medicine.* Berkeley, CA: University of California Press.

Knight, J. (2003). *Updating the definition of internationalization* (Retrieved from www.bc.edu/bc_org/avp/soe/cihe/newsletter/News33/text001. Accessed on August 15, 2008.). Center for International Higher Education, Boston College.

Kohn, L., Corrigan, J. M., & Donaldson, M. S. (1999). *To err is human: Building a safer health system.* Washington, DC: National Academy Press.

Konner, M. (1987). *Becoming a doctor.* New York, NY: Penguin.

Koop, A. J., & Borbasi, S. A. (1994). Towards enhanced OSCE in Australian nurse education: A contribution from South Africa. *Curationis, 17*(3), 40–43.

Kormos, J. (1999). Simulating conversations in oral-proficiency assessment: A conversation analysis of role plays and non-scripted interviews in language exams. *Language Testing, 16*, 163–188.

Kramer, M. (2005). The educational needs of international medical graduates in psychiatric residencies. *Academic Psychiatry, 29*, 322–324.

Kurtz, S., & Silverman, J. (1996). The Calgary-Cambridge referenced observation guides: An aid to defining the curriculum and organizing the teaching in communication training programmes. *Medical Education, 30*(2), 83–89.

Kurtz, S., Silverman, J., & Draper, J. (2005). *Teaching and learning communication skills in medicine.* Oxford: Radcliffe Publishing.

Labov, J., & Hanau, C. (2005). Effective pedagogy in improving L2 English speaking doctors' pronunciation. Paper presented at the Second Language Research Forum (SLRF), New York City, NY.

Labov, W. (1972). *Language in the inner city.* Philadelphia, PA: University of Pennsylvania Press.

Lang, F., McCord, R., Harvill, L., & Anderson, D. S. (2004). Communication assessment using the common ground instrument: Psychometric properties. *Family Medicine, 36*(3), 189–198.

Larkin, G. L., McKay, M. P., & Angelos, P. (2005). Six core competencies and seven deadly sins: A virtues-based approach to the new guidelines for graduate medical education. *Surgery, 138*(3), 490–497.

Le, T., Bhushan, V., Sheikh-Ali, M., & Abu Shahin, F. (2010). *First aid for the USMLE STEP 2 CS Clinical Skills* (3rd ed.). New York, NY: McGraw-Hill Medical.

Leape, L. L., Brennan, T. A., Laird, A. G., Lawthers, N., Localio, A. R., Barnes, B. A., Hebert, L., Newhouse, J. P., Weiler, P. C., & Hiatt, H. (1991). The nature of adverse events in hospitalized patients. Results of the Harvard Medical Practice Study II. *The New England Journal of Medicine, 324*, 377–384.

Lemann, N. (1999). *The big test*. New York, NY: Farrar, Straus, & Giroux.

Levinson, W., Roter, D. L., Mullooly, J. P., Dull, V. T., & Frankel, R. M. (1997). Physician-patient communication. The relationship with malpractice claims among primary care physicians and surgeons. *Journal of the American Medical Association, 277*, 553–559.

Likic, R., Dusek, T., & Horvat, D. (2005). Analysis and prospects for curricular reform of medical schools in Southeast Europe. *Medical Education, 38*, 833–840.

Linell, P., Adelswärd, V., Sachs, L., Bredman, M., & Lindstedt, U. (2002). Expert talk in medical contexts: Explicit and implicit orientation to risk. *Research on Language and Social Interaction, 35*(2), 195–218.

Lingard, L., Schryer, C., Garwood, K., & Spafford, M. (2003). "Talking the talk": School and workplace genre tension in clerkship case presentations. *Medical Education, 37*, 612–620.

Long, M. (2005). Stabilization and fossilization in second language development. In: C. J. Doughty & M. H. Long (Eds.), *The handbook of second language acquisition* (pp. 487–536). Oxford: Blackwell.

Macdonald, D., Yule, G., & Powers, M. (1994). Attempts to improve English L2 pronunciation: The variable effects of different types of instruction. *Language Learning, 44*(1), 75–100.

Madden, C., & Myers, C. (Eds). (1994). *Discourse and performance of international teaching assistants*. Alexandria, VA: TESOL Publications.

Maher, J. C. (1986). English for medical purposes. *Language Teaching, 19*, 112–145.

Maher, J. C. (1992). *International medical communication in English*. Ann Arbor, MI: University of Michigan Press.

Majumdar, B., Keystone, J. S., & Cuttress, L. (1999). Cultural sensitivity training among foreign medical graduates. *Medical Education, 33*, 177–184.

Maley, A. (2003). Creative approaches to writing materials. In: B. Tomlinson (Ed.), *Developing materials for language teaching* (pp. 183–198). London: Continuum International Publishing Group.

Martinez, W., & Lo, B. (2008). Medical students' experiences with medical errors: An analysis of medical student essays. *Medical Education, 42*(7), 733–741.

Massachusetts Coalition for the Prevention of Medical Errors. (2006). *When things go wrong: Responding to adverse events*. Retrieved from www.ihi.org/NR/rdonlyres/A4CE6C77-F65C-4F34-B323-20AA4E41DC79/0/RespondingAdverseEvents.pdf. Accessed on June 25, 2008.

Maynard, D. (1991). Interaction and asymmetry in clinical discourse. *American Journal of Sociology, 97*, 448–495.

Maynard, D. W., & Heritage, J. (2005). Conversation analysis, doctor-patient interaction and medical communication. *Medical Education, 39*, 428–534.

McCullagh, M. (2004). *Speaking the same language, a course in doctor patient communication*. Unpublished master's thesis. Leeds Metropolitan University, Leeds, UK.

McCullagh, M., & Wright, R. (2008). *Good practice: Communication skills in English for the medical practitioner*. Cambridge: Cambridge University Press.

McDonnell, L., & Usherwood, T. (2008). International medical graduates: Challenges faced in the Australian training program. *Australian Family Physician, 37*(6), 481–484.

McGrath, B. (2004). Overseas-trained doctors: Integration of overseas-trained doctors in the Australian medical workforce. *Medical Journal of Australia, 181*, 640–642.

McMahon, G. (2004). Coming to America—International medical graduates in the United States. *New England Journal of Medicine, 350*, 2435–2437.

Mehrabian, A. (1967). Orientation behaviours and nonverbal attitude communication. *Journal of Communication, 17*(4), 324–332.

Mercer, S., & Reynolds, W. (2002). Empathy and quality of care. *British Journal of General Practice, 52*, S9–S12.

Mishler, E. G. (1984). *The discourse of medicine. Dialectics in medical interviews.* Norwood, NJ: Ablex.

Mishler, E. G. (1997). The interactional construction of narratives in medical and life-history interviews. In: B.-L. Gunnarsson, P. Linell & B. Nordberg (Eds.), *The construction of professional discourse* (pp. 223–244). New York, NY: Longman.

Mistica, M., Baldwin, T., Cordella, M., & Musgrave, S. (2008). Applying discourse analysis data mining methods to spoken OSCE assessments. *Proceedings of the 22nd International Conference on Computational Linguistics (COLING 2008)*, Association for Computational Linguistics, East Stroudsburg, PA (pp. 577–584).

Mullan, F. (2005). The metrics of the physician brain drain. *New England Journal of Medicine, 353*, 1810–1818.

National Academy of Sciences, National Academy of Engineering, Institute of Medicine, Committee on Science, Engineering, and Public Policy. (2000). *Enhancing the postdoctoral experience for scientists and engineers: A guide for postdoctoral scholars, advisers, institutions, funding organizations, and disciplinary societies.* Washington, DC: National Academy Press.

Norcini, J. J., Blank, L. L., Arnold, G. K., & Kimball, H. R. (1995). The mini-CEX (Clinical Evaluation Exercise): A preliminary investigation. *Annals of Internal Medicine, 123*, 795–799.

Norcini, J. J., Boulet, J. R., Dauphinee, W. D., Opalek, A., Krantz, I. D., & Anderson, S. T. (2010). Evaluating the quality of care provided by graduates of international medical schools. *Health Affairs, 29*, 1461–1468.

Nyquist, J., Abbott, R., Wulff, D., & Sprague, J. (1991). *Preparing the professoriate of tomorrow to teach.* Dubuque, IA: Kendall Hunt Publishing Company.

O'Grady, C. (2011). *The nature of expert communication as required for the general practice of medicine: A discourse analytical study.* Unpublished doctoral dissertation, Department of Linguistics, Macquarie University, Sydney, Australia.

Olmstead-Wang, S. (2009). Medical doctors using authentic webcast lectures to learn lexical phrases. In: S. Rilling & M. Dantas-Whitney (Eds.), *Authentic materials in the language classroom and beyond: Adult learners* (pp. 231–238). Alexandria, VA: TESOL Publications.

Ong, L., de Haes, J., Hoos, A., & Lammes, F. (1995). Doctor-patient communication: A review of the literature. *Social Science and Medicine, 40*, 903–918.

Orion, G. (1999). *Pronouncing American English: Sounds, stress, and intonation.* Boston, MA: Heinle & Heinle.

Penner, J. (1995). Change and conflict: Introduction of the communicative approach in China. *TESL Canada Journal/Revue TESL du Canada, 12*(2), 1–17.

Pennycook, A. (1998). *English and the discourses of colonialism.* London: Routledge.

Pettigrew, T. (1998). Intergroup contact theory. *Annual Review of Psychology, 49*, 65–85.

Phillips, D. P., & Bredder, C. C. (2002). Morbidity and mortality from medical errors: An increasing serious public health problem. *Annual Review of Public Health, 23*, 135–150.

Phillips, P. D., Christenfield, N., & Glynn, L. M. (1998). Increase in U.S. medication-error deaths between 1983 and 1997. *Lancet, 351*, 643–644.

Pialorsi, F. (1984). Toward an anthropology of the classroom: An essay on foreign teaching assistants and U.S. students. In: K. Bailey, F. Pialoris & J. Zukowski-Faust (Eds.), *Foreign teaching assistants in U.S. universities* (pp. 16–21). Washington, DC: NAFSA.

Pickering, L. (2001). The role of tone choice in improving ITA communication in the classroom. *TESOL Quarterly, 35*, 233–255.

Pilcher, J. (2006). Case #10: Teaching speaking and listening to teachers in China. In: K. S. Folse (Ed.), *The art of teaching speaking* (pp. 83–84). Ann Arbor, MI: University of Michigan Press.

Pilotto, L., Duncan, G., & Anderson-Wurf, J. (2007). Issues for clinicians training international medical graduates: A systematic review. *Medical Journal of Australia, 187*(4), 225–228.

Plight of Foreign Doctors. (1960, December 5). *Time*. Retrieved from www.time.com/time/magazine/article/0,9171,895084-1,00.html. Accessed on September 3, 2008.

Polackova, G. (2008). Understanding and use of phrasal verbs and idioms in medical/nursing texts. *Bratislavské Lekárske Listy, 109*(11), 531–532.

Professional and Linguistic Assessments Board (PLAB). (2010). *Part 2 guidance*. Retrieved from www.gmc-uk.org/doctors/plab/advice_part2.asp. Accessed on January 3, 2011.

Pugno, P., McGaha, A., Schmittling, G., DeVilbiss, A., & Kahn, N. (2007). Results of the 2007 national resident matching program: Family medicine. *Family Medicine, 39*(8), 562–571.

Rao, N. R., Kramer, M., Saunders, R., Twemlow, S. W., Lomax, J. W., Dewan, M. J., Myers, M. F., Goldberg, J., Cassimir, G., Kring, B., & Alami, O. (2007). An annotated bibliography of professional literature on international medical graduates. *Academic Psychiatry, 31*, 68–83.

Raymond, M. R., Clauser, B. E., Swygert, K. A., & van Zanten, M. (2009). Measurement precision of spoken English proficiency scores on the USMLE Step 2 Clinical Skills Examination. *Academic Medicine, 84*, S83–S85.

Reader, T. W., Flin, R., & Cuthbertson, B. H. (2007). Communication skills and error in the intensive care unit. *Current Opinion in Critical Care, 13*, 732–736.

Roberts, C., & Sarangi, S. (2005). Theme-oriented discourse analysis of medical encounters. *Medical Education, 39*, 632–640.

Roberts, C., Sarangi, S., & Moss, B. (2004). Presentation of self and symptoms in primary care consultations involving patients from non-English speaking background. *Communication and Medicine, 1*(2), 159–169.

Roberts, C., Wass, V., Jones, R., Sarangi, S., & Gillett, A. (2003). A discourse analysis study of 'good' and 'poor' communication in an OSCE: A proposed new framework for teaching students. *Medical Education, 37*, 192–201.

Robertson, W. W. (2006). Opinion piece: The continuum of general competency. *ACGMEe Bulletin*. Retrieved from www.acgme.org/acWebsite/bulletin-e/e-bulletin03_06.pdf. Accessed on June 25, 2008.

Robinson, J. (1998). Getting down to business: Talk, gaze and body orientation during openings of doctor-patient consultations. *Journal of the Society for Human Communications Research, 25*(1), 97–123.

Rogers, C. (1961). *On becoming a person. A therapist's view of psychotherapy*. Boston, MA: Mifflin.

Ross, M., Carroll, G., Knight, J., Chamberlain, M., Fothergill-Bourbonnais, F., & Linton, J. (1988). Using the OSCE to measure clinical skills performance in nursing. *Journal of Advanced Nursing, 13*(1), 45–56.

Rothman, A. I., & Cusimano, M. (2000). A comparison of physician examiners', standardized patients', and communication experts' ratings of international medical graduates' English proficiency. *Academic Medicine, 75,* 1206–1211.

Rothman, A. I., & Cusimano, M. (2001). Assessment of English proficiency in international medical graduates by physician examiners and standardized patients. *Medical Education, 35,* 762–766.

Rounds, P. (1987). Characterizing successful classroom discourse for NNS teaching assistant training. *TESOL Quarterly, 21,* 643–671.

Rubin, D., Healy, P., Zath, R., Gardiner, T., & Moore, C. (1997). Non-native physicians as message sources: Effects of accent and ethnicity on patients' responses to AIDS prevention counseling. *Health Communication, 9,* 351–368.

Rughani, A., & Davangere, A. (2010). *Curriculum evaluation focused on the experience of IMG trainees in Yorkshire and the Humber Deanery.* Retrieved from www.yorksandhumberdeanery.nhs.uk/general.../IMGsurveyindetail.doc. Accessed on January 10, 2011.

Sacks, H., Schegloff, E., & Jefferson, G. (1974). A simplest systematic for the organization of turn-taking in conversations. *Language, 59,* 941–942.

Salsber, E., & Forte, G. (2002). Trends in the physician workforce, 1980–2000. *Health Affairs, 21,* 165–173.

Sarangi, S., Bennert, K., Howell, L., & Clarke, A. (2003). 'Relatively speaking': Relativisation of genetic risk in counseling for predictive testing. *Health, Risk and Society, 5*(2), 155–170.

Sarangi, S., & Clarke, A. (2002). Zones of expertise and the management of uncertainty in genetics risk communication. *Research on Language and Social Interaction, 35*(2), 139–171.

Sarangi, S., & Roberts, C. (1999). The dynamics of interactional and institutional orders in work-related settings. In: S. Sarangi & C. Roberts (Eds.), *Talk, work, and institutional order* (pp. 1–60). Berlin: Mouton de Gruyter.

Schim, S. M., Doorenbos, A. Z., Miller, J., & Benkert, R. (2003). Development of a cultural competence assessment instrument. *Journal of Nursing Measurement, 11*(1), 29–40.

Schön, D. (1983). *The reflective practitioner: How professionals think in action.* New York, NY: Basic Books.

Schuster, B. (2000). *Strengths and weaknesses of international medical graduates in U.S. programs: A chairperson's perspective.* Retrieved from www.acponline.org/img/shuster.htm. Accessed on September 1, 2008.

Scollon, R., & Scollon, S. W. (2001). *Intercultural communication* (2nd ed.). Cambridge, MA: Basil Blackwell.

Searight, H. R., & Gafford, J. (2006). Behavorial science education and the international medical graduate. *Academic Medicine, 81*(2), 164–170.

Selinker, L. (1972). Interlanguage. *International Review of Applied Linguistics, 10,* 209–230.

Sharifian, F. (2003). On cultural conceptualisations. *Journal of Cognition and Culture, 3*(3), 188–207.

Sharifian, F. (2007). L1 cultural conceptualisations in L2 learning. In: F. Sharifian & G. B. Palmer (Eds.), *Applied cultural linguistics: Implications for second language learning and intercultural communication* (pp. 53–63). Amsterdam: John Benjamins.

Shaw, P. (1994). Discourse competence in a framework for ITA training. In: C. Madden & C. Myers (Eds.), *Discourse and performance of international teaching assistants* (pp. 27–51). Alexandria, VA: TESOL Publications.

Shi, L. (2009). English for medical purposes. In: D. Belcher (Ed.), *English for specific purposes in theory and practice* (pp. 205–228). Ann Arbor, MI: University of Michigan Press.

Shi, L., Corcos, R., & Storey, A. (2001). Using student performance data to develop an English course for clinical training. *English for Specific Purposes, 20*, 267–291.

Sierles, F. S. (2005). Using film as the basis of an American culture course for first-year psychiatry residents. *Academic Psychiatry, 29*, 100–104.

Silverman, J., Kurtz, S., & Draper, J. (2005). *Skills for communicating with patients*. Oxford: Radcliffe Publishing.

Smith, B. R., Wells, A., Alexander, B., Bovill, E., Campbell, S., Dasgupta, A., Fung, M., Heller, B., Howe, J., Parvin, C., Peerschke, E., Rinder, H., Spitalnik, S., Weiss, R., & Wener, M.The Academy of Clinical Laboratory Physicians and Scientists. (2006). Curriculum content and evaluation of resident competency in clinical pathology (laboratory medicine): A proposal. *Human Pathology, 37*(8), 934–968.

Smith, R., Byrd, P., Nelson, G., Barrett, R., & Constantinides, J. (1992). *Crossing pedagogical oceans: International teaching assistants in U.S. undergraduate education*. ASHE-ERIC Higher Education Report no. 8. Washington, DC: The George Washington University, School of Education and Human Development.

Smith, R. V. (1998). *Graduate research: A guide for students in the sciences*. Seattle, WA: University of Washington Press.

Sonderen, M. J., Denessen, E., Ten Cate, O. T. J., & Splinter, T. A. W. (2009). The clinical skills assessment for international medical graduates in The Netherlands. *Medical Teacher, 31*, e533–e538.

Spencer, J. A., & Jordan, R. K. (1999). Learner centred approaches in medical education. *British Medical Journal, 318*(8), 1280–1283.

Spike, N. (2006). International medical graduates: The Australian perspective. *Academic Medicine, 81*, 842–846.

Stenson, N., Downing, B., Smith, J., & Smith, K. (1992). The effectiveness of computer-assisted pronunciation training. *Computer-Assisted Language Instruction Consortium (CALICO) Journal, 9*(4), 5–19.

Stern, H. H. (1992). *Issues and options in language teaching*. Oxford: Oxford University Press.

Stewart, M. (1995). Effective physician-patient communication and health outcomes: A review. *Canadian Medical Association Journal, 152*(9), 1423–1433.

Stewart, M., Brown, J., Donner, A., McWhinney, I., Oates, J., & Weston, W. (2000). The impact of patient-centred care on outcomes. *Journal of Family Practice, 49*(9), 796–804.

Stokoe, E. (2011). Simulated interaction and communication skills training: The "conversation analytic" role-play method. In: C. Antaki (Ed.), *Applied conversation analysis: Intervention and change in institutional talk*. London: Palgrave Macmillan.

Suchman, A., Markakis, K., Beckman, H., & Frankel, R. (1997). A model of empathic communication in the medical interview. *Journal of the American Medical Association, 277*(8), 678–682.

'Sufficient Checks' on locum GP. (2010). *BBC*. Retrieved from http://www.news.bbc.co.uk/1/hi/8461407.stm. Accessed on February 22, 2011.

The Economist. (2010). Sun, shopping, and surgery: Can the Gulf attract medical tourists? *The Economist*, December 11. Retrieved from http://www.economist.com/node/17680806?story_id=17680806. Accessed on June 5, 2011.

Sutnick, A. I., Kelley, P. R., & Knapp, D. (1972). The English language and the FMG. *Journal of Medical Education, 47*, 434–439.

Sutnick, A. I., Stillman, P. L., Norcini, J. J., Friedman, M., Regan, M. B., & Williams, R. G. (1993). ECFMG assessment of clinical competence of graduates of foreign medical schools. Educational Commission for Foreign Medical Graduates. *Journal of the American Medical Association, 270*, 1041–1045.

Swales, J. (1985). *Episodes in ESP*. Oxford: Pergamon Press.

Swales, J., & Feak, C. (2004). *Academic writing for graduate students: Essential tasks and skills*. Ann Arbor, MI: University of Michigan Press.

Swan, M., & Smith, B. (Eds). (2001). *A teachers' guide to interference and other problems*. New York, NY: Cambridge University Press.

Tannen, D. (1989). *Talking voices. Repetition, dialogue, and imagery in conversational discourse*. Cambridge: Cambridge University Press.

Tanner, M. (1991). *NNSTA-student interaction: An analysis of TAs' questions and student responses in a laboratory setting*. Unpublished doctoral dissertation, University of Pennsylvania, Philadelphia, PA.

The Joint Commission on Accreditation of Healthcare Organizations. (2007). *Improving America's hospitals: The Joint Commission's annual report on quality and safety*. Retrieved from www.jointcommissionreport.org/pdf/JC_2007_Annual_Report.pdf. Accessed on September 6, 2008.

The Joint Commission on Accreditation of Healthcare Organizations. (2008a). *Accreditation program: Hospital national patient safety goals*. Retrieved from www.jointcommission.org/assets/1/6/2011_NPSGs_HAP.pdf. Accessed on May 10, 2010.

The Joint Commission on Accreditation of Healthcare Organizations. (2008b). *Behaviors that undermine a culture of safety*. Sentinel event alert 40, July 9, 2008. Retrieved from www.jointcommission.org/sentinel_event_alert_issue_40_behaviors_that_undermine _a_culture_of_safety. Accessed on May 10, 2010.

The NHS Information Centre, NHS Staff 1999–2009 (General Practice). Retrieved from http://www.ic.nhs.uk/webfiles/publications/010_Workforce/nhsstaff9909/GP/General%20Practice %20%20Bulletin%20Tables%201999%20-%202009.pdf, Table 6. Accessed on July 3, 2011.

The NHS Information Centre, NHS Staff 1999–2009 (Medical and Dental). Retrieved from www.ic.nhs.uk/webfiles/publications/010_Workforce/nhsstaff9909/Medical/Medical_Den tal_Bulletin_1999-2009.pdf, Table 4. Accessed on July 3, 2011.

Thompson, N. (2003). *Communication and language: A handbook of theory and practice*. Basingstoke, UK: Palgrave Macmillan.

Tiersky, M., & Tiersky, E. (1992). *The language of medicine in English*. New York, NY: Pearson ESL.

Tipton, S. (2005). Improving international medical graduates' performance of case presentations. *Journal of Applied Linguistics, 2*, 395–406.

Tipton, S. (2008, April). The clinical skills (CS) test as threshold. Paper presented at the 42nd Annual TESOL Convention and Exhibition, New York City, NY.

Tiwari, A., Lai, P., So, M., & Yuen, K. (2006). A comparison of the effects of problem-based learning and lecturing on the development of students' critical thinking skills. *Medical Education, 40*, 547–554.

Tomlinson, B. (1998). *Materials development in language teaching*. Cambridge: Cambridge University Press.

Townsend, A. H., McLivenny, S., Miller, C. J., & Dunn, E. V. (2001). The use of an objective structured clinical examination (OSCE) for formative and summative assessment in a general practice clinical attachment as its relationship to final medical school examination performance. *Medical Education, 35*(9), 841–846.

Tsao, F. (2000). The language planning situation in Taiwan. In: R. E. Baldauf & R. B. Kaplan (Eds.), *Language planning in Nepal, Taiwan and Sweden* (pp. 60–106). Clevedon, UK: Multilingual Matters Ltd.

Turner, L. (2007). First world health care at third world prices: Globalization, bioethics and medical tourism. *BioSocieties, 2*, 303–325.

Tyler, A. (1992). Discourse structure and the perception of incoherence in international teaching assistants' spoken discourse. *TESOL Quarterly, 26*, 713–729.

U.K. Foundation Programme Office. (2009). *Rough guide to the academic foundation programme and compendium of academic competences.* Retrieved from www.foundation-programme.nhs.uk. Accessed on April 27, 2011.

United States Medical Licensing Examination (USMLE). (2009). *2009 USMLE Bulletin— Overview.* Retrieved from www.usmle.org/General_Information/bulletin/2009/overview.html. Accessed on June 23, 2009.

van Dijk, T. A. (1996). Discourse, power and access. In: C. R. Caldas-Coulthard & M. Coulthard (Eds.), *Texts and practices: Readings in critical discourse analysis* (pp. 84–104). London: Routledge.

van Zanten, M. (2008, April). Assessment of communication skills in entry. Paper presented at the 42nd Annual TESOL Convention and Exhibition, New York City, NY.

van Zanten, M., Boulet, J. R., & McKinley, D. W. (2003). Correlates of performance of the ECFMG Clinical Skills Assessment: Influences of candidate characteristics on performance. *Academic Medicine, 78*, S72–S74.

van Zanten, M., Boulet, J. R., McKinley, D. W., De Champlain, A., & Jobe, A. C. (2007). Assessing the communication and interpersonal skills of graduates of international medical schools as part of the United States Medical Licensing Exam (USMLE) Step 2 Clinical Skills (CS) Exam. *Academic Medicine, 82*, S65–S68.

van Zanten, M., Boulet, J. R., McKinley, D. W., & Whelan, G. P. (2003). Evaluating the spoken English proficiency of international medical graduates: Detecting threats to the validity of standardised patient ratings. *Medical Education, 37*, 69–76.

Vardanian, R. (1964). Teaching English intonation through oscilloscope display. *Language Learning, 14*, 109–117.

Wennerstrom, A. (1989). *Techniques for teachers. Workbook and videotape.* Seattle, WA: University of Washington Extension.

Whelan, G. P. (2006). Commentary: Coming to America: The integration of international medical graduates into the American medical culture. *Academic Medicine, 81*(2), 176–178.

Whelan, G. P., McKinley, D. W., Boulet, J. R., Macrae, J., & Kamholz, S. (2001). Validation of the doctor-patient communication component of the Educational Commission for Foreign Medical Graduates Clinical Skills Assessment. *Medical Education, 35*, 757–761.

Wilkinson, R. (2008). Locating the ESP space in problem-based learning. In: I. Fortanet-Gomez & A. Raisanen (Eds.), *ESP in European higher education* (pp. 55–73). Amsterdam: John Benjamins.

Willet, W. C. (2001). *Eat, drink and be healthy: The Harvard medical school guide to healthy eating.* New York, NY: Simon & Schuster Source.

Williams, J. (1992). Planning, discourse marking, and the comprehensibility of international teaching assistants. *TESOL Quarterly, 26*, 693–711.

Wilner, L. K. (2007). Communication skills training programs for doctors. *Academic Internal Medicine Insight, 5*(3), 14–15.

Wilner, L. K., & Whittaker, F. M. (2008). *Medical speaking rules and the medical speaking inventory*. Owings Mills, MD: ESL Rules, LLC.

Wodak, R. (1999). Critical discourse analysis at the end of the 20th century. *Research on Language and Social Interaction, 32*, 185–193.

Wood, A., & Head, M. (2004). 'Just what the doctor ordered': The application of problem-based learning to EAP. *English for Specific Purposes, 23*, 3–17.

Wu, W.-H., Chen, S.-F., & Wu, C.-F. (1989). The development of higher education in Taiwan. In: P. Altbach & V. Selvaratnam (Eds.), *From dependency to autonomy: The development of Asian universities* (pp. 117–136). Norwell, MA: Kluwer Academic Publishers.

Young, R. (Ed.). (1989). The training of international teaching assistants [special issue]. *ESP Journal, 8*(2).

Zeiger, M. (2000). *Essentials of writing biomedical research papers*. New York, NY: McGraw-Hill.

Zetkulic, M. (2008, April). Assessing workplace communication skills through objective skills clinical examination (OSCE) station diagnostics. Paper presented at the 42nd Annual TESOL Convention and Exhibition, New York City, NY.

Zoppi, K., & Epstein, R. (2002). Is communication a skill? Communication behaviors and being in relation. *Family Medicine, 34*(5), 319–324.